*dquarters*
Bartlett
s
e Drive
MA 01776
00
b.com
b.com

Jones and Bartlett
Publishers Canada
2406 Nikanna Road
Mississauga, ON L5C
2W6
CANADA

Jones and Bartlett
Publishers International
Barb House, Barb Mews
London W6 7PA
UK

n Credits
ns Editor: Penny M. Glynn
Manager: Amy Rose
Production Editor: Karen C. Ferreira
ssistant: Amy Sibley
Services Manager: Bret Kerr
d Binding: RR Donnelley Harrisonburg
ting: RR Donnelley Harrisonburg

the United States of America
4 03   10 9 8 7 6 5 4 3 2 1

# FUSZARD'S
# INNOVATIVE
# TEACHING
# STRATEGIES
# IN NURSING

## THIRD EDITION

Arlene J. Lowenstein

Martha J. Bradshaw

**JONES AND BARTLETT PUBLISH**
*Sudbury, Massachusetts*
BOSTON   TORONTO   LONDON   SINGA

*World H*
Jones ar
Publish
40 Tall
Sudbur
978-443
info@jb
www.jb

Produ
Acqui
Produ
Assoc
Editor
Produ
Printi
Cover

Printe
07 06

*To our colleagues, nursing educators*

# Table of Contents

# Contributors

**David J. Anna, RN, MSN**
Assistant Professor
School of Nursing
Department of Mental Health/
 Psychiatric Nursing
Medical College of Georgia
Augusta, Georgia

**Gayle W. Bentley, RN, MSN**
Assistant Professor
Department of Community Nursing
School of Nursing
Medical College of Georgia
Augusta, Georgia

**Ronald Borans, RN, MSN, ANP**
MGH Institute of Health Professions
Boston, Massachusetts

**Martha J. Bradshaw, RN, PhD**
Associate Professor
School of Nursing
Medical College of Georgia
Augusta, Georgia

**Christine Bridges, RN, DNSc**
Assistant Clinical Professor
Graduate Program in Nursing
MGH Institute of Health Professions
Boston, Massachusetts

**Billye Brown, RN, EdD, FAAN**
Professor Emeritus and Former Dean
School of Nursing
The University of Texas at Austin
Austin, Texas
and
Consultant
Tuft & Associates
Chicago, Illinois

**Pat Christensen, RN, MSN, PhD**
Professor
School of Nursing
University of South Carolina
Spartanburg, South Carolina

**Patricia R. Cook, RN, PhD**
Associate Professor
Assistant Head School of Nursing
University of South Carolina–Aiken
Aiken, South Carolina

**Inge Corless, RN, PhD**
Professor
Graduate Program in Nursing
MGH Institute of Health Professions
Boston, Massachusetts

**Connie F. Cowan, RN, MSN**
Clinical Education Specialist
Harris Methodist Fort Worth
Nursing Education Department
Fort Worth, Texas

**Elizabeth Crary, RN, MSN, ANP**
MGH Institute of Health Professions
Boston, Massachusetts

**Betty G. Davis, RN, BSN, MS**
Associate Professor
Mary Black School of Nursing
Baccalaureate Nursing Program
University of South Carolina
   Spartanburg
Spartanburg, South Carolina

**Sara E. Dolan, RN, MSN**
MGH Institute of Health Professions
Boston, Massachusetts

**Linda A. Ellis, RN, EdD**
Associate Professor and Associate
   Dean Emeritus
School of Nursing
Medical College of Georgia
Augusta, Georgia

**Barbara Fuszard, RN, PhD, FAAN**
Professor Emeritus
Medical College of Georgia
Augusta, Georgia

**Donna Gallagher, RN, CS, MS,
   ANP, FAAN**
Principal Investigator and Director
New England AIDS Education and
   Training Center
University of Massachusetts Medical
   and Nursing Schools
Boston, Massachusetts
and
Term Lecturer
MGH Institute of Health Professions
Boston, Massachusetts

**Beverly George-Gay, RN, MSN**
Formerly, Assistant Professor
Medical College of Georgia
School of Nursing—Department of
   Adult Nursing
Augusta, Georgia

**Glenda F. Hanson, RN, MSN, PhD**
Associate Professor
Learning Resource Coordinator
Georgia Baptist College of Nursing
Atlanta, Georgia

**Sandra M. Hillman, RN, PhD**
Associate Professor
Kennesaw State University
College of Health and Human
   Services
Department of Baccalaureate Nursing
Kennesaw, Georgia

**Charlotte James Koehler, RN, MN,
   IBCLC**
School of Nursing
University of South Carolina at
   Spartanburg
Spartanburg, South Carolina

**Veronica Kane, RN, MSN, CPNP**
Pediatric Nurse Practitioner
Nursing Program
MGH Institute of Health Professions
Boston, Massachusetts

**Sarah Kressy, RN, MSN, ANP**
MGH Institute of Health Professions
Boston, Massachusetts

**Clinton E. Lambert, Jr., RN, CS,
   PhD**
President and Counselor
Lambert Counseling Services, Inc.
Thomson, Georgia

**Vickie A. Lambert, RN, DNSc, FAAN**
Dean and Professor
Medical College of Georgia
School of Nursing
Augusta, Georgia

**Arlene J. Lowenstein, RN, PhD**
Professor and Director
Graduate Program in Nursing
MGH Institute of Health Professions
Boston, Massachusetts

**Alfred E. Lupien, PhD, CRNA**
Coordinator and Associate Professor
Nursing Anesthesia Program
Medical College of Georgia
Augusta, Georgia

**Hollie T. Noveletsky-Rosenthal, PhD, RNC**
Assistant Professor
Graduate Program in Nursing
MGH Institute of Health Professions
Boston, Massachusetts

**Katherine E. Nugent, RN, PhD**
Professor and Associate Dean,
    Academic Programs
Medical College of Georgia—School
    of Nursing
Augusta, Georgia

**Carol Picard, RN, PhD**
Associate Professor and Associate
    Director
Graduate Program in Nursing
MGH Institute of Health Professions
Boston, Massachusetts

**Judith Schurr Salzer, RN, MS, MBA**
Assistant Professor
Parent-Child Nursing
Medical College of Georgia
Augusta, Georgia

**Richard L. Sowell, RN, PhD, FAAN**
Professor and Chair
Administrative and Clinical Nursing
University of South Carolina,
    Columbia
Columbia, South Carolina

**Laurie Jowers Taylor, MSN, PhD**
Associate Professor
Florida State University
School of Nursing
Tallahassee, Florida

**Martha S. Tingen, RN, CS, ANP, PhD**
Associate Professor
School of Nursing
Medical College of Georgia
Augusta, Georgia

**Astrid Hellier Wilson, RN, DSN, CNS**
Associate Professor of Nursing
Clayton College and State University
Morrow, Georgia

**Barbara C. Woodring, RN, MS, MN, EdD**
Associate Dean
School of Nursing
University of Alabama at Birmingham
Birmingham, Alabama
Formerly, Professor and Chair
Department of Parent-Child Nursing
School of Nursing
Medical College of Georgia
Augusta, Georgia

**Elaine W. Young, RN, PhD**
Associate Professor
Graduate Program in Nursing
MGH Institute of Health Professions
Boston, Massachusetts

# Foreword

The first and second editions of this book were prepared and written by Barbara Fuszard. Those two publications prepared the groundwork for this excellent publication. The contributors to this text are individuals who are skilled in their respective specialties. The book is written for teachers who teach at any level and in any discipline. It is applicable for graduate or undergraduate students. I like that. I have read the page proofs for this book and have found it interesting and useful. Although my formal teaching days are now history, I found the information provided in this book by these experts to be immensely absorbing.

The reason for a book of this type is to provide a reference for teachers to enable them on their journeys to becoming excellent teachers. This book provides information for them to study and use in their effort to make their class one that all students want to attend. The teacher will direct a class in which students are stimulated to learn through innovative and diverse methods of teaching.

Teachers are performers. One has to mount a "production" while teaching important and pertinent information to gain the interest of some students. This is not intended to say that the teacher is playing a role, but that the teacher is providing an amiable environment in which learning can happen. This reflects the strategy of role-playing as a strategy for teaching. Humor is important in the classroom. One chapter discusses how humor facilitates learning. Teachers need to ascertain how their students best learn and shape their teaching style to that method. This book provides many suggestions for making the teaching process interesting, and the learning process entertaining and engaging while providing consequential information.

For many years, authors have written about teaching and about the teaching/learning strategies; however, in this book, the contributing authors, under the attentive direction of Arlene Lowenstein and Martha Bradshaw, have brought us a wealth of information about innovative teaching strategies. The experts writing about each strategy have contributed their cognizance of the topic and their vision of what can be accomplished by the teacher utilizing innovative teaching strategies.

Lowenstein and Bradshaw have made some modifications in the book from the previous two editions. They have introduced some subjects that were not as much in the forefront of teaching/learning even five years ago. They have expanded on some of the tried-and-true concepts of teaching/learning. Some topics simply cannot be improved, although permutation of content is constant when the excellent teacher is preparing to teach. Many examples of realistic situations are used to illustrate the strategies cited. These examples include strategies for innovative teaching, such as reflective practice, high-fidelity patient stimulation, distance learning, and Web-based learning, to list only a sample of the suggestions.

Who should read this text? Any serious teacher of students, at any level, and in any discipline.

*Billye Brown, RN, EdD, FAAN*
*Professor Emeritus and Former Dean*
*The University of Texas at Austin*
*School of Nursing*
*Manchaca, Texas*

# Acknowledgments

This Third Edition is the result of much gracious guidance and encouragement from Dr. Barbara Fuszard. We appreciate our contributors who willingly and promptly developed the foreword and chapters. It is to them that this quality work can be attributed.

*Arlene J.Lowenstein*
*Martha J. Bradshaw*

# PART I

# Introduction

Creating an effective learning environment is not an easy task in today's world, and is even more complex in nursing education. Nursing is taught in many different types and levels of post secondary educational settings. In addition, nursing students are extremely diverse. Traditional undergraduates, entering nursing directly from high school, sit side by side with a vast variety of nontraditional students returning to school. There is a wide range of age and experience within the student body. Nontraditional students may be RNs returning to school for a baccalaureate or graduate degree, while other students may be embarking on nursing as a second career. Nurse educators are challenged to recognize different learning needs, and respect and utilize the knowledge and experiences, nursing and non-nursing, that students bring to the classroom. The teaching strategies and examples throughout this book may be adapted for use in a variety of settings, at undergraduate and graduate levels, taking into account the diversity of learning needs.

The chapters in Part I provide a foundation for understanding, selecting, and adapting specific teaching strategies to the nurse educator's setting and student body. The contributors provide a theory base for learning and critical thinking and bring in various dimensions of effective learning that include creativity, humor, and innovation.

# CHAPTER 1

# Effective Learning:
# What Teachers Need To Know

*Martha J. Bradshaw*

*Knowing is a process, not a product—Jerome Bruner[1]*

What brings about effective learning in nursing students? Is it insight on the part of the student? A powerful clinical experience? Perhaps it is the dynamic, creative manner in which the nurse educator presents information or structures the learning experience. Effective learning likely is the culmination of all of these factors, in addition to others. In this chapter, dimensions of effective learning will be explored as a foundation for use of the innovative teaching strategies presented in subsequent chapters.

## THEORIES OF LEARNING

We approach learning individually, based largely on cognitive style (awareness of and taking in of relevant information) and preferred approaches to learning, or learning style. Some students are aware of their style and preference, some gain insight into these patterns as they become more sophisticated learners, and some students have never been guided to determine how they learn best.

Theoretical underpinnings classify learning as *behavioristic* or *cognitive*. Behavioristic learning was the earliest pattern identified through research. Psychologists such as Skinner and Thorndike described learning as a change in behavior and used stimulus response actions as an example. Subsequent theorists have described more complex forms of behaviorist learning. Bandura's[2] Theory of Social Learning describes human learning to come from others through observation, imitation, and reinforcement. We learn from society and we learn to be social. This type of learning is evident when we describe the need to "socialize" students to the profession of nursing.

Robert Gagne formulated suggestions for sequencing of instruction, conditions by which learning takes place, and outcomes of learning, or categories in which human learning occurs.[3] These learning categories are based on a hierarchical arrangement of learning theories, moving from simple to complex learning, and include intellectual and motor skills, verbal information, cognitive strategies, and attitudes. For example, within the category of intellectual skills are the following stages:

- *Discrimination learning*—distinguishing differences, in order to respond appropriately
- *Concept learning*—detecting similarities, in order to understand common characteristics
- *Rule learning*—combination of two or more concepts, as a basis for action in new situations

Gagne's ideas seem to combine behaviorism and cognitive theories. Use of behaviorism in nursing education was especially popular in the 1970s and early 1980s through the use of concrete, measurable, specific behavioral objectives. Even though nursing education has moved away from the concrete methods of learning and evaluation, use of the hierarchical arrangement is seen in curriculum development and learning outcomes.

Cognitive theories address the perceptual aspect of learning. Cognitive learning results in the development of perceptions and insight, also called *gestalt*, that brings about a change in thought patterns ("Aha") and related actions. Jerome Bruner[4] described cognitive learning as processes of conceptualization and categorization. He contended that intellectual development includes awareness of one's own thinking, the ability to recognize and deal with several alternatives and sequences, and the ability to prioritize. Bruner also saw the benefit of discovery learning to bring about insights.[5] Ausubel's assimilation theory focused on meaningful learning, in which the individual develops a more complex cognitive structure by associating new meanings with old ones that already exist within the learner's frame of reference.[6] Ausubel's theory relies heavily on the acquisition of previous knowledge. Meaningful learning occurs either by rote or discovery.[7]

Gardner's theory of multiple intelligences recognizes cognition as more than knowledge acquisition. Based on his definition of intelligence as "the ability to solve problems or fashion products that are valued in more than one setting,"[8(p.5)] Gardner has described seven forms of intelligence:

1. *Linguistic*—related to written and spoken words and language, and use and meaning of language(s)
2. *Musical/rhythmic*—based on sensitivity to rhythm and beat, recognition of tonal patterns and pitch, and appreciation of musical expression
3. *Logical/mathematical*—related to inductive and deductive reasoning, abstractions, and discernment of numerical patterns
4. *Visual/spatial*—ability to visualize an object or to create internal (mental) images, thus able to transform or re-create

5. ***Bodily kinesthetic***—the taking in and processing of knowledge through use of bodily sensations. Learning is accomplished through physical movement or use of body language
6. ***Interpersonal***—emphasizes communication and interpersonal relationships, recognition of mood, temperament, and other behaviors
7. ***Intrapersonal***—related to inner thought processes, such as reflection and metacognition, includes spiritual awareness and self-knowledge[9]

Cognitive theories that address learning stages appropriate for college students include Perry's model of intellectual and ethical development.[10] This model recognizes four nonstatic stages in which students progress: (1) dualism (black vs. white), (2) multiplicity (diversity and tolerance), (3) relativism (decision made by reasoned support), and (4) commitment to relativism (recognition of value set for decision making). Sheahan sees this as the culmination of education, in which the learner has integrated information, values, and attitudes to such an extent that they become one's own.[11] Perry's ideas can serve to explain how critical thinking is developed over time.

Belenky and colleagues formulated learning stages for women.[12] This model, based on feminist theory, recognizes the perceptual differences between men and women and points to the notion that nursing and educational practices have been traditionally male oriented.[13] For example, approaches to learning and solving problems in health care traditionally have been scientific. Thus, professionalism has been equated with the scientific, or medical, model, rather than a holistic or qualitative one.[14] Nursing also embraces a feminist perspective that emphasizes connectedness, caring, recognition of oppression, and a heightened understanding of others.

## APPROACHES TO LEARNING

Emerging from learning theories are descriptions of preferred styles or approaches to learning. Categorized as *cognitive styles* and *learning styles*, these approaches to learning are the ways that individuals acquire knowledge, which are concerned more with form or process than content.[15] Cognitive style deals with information process, the natural, unconscious internal process concerned with thinking and memory. It is the consistent way in which individuals organize and handle information.[16] The most common example of cognitive style is Witkin and colleagues' field dependent-field independent style.[17]

The field dependent-field independent style describes one's field of perception, or how one takes in information or data. Whereas one style generally predominates, people possess the capacity for both styles. Field-dependent individuals are more global, are open to external sources of information, are influenced by their surroundings, and therefore see the situation as a whole, rather than identifying and focusing on the separate aspects of it. Field-dependent people tend to be social, people-oriented, and sensitive to social cues. Learners in which the field-dependent style predominates may be externally motivated and therefore take a more spectator or passive role in the learning process, preferring to be "taught" rather than to actively participate.[18] Field-independent individuals are less sensitive to the social environment and thus take on a more analytical approach to information. By identifying aspects of the situation separately, they are able to restructure information and to develop their own system of classification. Field-independent learners enjoy concepts, challenges, and hypotheses, and are task oriented.[19]

An aspect of learning style related to student behavior is *response style*. Kagan (1965) pioneered work, with school-age children, on the concepts of reflection and impulsiveness.[20] These dimensions of cognitive response style describe personal tendencies regarding possibilities to solutions and choice selection. Individuals who have the impulsivity tendency prefer the quick, obvious answer, especially in highly uncertain problems, thus selecting the "nearly correct" answer as first choice. Reflective individuals identify and carefully consider alternatives before making a decision or choice. The implications for nursing education are apparent and will be discussed further. One problem that emerges with individuals who have a strong tendency in one of these dimensions is that the impulsive individual acts too quickly, based on an instant decision. On the other hand, the reflective individual may be immobilized in decision making, which has outcomes implications.[21]

Reflection, as associated with learning, was described as early as 1916 by Dewey as being a process of inquiry.[22] To reflect on a situation, experience, or collection of information is to absorb, consider, weigh, speculate, contemplate, and deliberate. Such reflection serves either as a basis for reasoned action or to gain understanding or attach meaning to an experience. The most notable descriptions of reflection, especially as related to nursing, have been presented by Schon.[23] In his work, Schon related reflection to problem solving. He pointed out that traditional means of teaching and learning result in structured problem solving where the ends are clear and fixed. In the reality of health care, such ends are not always so concrete.

Schon also believes that professionals in practice demonstrate a unique proficiency of thinking, and he has described three aspects of this thinking: (1) knowing-in-action (use of a personally constructed knowledge base), (2) reflection-in-action (conscious thinking about what one is doing, awareness of use of knowledge), and (3) reflection-on-action (a retrospective look at thoughts and actions, to conduct self-evaluation and make decisions for future events).[24] Reflection results in synthesis. This outcome is evident when the individual carries over thoughts, feelings, and conclusions to other situations. Thus, reflection is the foundation for growth through experience. Reflection, as a form of thinking and learning, can be cultivated.

One of the best known descriptions of learning styles is Kolb's,[25] which emerged from John Dewey's seminal theory on experiential learning. Dewey pio-

neered educational thinking regarding the relationship between learning and experience. The relationship between the learning environment and personal factors
such as motivation and goals can lead the learner through a stream of experiences
that, once connected, bring about meaningful learning.[26] Using these ideas, Kolb[27]
went on to describe learning as occurring in stages: concrete experiences, observation and reflection on the experience, conceptualization and generalization, then
theoretical testing in new and more complex situations. Learning is cyclical, with
new learning coming from new experiences. Consequently, learning occurs in a
comprehensive means, beginning with performance (concrete experience) and
ending with educational growth. Kolb further explained that individuals go about
this learning along two basic dimensions: grasping experiences (prehension) with
abstract-concrete poles and transforming, with action-reflection poles.[28] Applying
his experiential learning theory to his dimensions, Kolb identified four basic
learning styles:

1. *Converger*—prefers abstract conceptualization and active experimentation.
   These individuals are more detached and work better with objects than
   people. They are problem solvers and apply ideas in a practical manner.
2. *Diverger*—prefers concrete experience and reflective observation. Individuals with this tendency are good at generating ideas and displaying emo-
   tionalism and interest in others. Divergers are imaginative and can see the
   "big picture."
3. *Assimilator*—prefers abstract conceptualization and reflective observation.
   Assimilators easily bring together diverse items into an integrated entity,
   sometimes overlooking practical aspects or input from others. Theoreticians
   likely are assimilators.
4. *Accommodator*—prefers concrete experience and active experimentation.
   These individuals, while intuitive, are risk takers and engage in trial-and-
   error problem solving. Accommodators are willing to carry out plans, and
   they like and adapt to new circumstances.[29, 30]

Svinicki and Dixon report that average learning style scores for undergraduate
nursing majors are predominantly in the Converger category, with a tendency toward the Accommodator category.[31] Among nursing faculty, however, the average style is that of Diverger. Implications for teaching-learning and professional
development will be discussed further.

Gregorc's categorization of learning styles is similar to Kolb's, except that
Gregorc believes that an individual's style is static, even in light of the changing
educational setting.[32] Thus, even through maturity and further learning, an individual still approaches learning in the same way. Gregorc uses the learning style
categories of Concrete Sequential, Concrete Random, Abstract Sequential, and
Abstract Random. In his research, Gregorc determined that individuals have preferences in one or two categories. In studying both first-year and fourth-year baccalaureate nursing students, Wells and Higgs discovered that these students have

preferences in the concrete sequential and abstract random categories (total 81 percent of first-year students, 74 percent of fourth-year students).[33]

## USE OF LEARNING STYLES AND PREFERENCES: APPLICATION OF RESEARCH

Theoretical foundations regarding learning and descriptive studies of cognitive and learning styles provide insight and understanding of self. It would be difficult to address research on all modes of learning in this one chapter. A summary application of information from the vast field of knowledge about learning theory and cognitive and learning styles has been developed by Svinicki (1994) as six operating principles:

1. If information is to be learned, it must first be recognized.
2. During learning, learners act on information in ways that make it more meaningful.
3. Learners store information in long-term memory in an organized fashion related to their existing understanding of the world.
4. Learners continually check understanding, which results in refinement and revision of what is retained.
5. Transfer to new contexts is not automatic but results from exposure to multiple applications.
6. Learning is facilitated when learners are aware of their learning strategies and monitor their use.[34(p.275)]

To understand one's own learning styles is to help understand one's own thinking, to be aware of a fit between style and strategies for learning, and thus to select the most effective and efficient means to go about learning. Some students are aware of how they learn best and gravitate toward that strategy. Nursing instructors see this process in students who choose to sit in the front row of the class, take many notes, and feel involved with the topic, or students who choose to not come to class but instead read course material, watch videos, and acquire information as it pertains to a clinical assignment. Some students adhere to tradition-bound forms of learning, such as lecture and reading, yet do not maximize their learning. This result explains why these students benefit more from direct clinical experiences. Many students find learning to be more powerful when they experience something new or significant in a clinical environment, then explore information and reflect on the experience. Learning experiences can be adapted to the environment and are influenced by the environment in which they occur. Awareness and comprehension of one's style of learning enables one to tailor the learning environment for optimal outcomes. A simple test that will guide the student in discovering his or her learning style(s) is presented in the Example.

Feedback from an observer, such as the instructor, can heighten awareness of personal styles. The knowledgeable educator also can guide the student in enhancing predominant styles or in beginning to cultivate additional dimensions of thinking and responding. For example, a student who is predominantly impulsive in decision making should be guided to explore outcomes of decisions and encouraged to increase reflection time as appropriate. Conversely, the student who is highly reflective may need to explore reasons that bring about hesitancy or prolonged deliberation and the outcomes of such behaviors.

## EFFECTIVE TEACHING FOR EFFECTIVE LEARNING

A knowledgeable and insightful educator is the key to effective learning in many situations. Consequently, nursing faculty should call upon a knowledge base in learning and teaching as well as an extensive repertoire of useful strategies to reach learning goals. Of course, each strategy will have different effects on the attainment of learning outcomes in each student, based on the attributes and use of the strategy, in addition to learning and cognitive styles and learning preferences.[35] Here are some broad suggestions for applying information about learning in teaching situations. The specific strategies addressed in subsequent chapters provide detailed information that enable faculty to use each method in an optimal way.

Underlying assumptions regarding the nature of nursing education are derived in part from principles on adult learning, as formulated by Knowles.[36] Key principles include assuming responsibility for one's own learning and recognition of meaning or usefulness of information to be learned. Students in health professions are career-oriented and need to see practical value in their educational endeavors. As consumers, adult students need to believe that they are receiving the maximum benefit from learning experiences. Furthermore, taking charge of one's own learning is empowering. Students who gain a sense of self-responsibility can feel empowered in other areas of their lives, such as professional practice. Faculty, in turn, have the responsibility to cultivate empowerment and to effect learning outcomes.

The classroom environment should be fresh and challenging each time the class meets. Faculty should endeavor to provide variety in the manner in which they teach, rather than the same, predictable, albeit comfortable method of "telling," rather than teaching. As providers of information, instructors need to remember that learning is best brought about by a combination of motivation and stimulation. Effective learning goes beyond the role of the faculty as "performer" and provider of knowledge.[37] The effective instructor should be the facilitator of learning in the students. In professional education, motivation is gained when the relationship to the well-being of the client is pointed out. The value of faculty experience is evident when the nurse-teacher shares from his or her own professional experiences and uses these anecdotes as examples for client outcomes.

Students are more likely to remember information with which they can agree or relate, and forget that with which they disagree.[38] Disagreement or disharmony should be explored in an objective fashion. Viewpoints can then be strengthened or altered. Questioning and discussion should be based on the diversity that exists among the students. An openness to and acceptance of others (emerging from feminist theory), along with Perry's stage of multiplicity,[39] benefits male students who are incorporated into a female-dominated profession. Conversely, female students who are accustomed to a male-dominated world may have difficulty expressing openness about their own learning experiences. An instructor who is able to establish a sense of trust and confidence with the students can promote the expression of different perspectives likely to be found in the group. Nurse educators should support students who are at various levels of cognitive growth, looking upon students from a criterion framework, rather than a normative one. Faculty should show that various viewpoints are welcome, legitimate, and worthy of discussion. Teachers can cultivate further development in the individual learners by demonstrating how to critique a theory, develop a rationale, or work through the steps of problem solving. These strategies will facilitate growth in students who are in an early cognitive stage such as dualism, or will challenge more advanced students to a commitment to realism.[40]

Delivery of information should be based on instructional theory in addition to content expertise. Using Ausubel's principles of advanced organizer, the teacher can develop inductive discovery by which students can build on previously acquired, simplistic knowledge to develop new or broader concepts.[41] This strategy operationalizes some of Svinicki's cognitive principles.[42]

Effective learning experiences that emerge from identified styles should be developed and used in both class and clinical settings. Information from Kolb's four dimensions serves as an excellent example.[43] Students who are **convergers** readily become bored with "straight lecture," especially with topics that are abstract in nature. These individuals work better by themselves, so they are less likely to participate well in group projects. Learners with the **diverger** style learn from case studies and will actively participate in discussion, but they may have difficulty detaching personal values from the issue. These students often are visionary group leaders. Individuals with the **assimilator** style manipulate ideas well, so they will participate well in discussion or write comprehensive papers; however, these students may be less practical and have difficulty with some of the realism of nursing practice. **Accommodators** usually enjoy case studies, new or unusual teaching strategies, skills lab, and "tinkering" with new equipment. These learners will be most responsive to a challenging, complex client.

In the clinical setting, the instructor may wish to provide introductory motivation through discovery learning. One way to accomplish this goal is to have each student observe or follow a registered nurse to gain exposure to the myriad tasks and responsibilities of a professional health care provider. Whereas students may have some rudimentary ideas of "what nurses do," they "discover" the depth and demands required in day-to-day work by observing actual practice. This strategy should broaden their perspective and set the stage for meaningful learning, which includes increased retention of material and greater inquiry.[44]

As students develop clinical written summaries about their clients, instructors should be flexible with the type of written work submitted. Traditionally, nursing students develop some form of a care plan based on the Nursing Process. The structured, linear method has taken criticism as "the only way" to look at clients. As a concrete, methodical strategy, the Nursing Process care plan is effective for students who are field-independent and who can readily discern the data and related information needed for each step.

Additional methods of client summary or analysis should be introduced, and students should be encouraged to try each method. In doing so, students may broaden their ways of seeing clients and nursing problems, thus setting the stage for increased insight, analysis, and confidence. For example, use of the concept map is a way in which a student can envision the client or care situation in a holistic manner. Concept maps provide a fluidity that enhances the ability to determine relationships and make connections. Therefore, this strategy likely will be used positively by students who demonstrate Gardner's categories of visual/spatial or interpersonal intelligence. Learners who are field-dependent also should do well with the concept map strategy because of their tendency to see the situation as a whole.[45] Concept mapping should be effective for learners with all of Kolb's styles but for different reasons and with different outcomes.

Guided reflection, especially reflection-on-action, helps the student bring closure to the clinical experience, as well as conduct self-evaluation and gain from the experience. Journal writing is one of the most effective means by which the student can capture thoughts and responses and preserve these ideas in writing for subsequent consideration. This strategy is particularly useful as a means by which students can identify and modify impulsive-reflective tendencies. Journal writing will have the best results with divergers and assimilators, and some students may benefit from open discussion about the experiences entered into their journals. Again, feedback from the faculty is crucial and should be as thoughtful as the entries provided by the student. Faculty reading journals should guide the student in growth of insight and patterns of reflection.

One of the greatest challenges for faculty is in developing the blend of strategies to bring about effective learning in all students. Part of the challenge is the "fit" between the faculty's styles and learning preferences and that of each of the learners. Faculty should become aware of their approaches to learning and how these approaches enhance or hinder the learning of others.[46] Faculty especially should be on guard against favoritism to students who possess the same attributes as the instructor. Conversely, the congruency between styles of the teacher and of the student may enhance a relationship that is especially meaningful and may evolve into professional mentoring.

## FUTURE CONSIDERATIONS

From this chapter, many ideas emerge that are worthy of more detailed scrutiny. A study by Ostmoe and colleagues in 1984 indicated that baccalaureate nursing students prefer traditional, teacher-directed teaching strategies and are less interested in innovative, "alternative" strategies.[47] It would be interesting to see if this view persists in light of vast curriculum and teaching revisions that have occurred as an answer to the monumental changes in health care and professional practice. The foci on critical thinking, decision making, and active learning have changed the nature of nursing education to such an extent that innovative strategies are selected as the best approach to meet the learning outcomes. One factor that Moffett and Hill have discovered as having a positive influence on learning outcomes was preparation for class.[48] Student preparation may be linked to motivation and interest in the subject. The vast amount of available material on student learning styles may lead faculty to wonder if they should actively assess learning styles and develop teaching methods accordingly and individually. Perhaps preliminary studies should be conducted on congruency between faculty learning styles and how these styles are translated into approaches for teaching.

More research with professional health care students is needed on development of insight, intuition, and roles of reflection and women's ways of knowing. Kelly and Young suggest that studies regarding learning styles need stronger methodology, such as sample size, better control of variables, and evaluation with practical application.[49]

## CONCLUSION

Effective learning is more than merely the results of good teaching. It is enhanced by a learning environment that includes active interactions among faculty, students, and student peers. Effective learning is achieved through the use of creative strategies designed not to entertain but to inform and stimulate. The best ways faculty can bring about effective learning are by recognizing students as individuals, with unique, personal ways of knowing and learning, by creating learning situations that recognize diversity, and by providing empowering experiences in which students are challenged to think.

---

## EXAMPLE
## How Do I Learn Best?[50]

This instrument typically takes four to six minutes to complete and can be self-scored. The style categories are visual, aural, read/write, and kinesthetic, which correspond with categories found in Gardner's multiple forms of intelligence. Students are directed to complete the brief questions, then are shown the learning modalities that best fit predominant styles.

## HOW DO I LEARN BEST?

This test is to find out something about your preferred learning method. Research on left brain/right brain differences and on learning and personality differences suggests that each person has preferred ways to receive and communicate information.

Choose the answer that best explains your preference and put the key letter in the box. If a single answer does not match your perception, please enter two or more choices in the box. Leave blank any question that does not apply.

☐ 01. You are about to give directions to a person. She is staying in a hotel in town and wants to visit your house. She has a rental car. Would you:
V) draw a map on paper?
R) write down the directions (without a map)?
A) tell her the directions by phone?
K) collect her from the hotel in your car?

☐ 2. You are staying in a hotel and have a rental car. You would like to visit a friend whose address/location you do not know. Would you like them to:
V) draw you a map on paper?
R) write down the directions (without a map)?
A) tell you the directions by phone?
K) collect you from the hotel in their car?

☐ 3. You have just received a copy of your itinerary for a world trip. This is of interest to a friend. Would you:
A) call her immediately and tell her about it?
R) send her a copy of the printed itinerary?
V) show her the itinerary on a map of the world?

☐ 4. You are going to cook a dessert as a special treat for your family. Do you:
K) cook something familiar without need for instructions?
V) thumb through the cookbook looking for ideas from the pictures?
R) refer to a specific cookbook where there is a good recipe?
A) ask for advice from others?

☐ 5. A group of tourists has been assigned to you to find out about national parks. Would you:
K) drive them to a national park?
R) give them a book on national parks?
V) show them slides and photographs?
A) give them a talk on national parks?

☐ 6. You are about to purchase a new stereo. Other than price, what would most influence your decision?
A) A friend talking about it.
K) Listening to it.
R) Reading the details about it.
V) Its distinctive, upscale appearance.

☐ 7. Recall a time in your life when you learned how to do something like playing a new board game. Try to avoid choosing a very physical skill, e.g., riding a bike. How did you learn best? By:
V) visual clues—pictures, diagrams, charts?
A) listening to somebody explaining it?
R) written instructions?
K) doing it?

☐ 8. Which of these games do you prefer?
V) Pictionary
R) Scrabble
K) Charades

☐ 9. You are about to learn to use a new program on a computer. Would you:
K) ask a friend to show you?
R) read the manual that comes with the program?
A) telephone a friend and ask questions about it?

☐ 10. You are not sure whether a word should be spelled "dependent" or "dependant." Do you:
R) look it up in the dictionary?
V) see the word in your mind and choose the best way it looks?
A) sound it out in your mind?
K) write both versions down?

☐ 11. Apart from price, what would most influence your decision to buy a particular textbook?
K) Using a friend's copy.
R) Skimming parts of it.
A) A friend talking about it.
V) It looks OK.

☐ 12. A new movie has arrived in town. What would most influence your decision to go or not go?
A) Friends talked about it.
R) You read a review about it.
V) You saw a preview of it.

☐ 13. Do you prefer a lecturer/teacher who likes to use:
R) handouts and/or a textbook?
V) flow diagrams, charts, slides?
K) field trips, labs, practical sessions?
A) discussion, guest speakers?

## LEARNING MODALITY

| | In Class | When Studying | For Exams |
|---|---|---|---|
| **Visual** | Underlining<br>Use different colors<br>Use symbols, charts, arrangements on a page | Recall visual aspects of presentation<br>Reconstruct images in different ways<br>Redraw pages from memory<br>Replace words with symbols and initials | Recall the pictures on the pages<br>Draw, use diagrams where appropriate<br>Practice turning visuals back into words |
| **Aural** | Attend lectures and listen<br>Discuss topics with students<br>Use a tape recorder<br>Discuss overheads, pictures, and other visual aids<br>Leave space in notes for later recall | May take poor notes because of preference for voices<br>Expand your notes by talking out ideas<br>Explain new ideas to another student<br>Read assignments out loud | Speak your answers/Tutorials<br>Practice writing answers to an old exam<br>Read questions to self or have someone read them to you |
| **Reading/ Writing** | Use lists, headings<br>Write out lists and definitions<br>Use handouts and textbooks | Write out the words<br>Reread notes silently<br>Rewrite ideas into other words<br>Use lecture notes/Read | Practice with multiple-choice questions<br>Write paragraphs, beginnings, endings<br>Organize diagrams into statements |
| **Kinesthetic: use all your senses** | May take notes poorly because topics do not seem relevant<br>Go to lab, take field trips<br>Use trial-and-error method<br>Listen to real-life examples | Put examples in note summaries<br>Talk about notes, especially with another K person<br>Use pictures and photos to illustrate | Write practice answers<br>Role-play the exam situation in your head |

## NOTES

1. J. Bruner, *Toward a Theory of Instruction* (New York: W.W. Norton & Co., 1966).

2. A. Bandura, *Social Learning Theory* (Morristown, NJ: General Learning Press, 1977).

3. G. LeFrancois, *Psychology for Teaching*, 6th ed. (Belmont, CA: Wadsworth Publishing, 1988).

4. Bruner, *Theory of Instruction*, 2.

5. Bruner, *Theory of Instruction*, 96.

6. D.P. Ausubel, *Educational Psychology: A Cognitive View* (New York: Holt, Rinehart and Winston, 1968).

7. B. Norton, From Teaching to Learning: Theoretical Foundations, in *Teaching in Nursing,* eds. D.M. Billings and J.A. Halstead (Philadelphia: Saunders, 1988), 211–245.

8. H. Gardner and T. Hatch, *Multiple Intelligences Go To School: Educational Implications of the Theory of Multiple Intelligences* (Technical Report No. 4) (New York: Center for Technology in Education, 1990, March).

9. Gardner and Hatch, *Multiple Intelligences,* 5.

10. W.G. Perry, *Forms of Intellectual and Ethical Development in the College Years: A Scheme* (New York: Holt, Rinehart and Winston, 1970).

11. J. Sheahan, Some Aspects of the Teaching and Learning of Nursing, *Journal of Advanced Nursing* 5 (1980):491–511.

12. M.F. Belenky, B.M. Clinchy, N.R. Goldberger, and J.M. Tarule, *Women's Ways of Knowing* (New York: Basic Books, 1986).

13. Norton, From Teaching to Learning, 234.

14. G.L. Dickson, The Unintended Consequences of Male Professional Ideology for the Development of Nursing Education, *Advances in Nursing Science* (1993):67–83.

15. M.A. Miller and D.E. Babcock, *Critical Thinking Applied to Nursing* (St. Louis: Mosby, 1996).

16. S. DeYoung, *Teaching Nursing* (Redwood City, CA: Addison-Wesley, 1990).

17. H.A. Witkin, C.A. Moore, D.R. Goodenough, and P.W. Cox, Field-Dependent and Field-Independent Cognitive Styles and Their Implications, *Review of Educational Research* 47 (1977):1–64.

18. Miller and Babcock, *Critical Thinking*, 39.

19. Miller and Babcock, *Critical Thinking*, 39.

20. J. Kagan, Reflection-Impulsivity and Reading Ability in Primary Grade Children, *Child Development* 36, no. 3 (1965):609–628.

21. R. Partridge, Learning Styles: A Review of Selected Models, *Journal of Nursing Education* 22 (1983):243–248.

22. Miller and Babcock, *Critical Thinking*, 95.

23. D.A. Schon, *The Reflective Practitioner: How Professionals Think in Action* (New York: Basic Books, 1983).

24. Schon, *The Reflective Practitioner.*

25. D.A. Kolb, *Experiential Learning Theory* (Englewood Cliffs, NJ: Prentice-Hall, 1984).

26. E. Kelly and A. Young, Models of Nursing Education for the 21st Century, in *Review of Research in Nursing Education,* vol. vii, ed. K. Stevens (New York: National League for Nursing, 1996), 1–39.

27. Kolb, *Experiential Learning*, 38.

28. Kelly and Young, Models of Nursing Education, 17.

29. Miller and Babcock, *Critical Thinking*, 43–44.

30. Partridge, Learning Styles, 245.

31. M.D. Svinicki and N.M. Dixon, The Kolb Model Modified for Classroom Activities, *College Teaching* 35, no. 4 (1987):141–146.

32. A.F. Gregorc, Learning/Teaching Styles: Their Nature and Effects, in *Student Learning Styles* (Reston, VA: National Association of Secondary Principals, 1979), 19–26.

33. D. Wells and Z.R. Higgs, Learning and Learning Preferences of First and Fourth Semester Baccalaureate Degree Nursing Students, *Journal of Nursing Education* 29, no. 9 (1990):385–390.

34. M.D. Svinicki, Practical Implications of Cognitive Theories, in *Teaching and Learning in the College Classroom,* eds. K.A. Feldman and M.B. Paulsen (Needham Heights, MA: Ginn Press, 1994), 274–281.

35. P.M. Ostmoe, H.L. Van Hoozer, A.L. Scheffel, and C.M. Crowell, Learning Style Preferences and Selection of Learning Strategies: Consideration and Implication for Nurse Educators, *Journal of Nursing Education* 23, no. 1 (1984):27–30.

36. M.A. Knowles, *The Adult Learner: A Neglected Species,* 2nd ed. (Houston: Gulf Publishing, 1978).

37. B.S. Moffett and K.B. Hill, The Transition to Active Learning: The Lived Experience, *Nurse Educator* 22, no. 4 (1977):44–47.

38. DeYoung, *Teaching Nursing*, 29.

39. Perry, *Forms of Intellectual and Ethical Development.*

40. Perry, *Forms of Intellectual and Ethical Development.*

41. DeYoung, *Teaching Nursing.*

42. Svinicki, Kolb Model Modified, 275.

43. Kolb, *Experiential Learning Theory*, 38.

44. DeYoung, *Teaching Nursing.*

45. Witkin, Moore, Goodenough, and Cox, Field Dependent and Field Independent Styles.

46. Kelly & Young, Models of Nursing Education, 31.

47. Ostmoe, Van Hoozer, Scheffel, and Crowell, Learning Style Preferences, 29.

48. Moffett and Hill, Transition to Active Learning, 45.

49. Kelly and Young, Models of Nursing Education, 34.

50. Gardner and Hatch, *Multiple Intelligences.*

# CHAPTER 2

# Strategies for Innovation

*Arlene J. Lowenstein*

The scope of change in health care has been enormous, and the rate at which change occurs continues to accelerate. Today's technology and therapeutics were inconceivable even a few decades ago. Over time, the growth of the nursing profession has been influenced by many factors, including those new technologies and therapeutics. But there are many other influencing factors and forces, including, but not limited to:

- The appearance of new diseases, such as HIV/AIDS and Lyme disease.
- War and its consequences, which brought new techniques to care for burns and radiation, growth of the use of penicillin and other antibiotics, treatments for posttraumatic stress syndrome, and nursing in the military and veterans' systems.
- Sociocultural issues, including the civil rights movement, the feminist movement, the consumer revolution of the late 1960s and 1970s, and changing immigration and demographic patterns, which brought dramatic changes in maternity care from shortened length-of-stay to sibling visitation, brought increased diversity in nursing education, and created more emphasis on culturally competent care.
- Religion, which brought in ethical components of care and the development of Parish Nursing.
- Changing economics and political/legal issues, which brought us Medicare, Medicaid, managed care, and legalized abortion.
- Changes in education that brought nursing into academic settings and gave rise to nursing science and nursing research, thereby changing practice and creating new roles, such as advanced practice nursing.

These forces are not isolated but are part of the total environment in which we live and work. They are ever-changing and interacting, challenging nurse educators to keep on top of the trends, technologies, and resources, while enabling self-directed student learning. Graduates who are self-directed learners understand and are responsive to health care system changes when they are in practice and out of the school setting, where there are no faculty members with whom to consult.

Nurse educators straddle the fields of health care practice and education. They need to be knowledgeable about changes in practice and technology in both fields. What nurses learn, as well as how they are taught, must keep pace with the changing milieu. The field of education has also changed over the years through many of the same forces that affected health care. Technology and therapeutics in health care can be compared to a new understanding of learning theories and teaching methods in education. The student entering nursing from high school today is most likely much more comfortable with the use of computers than the RN returning to school or an older student who has chosen nursing as a second career. The nursing classroom is also more culturally diverse than ever before, and more men are entering the profession. Younger students may have had very different cultural experiences in the secondary schools than did older students. Different cultures and experiences may produce different expectations of teaching and learning. Respecting learning-need differences and establishing an innovative climate in the classroom can help to prepare students for the changes they will face in practice. An educational climate that values different viewpoints and experiences among students encourages those students to create their own innovations. Those innovations will serve them in good stead by enhancing positive interactions with the wide variety of persons for whom they will be caring and with whom they will be working.

Sources of information have multiplied. The Internet has laid at our doors the possibility of learning over long distances. The barrier of geography has been breached. Even nurses in rural communities have access to continued learning by highly qualified nurse educators. Innovative computer-based materials can provide technical training within the classroom—audio and video combining to offer a breadth of exposure previously only available through many hours at the bedside. This capability is becoming much more important as productivity pressures make clinical sites for student experience harder and harder to find.

How do we teach more and more information to our students without overwhelming them? And how do we maintain the underlying paradigm of care and compassion? How do we maintain the threads of classical nursing as patient-centered, holistic, and compassionate within the complex scientific information our students must master? In this textbook, we hope to provide nurse educators with ideas and examples that have been used to allow students to master the facts and theory as well as the perspective of a caring professional. Implementing and adapting these methods will lead to further discovery of successful teaching strategies to keep pace with changes in the profession.

## EXAMPLES OF INNOVATION

Innovative teaching strategies can range from simple to complex. Innovations can be developed for an exercise within a course to the method by which the entire course is taught. Teaching innovations can be developed for whole programs, or even whole schools. They can be developed by one faculty member or by groups of faculty members. The prime objective is that the teaching strategies selected must address what needs to be learned in relation to the learning needs of students.

Think back to a favorite teacher or any strongly remembered event. Why does it stand out? What makes it unique among similar events? A major factor can be the realization that one object was completely different or out of its usually defined place, whereas the surrounding objects appeared normal. The teachers we remember often stood apart from our perception of others by only one or two details, but these details were out of the normal range. We remember the different much more than the normal, yet we can grasp only a small amount of different and a large amount of the usual. The occasional nondigestible, completely different bit in the sea of the expected forces our energies on analyzing not just the different bit but also the other 99 percent rote material normally not given much attention and easily forgotten.

Kirp, a professor of public policy, asked a former student, who was now a college professor, what she remembered about his teaching. He was astonished to hear that she remembered his baseball stories. She elaborated that the baseball anecdotes prodded her into thinking of him as more approachable and more human. Once she felt that way, she began to pay attention.[1] Exhibit 2–1 is an example

---

**Exhibit 2–1** Analogy: Pain Management and the Sinking of the Titanic

Bone surgery, such as ankle fusion, is a very painful procedure for patients. To create a more dynamic understanding of a patient's experience with pain and the need for appropriate pain relief measures, an analogy was used to discuss the issues involved. The choice of the Titanic disaster as an analogy actually came from a patient's description of the pain he felt in the postoperative period and his feeling that the nursing staff needed to pay more attention to pain relief. He felt there were times when he was totally immersed with the pain, and relief could have been started sooner and on a more even keel.

The Titanic was constructed with six watertight compartments that were expected to withstand a breach and keep the ship afloat. The compartments had very high walls but, unfortunately, no top. The design was appropriate for most possibilities, except the accident that actually happened. Students were told to think of the walls as the job of the pain medication and water as the pain. The wall of the pain medication isolates the water from the ship and the passengers' realization that they are sur-

*continues*

**Exhibit 2–1** continued

rounded by water. The pain is hidden. The danger lies in what happens if the water in the first compartment overflows its limit and then starts filling the second compartment. If up to three of these compartments fill with water (pain), it may not interfere with the ship's normal function; however, as the effect cascades, the ship sinks by the bow until it's "all hands lost."

Patients initially don't understand that a sea of pain surrounds them. As the pain relief diminishes and they suddenly (perhaps by waking from sleep) find themselves immersed, a fear of this unexpected and uncomfortable situation is formed. This fear becomes a constant presence even after pain relief is restored, leading to anxiety and apprehension over the possibility of a repeat experience. In very painful procedures, this fear can result in "clock watching" over the medication schedule as well as a compulsion to do anything to stay ahead of the pain curve. Appropriate pain relief measures, timing of administration, and other nursing measures can be discussed, continuing use of the analogy (i.e., use of lifeboats in the pain relief cycle.) Students can also be taught to develop and share their own analogies to improve learning retention.

of using something different in a lesson: an analogy of pain management to the sinking of the Titanic. The objective is to allow students to discover how what they know applies to other situations. Students will remember more if they can make the discovery.

An example of an innovative strategy at the school level was the introduction of interdisciplinary case studies to health profession students. Health care providers interact daily with members of other disciplines. The mission statement of the health professions school, with programs in nursing, physical therapy, and communications sciences disorders, included the following:

> While health professionals must be prepared to provide expert care within their respective disciplines, they contribute to evaluating and improving health care delivery by working in close cooperation with professionals from other disciplines. Students educated in an interdisciplinary setting, one that integrates academic and clinical pursuits, will be well-equipped to function as members of the health care team. The involvement of active practitioners from different fields in program planning, student supervision, and teaching supports such an integrated program.[2(p.13)]

Faculty members and administrators felt the need to strengthen the manner in which that portion of the mission statement was being addressed. Although students were exposed to a few multidisciplinary courses such as research and ethics, there was overall agreement that they needed more useful exposure to other disciplines within a clinical context. An interdisciplinary faculty task force was developed to explore possibilities. The academic dean staffed the task force and provided administrative support. After much discussion, the task force settled on a series of four required interdisciplinary clinical seminars as the preferred method.

The mechanics of developing and implementing the program were daunting, but the group was committed to the project. They enlisted other members of their departments to develop four case studies—one for each seminar. The subject of the case study would require care from each of the three disciplines. Thought was given to the need for students to be involved with different age groups and various clinical settings. Teams of faculty members with expertise in each area developed the following cases:

- Seminar Case 1. Pediatric patient with cerebral palsy who is starting school.
- Seminar Case 2. Elderly patient with cerebral vascular accident and dysphagia in an acute care setting.
- Seminar Case 3. Middle-aged adult with HIV and family issues in the community (end stages of illness).
- Seminar Case 4. Young teen with traumatic brain injury in a rehabilitation center.

The intensive involvement of many faculty members in the development of the cases had some very beneficial effects. Interdisciplinary cooperation was necessary as the cases were developed. Faculty members were able to learn from each other and appreciate the role of the other disciplines. The faculty members who developed the cases were now invested in the project and were able to support and commend it to other faculty members and to students in their classes, which reduced some resistance.

Each program was responsible for determining which students would be required to attend the seminars. The nursing program selected students who were in the spring semester of the second year of an entry-level master's program and were enrolled in the Primary Care I course. Nursing students in this program held a baccalaureate in any field prior to entry into the program. They had completed the first year and second fall semester in the generalist level of the nursing program. They were in the process of taking the RN licensing exam during this semester (they all passed). They were now in advanced-level coursework that would lead to a Master's of Science in Nursing degree and eligibility to sit for certification as a nurse practitioner. Interdisciplinary seminar attendance was mandatory and counted as part of the clinical component in the Primary Care I course, so that students would not be required to add hours to the course. Compromise and negotiation were needed on the part of the course faculty to recognize and accept that the interdisciplinary seminar was a legitimate learning experience appropriate to the course.

Scheduling the seminars was a major problem. Coordinating three programs with students in different classes and in clinical sites was very difficult. The seminars were held in the late afternoon, and students in clinical placements were asked to leave their clinical site early enough to return to the school. There is no easy answer to this problem. Each student was sent a letter outlining the purpose of the seminars and given the dates and times. The letter explained that attendance was mandatory and that the seminar would count as class hours.

Approximately 60 students were expected to attend the seminars. Four faculty members from each department were recruited to facilitate each seminar. In smaller departments, this meant that department faculty members participated in more than one seminar. The case discussions were designed so that students had an opportunity to participate in multidisciplinary groups, meet with their own specialty, and meet as a total group. The sessions were planned to last two hours each.

The role of the faculty members was to facilitate but not to lead the discussion among students. Faculty members were available to correct wrong information, but the focus was to have students take responsibility for explaining their discipline's role in working with the patient. Faculty members were not expected to be experts in the area under discussion or to introduce new material. The faculty role was explained to the students at the beginning of the session.

Preprepared case materials presented assessment tools used by each discipline and questions to be addressed. The goals of the seminar were presented and clarified to all of the students before breaking students into groups. Students presented their assessments and plans for working with the patients, defining priorities of care. Faculty facilitators encouraged participation by all. Each small group took notes to be presented to the entire group for general discussion.

Evaluations of the seminars from both faculty members and students were excellent. The time selected for the seminars was problematic for many participants and seemed to be the major concern of students. Some students had various excuses for not being able to attend. Snow forced the cancellation of one session. All students attended a minimum of one seminar, but most attended the sessions as scheduled. Students remarked that the discussions were excellent and that they had learned new knowledge from each other as the different disciplinary approaches were presented. Faculty members also benefited from the discussions, and interdepartmental communications were enhanced. Some faculty members were uncomfortable at first with the expectation of their role and were concerned that they did not know enough about specific cases; however, most soon realized that the objectives of the session were valid for the level of their expertise and the expectation of facilitation, not instruction. Overall, the project was deemed a strong success and will be presented again, with minor changes.

## DEVELOPING INNOVATIVE STRATEGIES

Innovation can occur at all levels of an educational organization. Support for innovation in education may begin at the top of the organization or be developed and implemented at program or individual class levels. Success is enhanced when administrators and faculty members work side by side to plan strategically and implement changes to improve the educational milieu.[3] Innovation at the school level is demonstrated by business school educators. These schools chose to focus more on entrepreneurship and to move away from the traditional management that prepared students to work in large organizations. This strategic innovation recognized the realities of the marketplace in a changing world. These schools set the pace for others to follow.[4]

Nursing education has grown through innovation. Mildred Montag's introduction of the associate degree program in nursing, developed through research to meet an assessed need, changed the landscape of nursing education. The introduction of nurse practitioner programs also created a revolution in the profession. The introduction of distance learning is the latest revolution and is growing rapidly, offering students different choices that are unfettered by the barrier of geography.

Successful innovation does not come easily and requires creativity, planning, and evaluation. Exhibit 2–2 describes a process for educators to work through to develop innovative teaching strategies.

Just as the nursing process calls for assessment, so does the educational process. *Assessment* of a course requires a look at both strengths and problems. How can the strengths be enhanced? What needs to be changed? Educators must focus on what the expected learning outcome should be. Specific content requirements change often in health care, as new techniques, technologies, and research bring new knowledge needs. With the overwhelming amount of information available in today's health care world, it will not be possible to include everything students need. They will need to have appropriate resources to supplement classroom or clinical learning. The instructor must decide what and how much content will be needed; this decision is often difficult. While addressing the content to be learned, it is also important to consider student learning needs. An understanding of the diversity in learning needs provides a foundation for the development of effective strategies.

To *define options,* the literature should be searched for suggestions or techniques that could address the identified needs. Asking students or other faculty members for suggestions can also be helpful. This is the place where creativity reigns. It is important to look at many different ways to address the learning objective, before selecting one. Asking the question "Is there another way to look at this?" can be fun and lead to additional options.

Once a strategy has been selected, *planning* is all-important. Understanding who the stakeholders are and what their investment is in the status quo or in change can be helpful in planning strategies to bring them on board. Many stakeholders, including students, do not like change and will resist new approaches. Using change theory can assist in demonstrating need and provide information that can make resisters more amenable to change. Some strategies will require curricular change, which is a complicated process and one that needs to be started

**Exhibit 2–2**  The Process of Innovation

*Assessment*

  What is the content to be learned? What are the student learning needs? How are those needs being met?—What is working and what is not?

*Defining options*

  How else can I look at this? Does the literature provide suggestions or techniques that would address the identified needs? Do students or other faculty members have suggestions that I could utilize?

*Planning*

  1. Does this change require working with curriculum committees, collaborating with other faculty members, or individual instructor planning? How should this change be approached?
  2. Will there be a need to work with technical specialists in the use of computer technology? Do I need additional technological knowledge to carry out this change?
  3. How can I best use change theory in this planning? Who are the stakeholders that need to be considered? How and where will I meet resistance? How will I develop support?
  4. How will I plan to evaluate the effectiveness of this innovation?

*Gaining support for innovation*

  What resources will be needed? How will they be acquired and funded? What is the level of administrative support required and available? What strategies will I use to gain additional support if needed?

*Preparing students for the innovation*

  Do I need written student instructions? If so, are they clear? Have I provided a mechanism for troubleshooting problems, and do students know how to address problems?

*Preparing faculty members for the innovation*

  If other faculty members are involved, do they need additional education? How will that be carried out? Is everyone in agreement as to how the strategy will be run? Is rehearsal time needed?

*Implementing the innovation*

  How much flexibility is available if the intervention is not going well? Will follow-up be needed?

*Evaluating the outcome*

  How will I measure the learning outcome? How have students reacted to the strategy, and can they provide input for change or improvement? If other faculty members are involved, can a consensus be reached about the direction for needed change and/or support for continuation?

early to avoid implementation delays. It is important to take time to develop support for the strategy. If this is a simple change within a course, then the instructor will need the support of students to participate effectively and not sabotage the effort. In more complex strategies, other faculty members or administrators may be the ones to bring in.

Some strategies will need help from technical specialists, who may be able to offer support and/or instruction for using the required equipment. Time must be allotted for adequate instruction to enable faculty members and students to reach a comfort level. Most important, the technical staff must be available to help solve problems, which are bound to occur. Planning strategies for troubleshooting and providing access for problem solving for both faculty members and students need to be thought out in advance of implementation.

Another phase of the planning process is planning for the evaluation of the strategy. This is the time to decide what needs to be evaluated and how it should be done. This phase can range from how the strategy will be used in student grading to evaluating learning outcomes for the class as a whole and needs to be developed to allow student and faculty input for future development. This can also be the time to develop an educational research project, if appropriate. Educational research and publication of results are needed and can assist all of us in understanding and applying an effective educational process.

*Gaining support for the innovation* is the next step. Some strategies require little or no resources to implement, whereas others require significant physical and/or financial resources. If resources are needed, then gaining support for acquisition of those resources is essential. Looking at alternative sources of funding is helpful. Grants can provide a good funding source but require time and effort to secure. Administrative support may be required, but administrators may also be an excellent resource to tap to discuss potential funding or acquisition of physical resources. Once the project has been developed, it is important to validate the support of stakeholders.

Class preparation is a given in education. *Preparing students for the innovation* is an important step. Student instructions need to be clear and specific. This is the time for motivating students to want to try this process, and for gaining their support. Students need to know how to address problems, especially when technology is involved. There may be a learning curve required with some strategies. Evaluation methods or grading must be made clear.

Students need to feel comfortable that they will not be punished for mistakes, but rather will benefit from those mistakes as part of the learning process.

*Faculty members may also need preparation for the innovation.* This is the time to be sure that everyone agrees about how the strategy will be run. Use of perception, validation, and clarification can be valuable here. Too often, people interpret statements differently. Checking that everyone has the same perceptions and clarifying differences can provide unity in approach to students and reduce problems of students playing one instructor against another. For some strategies, rehearsal time may be needed, or additional education may be required. Planning sufficient time for those activities will increase everyone's comfort level with the process.

The best part of the process is ***implementing the innovation.*** It is hoped that things will go well, but flexibility may be required if problems arise. Sometimes, unintended consequences, such as surfacing of emotional issues, can occur. Instructors should be alert to the need for follow-up or referral if problems arise.

***Evaluating the outcome*** is the final step in the process. Remember that learning can continue to occur long after implementation of the strategy. It may be possible to measure short-term attainment of learning outcomes, but it may or may not be possible to explore long-term effects. For certain strategies that were developed to provide a foundation for other learning experiences, it may be possible to remeasure students at the end of their program. Students and faculty members should be able to provide input for future development and use of the strategy. A strong evaluation process provides an opportunity to participate in educational research. Even if a strategy is not suitable for research, it still may be appropriate for publication.

Sharing teaching strategies presents the opportunity to improve the educational process. A catchword in health care today is "evidence-based practice." We also need evidence-based practice in education.

## CONCLUSION

In summary, innovative teaching strategies must be based on both learning objectives and student learning needs. The wide diversity of student learning needs means that educators must recognize that, although most students will benefit from the new approaches, some will not. This perspective can be disappointing, but it is realistic, and educators must take pride in what they have accomplished. Problems will occur that no amount of planning could foresee. These problems, although disturbing at the time, are often humorous memories in the future and can be addressed to improve future offerings. Developing effective teaching strategies is challenging and requires effort and persistence but can also be exceedingly rewarding and fun. Sharing those strategies with others will benefit students and faculty alike. We hope you will take advantage of the strategies presented in this book and go on to develop, implement, and share your own innovative strategies.

---

### NOTES

1. D.L. Kirp, Those Who Can't: 27 Ways of Looking at a Classroom, *Change* 29, no. 3 (1997):10–19.
2. MGH Institute of Health Professions, Mission Statement, Self-Study 2000, 13.

3. D.R. Woods, Getting Support for Your New Approaches, *Journal of College Science Teaching* 27, no. 4 (1998):285–286.

4. They Create Winners. *Success* 41, no. 7 (1994):43–46.

---

## SUGGESTED READINGS

Innovations in Master's Nursing Education: New Ways of Learning for the Marketplace. 1997. Proceedings of the American Association of Colleges of Nursing Annual Conference on Master's Education (San Antonio, Texas, December 4–6, 1997). Eric Document ED433736.

Kirp, D.L. 1997. Those who can't: 27 ways of looking at a classroom. *Change* 29, no. 3:10–19.

Travis, L., and P.F. Brennan. 1998. Information science for the future: An innovative nursing infomatics curriculum. *Journal of Nursing Education* 37, no. 4:162–168.

Woods, D.R. 1998. Getting support for your new approaches. *Journal of College Science Teaching* 27, no. 4:285–286.

# CHAPTER 3

# Critical Thinking in Nursing Education

*Patricia R. Cook*

## INTRODUCTION

Let's set the stage: The patient is a 62-year-old female admitted with "anemia." Twenty-four hours prior to admission the patient fainted in the grocery store. Because of the patient's history of uterine cancer six years ago and the possibility of metastasis, she is admitted for a comprehensive evaluation. You admit the patient to the unit and conduct your initial interview. The patient informs you that her stools have been very dark and that she has been taking an anti-inflammatory for her swollen knee. Is this information related to her admitting diagnosis? What components of the patient's history should the nurse consider as relative to the current situation?

Each day nurses are faced with situations such as this example. Nurses are required to think critically in order to deliver safe and competent nursing care. The challenge facing nursing education today is to develop a nursing curriculum that contains effective teaching/learning strategies for students to develop skills in critical thinking. Utilization of critical thinking provides a nurse with the advantage of looking at things from a point of view that is grounded in purposeful and methodical thinking. This challenge seems at face value to be fairly simple, but this task is difficult and complex for those responsible for educating tomorrow's nurses.

## DEFINITION OF CRITICAL THINKING

Scholars from various disciplines have examined the concept of critical thinking to gain a better understanding of this process. In an early discussion by Dewey,[1] he used the phrase *reflective thinking* to describe this process. Following Dewey's contributions to understanding critical thinking, Watson and Glaser[2] looked at critical thinking and identified three elements that make up this thinking process, namely attitude, knowledge, and skill. First, the critical thinker must have the attitude or desire to approach the problem and to accept that the problem needs to be solved. Next, the critical thinker must have knowledge of the problem's subject matter. The critical thinker then must have the necessary skills to use and manipulate this knowledge in the problem-solving process.

Ennis studied critical thinking and defined it as "reflective and reasonable thinking that is focused on deciding what to believe or do."[3(p.45)] He added that critical thinking is a practical activity that requires creativity in identifying hypotheses, questions, options, and ways of experimentation. Based on a philosophy background and an in-depth study of critical thinking, Paul identified critical thinking as thought that is "disciplined, comprehensive, based on intellectual standards, and as a result, well-reasoned."[4(p.20)] Paul related seven characteristics of the critical thinker:

1. It is thinking which is responsive to and guided by intellectual standards such as relevance, accuracy, precision, clarity, depth, and breadth.
2. It is thinking that deliberately supports the development of intellectual traits in the thinker, such as intellectual humility, intellectual integrity, intellectual perseverance, intellectual empathy, and intellectual self-discipline, among others.
3. It is thinking in which the thinker can identify the elements of thought that are present in all thinking about any problem, such that the thinker makes the logical connection between the elements and the problem at hand.
4. It is thinking that is routinely self-assessing, self-examining, and self-improving.
5. It is thinking in which there is integrity to the whole system.
6. It is thinking that yields a predictable, well-reasoned answer because of the comprehensive and demanding process that the thinker pursues.
7. It is thinking that is responsive to the social and moral imperative to not only enthusiastically argue from alternate and opposing points of view, but also to seek and identify weaknesses and limitations in one's own position.[5(pp.20–23)]

Probably, the most substantial definition of critical thinking was developed in the late 1980s by a group of theoreticians and published by the American Philosophical Association (APA) in 1990.[6] This group identified the critical thinker as one who is:

> habitually inquisitive, well-informed, trustful of reason, open-minded, flexible, fair-minded in evaluation, honest in facing personal biases, prudent in making judgments, willing to reconsider, clear about issues, orderly in complex matters, diligent in seeking relevant information, reasonable in the selection of criteria, focused in inquiry, and persistent in seeking results which are as precise as the subject and the circumstances of inquiry permit.[7(p.3)]

Nursing has used these critical thinking definitions from education and philosophy to formulate its own view of this important concept. Facione and Facione[8] described critical thinking as purposeful, self-regulatory judgment that gives reasoned consideration to evidence, content, conceptualization, methods, and criteria. Using the APA's definition of critical thinking, Facione and Facione identified the role of one's disposition in this thinking process. Within one's disposition there are seven elements: truth-seeking, open-mindedness, analyticity, systematicity, self-confidence, inquisitiveness, and maturity.[9] Using these seven elements, Facione and Facione developed *The California Critical Thinking Disposition Inventory (CCTDI) Test Administration Manual.*[10] This inventory was specifically put together to assess "one's opinions, beliefs, and attitudes."[11(p.3)]

Bandman and Bandman[12] discussed the issue of critical thinking and the role of reasoning in this thinking process. If individuals are critically thinking, then they will "examine assumptions, beliefs, propositions, and the meaning and uses of words, statements, and arguments."[13(p.4)] They continued by identifying four types of reasoning that constitute critical thinking, namely deductive, inductive, informal, and practical reasoning.

Alfaro-LeFevre discussed critical thinking and noted that critical thinking is a synonym for "reasoning . . . that involves distinct ideas, emotions, and perceptions."[14(p.8)] She delineated a description of critical thinking and noted that critical thinking in nursing:

1. Entails purposeful, outcome-directed (results-oriented) thinking.
2. Is driven by patient, family, and community needs.
3. Is based on principles of nursing process and scientific method.
4. Requires knowledge, skills, and experience.
5. Is guided by professional standards and ethics codes.
6. Requires strategies that maximize human potential (e.g., using individual strengths) and compensate for problems created by human nature (e.g., the powerful influence of personal perspectives, values, and beliefs).
7. Is constantly reevaluating, self-correcting, and striving to improve.[15(p.9)]

## IMPORTANCE IN NURSING

Enter any health care setting today, and the need for critical thinking is clearly evident. Situations in typical health care settings present a level of complexity that requires nurses to make rational and responsible decisions. Specific reasons critical thinking is needed in health care today include:

1. Situations require the nurse to process and utilize a great deal of information.
2. Information related to health care continues to expand on a daily basis.
3. Trends in health care have forced sick patients home prematurely, requiring extensive and complex home health care.

4. Changing staffing patterns in acute care facilities challenge nurses to care for high acuity patients.
5. Changes in health care will continue to occur—many of which we cannot begin to imagine.
6. Trends in technology show continued advances in diagnostics and treatment modalities.
7. Society continues to grow in complexity, with many diverse cultures represented in American society—a trend that is expected to continue.

Today's nurse and the nurse of the future must have the ability to use valuable time to think in an effective, organized, goal-directed, and open-minded manner. Nurses must solve problems using a variety of mental processes, such as reasoning, reflection, judgment, and creativity. Nursing education has the responsibility to produce graduates who possess and utilize critical thinking. The future of the graduate depends on nursing programs that continuously evaluate their programs and implement needed changes to ensure graduates' success on the National Council Licensure Examination for Registered Nurses (NCLEX-RN) and success as a member of the nursing work force. Therefore, teaching/learning strategies that promote the development of critical thinking need to be identified.

## THE ROLE OF NURSING EDUCATION

In nursing education, the challenge of producing students who think critically needs to be met by first examining all components of the teaching/learning process—curriculum, teaching/learning strategies, and evaluation measures. If nursing education implements an effective and comprehensive curriculum, identifies useful teaching/learning strategies to teach critical thinking, and applies appropriate evaluation measures, then students will be assured that they are leaving nursing programs with skills in critical thinking. Teaching/learning strategies can be identified based on Watson and Glaser's[16] key elements of critical thinking, namely attitude, knowledge, and skill.

### Attitude

Given any situation in nursing, students must first recognize that a problem exists and is worthy of solving. Faculty must utilize teaching/learning strategies that instill an attitude of curiosity and caring. From the first day of class until graduation, nursing faculty present common health care problems and relate them to needed nursing interventions. Clinical experiences provide students with opportunities to apply the concepts of nursing care in "real-life" situations. This introduction to real-life situations promotes the interest of students and develops beginning awareness of the many problems to be solved. Instructors play an important part in developing an attitude of inquiry by guiding students to ask questions, look for answers, and evaluate various factors in the delivery of nursing care.

## Knowledge

The issue of what to include in a nursing curriculum continues to frustrate nursing faculty. Today's knowledge of disease and illness has never been greater. Therefore, nursing faculty must evaluate the content of their curricula and include concepts that focus on developing a knowledge base that is applicable to multiple situations. Curriculum forms the structure for presenting concepts that provide the foundation for the development of critical thinking in nursing.

With a sound curriculum in place, nursing education is faced with identifying teaching/learning strategies that promote learning and the development of critical thinking. Unfortunately, there is no simple answer to developing the skill we call critical thinking. In her discussion of teaching methods, Klaassens[17] identified four principles for teaching critical thinking: First, the teaching method should move systematically through the stages of readiness, introduction, reinforcement, and extension. Second, it should be focused, moving from introduction of task and explanation of steps to presentation, supervised practice, and return demonstration by the student. Third, this method should blend with the typical topics, and fourth, guide students through the steps of knowledge acquisition—ending in formal thinking.

The traditional strategy for "imparting" knowledge in a nursing classroom has been lecture. Although students often prefer this teaching strategy, it does little to stimulate critical thinking. Today, nursing education has many teaching/learning strategies that promote the development of critical thinking. Using a variety of tools assists students with various learning styles to be effective learners. Selection and utilization of a variety of teaching/learning strategies requires the commitment of instructors to seek teaching/learning strategies that match students' cognitive level as well as the content being presented.

In 1979, Steinaker and Bell[18] identified an experiential taxonomy for use in planning and evaluating educational programs. Using a taxonomy reinforces that teaching/learning strategies should be evaluated and implemented based on the strategy's ability to reinforce learning "where the student is" at the time of the expected learning. The taxonomy developed by Steinaker and Bell has five categories, with varying levels within each category. These categories include exposure, participation, identification, internalization, and dissemination. The categories of exposure, participation, and identification are used to discuss the framework for appropriate teaching/learning strategies. The categories of internalization and dissemination are not being used because they require more experience within the practice of nursing following graduation from nursing programs.

*Exposure*

The category of exposure is used at the introduction level, where the student is aware of the experience, begins to form mental reactions to the stimuli, and becomes prepared for more experience. At this level, the instructor is setting the stage for learning—in other words, presenting basic concepts. Our goal is to develop skill in applying knowledge in the delivery of nursing care, but students must acquire knowledge prior to application. At this stage in learning, lecture is an effective strategy for the introduction of the content; however, students need additional teaching/learning strategies that offer them the opportunity to manipulate and process basic content.

*The following strategies are effective tools in applying basic concepts:*

1. *Study Guides:* In this strategy, students seek out basic information related to the subject topic. The guide directs students to answer questions about the subject. Instructors can be creative in developing study guides and can use patient scenarios to promote beginning "application" thinking. Use of study guides encourages students to independently seek out information. For many students, this beginning level of "empowerment" encourages them to be more responsible for their learning—a basic need for the critical thinker. With instructor-developed study guides, ample opportunity is available to include questions related to "why." Students must get in the mindset to ask "why" in order to begin understanding that all concepts do not apply to every situation.

2. *Computer-Assisted Instruction (CAI):* Using CAI to supplement the classroom lecture is an effective tool to reinforce basic concepts. Today, nursing education has access to a variety of CAI materials that offer students the opportunity to review and apply basic concepts. When selecting CAI programs, programs that are "basic" and that do not frustrate or overwhelm students should be identified. Use of CAI programs enhances "the logical processing of information, a feature that can help students make decisions."[19(p.19)]

3. *Case Studies:* Using case studies to apply concepts is nothing new to nursing education. Using examples of how concepts are applied in a clinical setting encourages students to think about how concepts relate to real-life situations. Case studies can be developed with varying levels of difficulty—ranging from the simple application of principles of hot and cold to the application of multiple concepts in the care of the burn patient. When using case studies at the exposure level, simple situations, focusing on specific focus concepts, should be included. Although case studies are often used as independent work for the student, they also are useful in the classroom. Case studies can be used as a class activity to teach students to "think on their feet" and to reinforce the need to understand the concepts in real-life situations.

4. ***Group Discussions:*** With the participation of students in classroom discussions, students learn from other students while developing their personal thinking skills. In this setting, students challenge each other's ideas and opinions, which is an important component to critical thinking.[20] When using an in-class activity such as group discussions, faculty need to continuously monitor the use of thinking and thoughtfulness and intervene as appropriate to redirect the group—if necessary.

5. ***Writing:*** Writing provides students with the opportunity to process concepts using mental imagery.[21] Students at all levels of a nursing curriculum can benefit from writing. At the basic level, students use concepts and build them into current knowledge as well as previous experiences. Using writing assignments provides the faculty with an opportunity to assess what students are learning and how well they process the new concepts.

### Participation

At the second level of the taxonomy, students have purposeful interaction with the experience. Many of the exposure strategies also are suitable for the participation level, namely writing, case studies, and CAI programs. Teaching/learning strategies at the participation level require recurrent thinking, however, because previously learned foundational concepts need to be used as students build on and learn beyond the basics. Writing, for example, requires students to move beyond the basic concepts and to use or apply them to a situation.

Writing at the participation level promotes student recognition that patient situations are not "textbook" and that they require the selection of interventions appropriate to that specific patient. In her discussion of a writing project conducted in California, Olson[22] identified four levels or domains of writing—sensory/descriptive, imaginative/narrative, practical/informative, and analytical/expository. The domain of sensory/descriptive is writing built on concrete concepts or points. The goal at this level is to center and focus on basic information. At the next level, students construct a story by means of identifying, sequencing, and capturing significant details. At the practical/informative level, students "learn accuracy, clarity, attention to facts, appropriateness to tone, and conventional forms."[23(p.23)] At the last level of the domain, students are expected to use the tasks of analysis, interpretation, and persuasion. Olson noted that these domains are not completely separate, and interdependency does exist among the levels.

CAI programs are effective tools to reinforce concepts. At the participation level, students using CAI programs are called on to problem solve using skills such as reasoning, questioning, prioritization, and discrimination. CAI programs that are appropriate for the students' knowledge and problem-solving level should be selected.

Case studies used at the participation level should involve more creativity and reasoning than those used at the exposure level. With more knowledge, students can be challenged to bring together concepts that have an increasing number of variables. For example, at the exposure level, students learn to identify the role of vital signs in the assessment of their patients. At the participation level, students should begin identifying the alterations in vital signs that occur when diseases affect the body and should identify needed interventions.

*Other teaching/learning strategies appropriate for the participation level include:*

1. ***Problem-Solving Team:*** Using groups to work as a team provides an opportunity for the students to share ideas and knowledge while working on a common goal or outcome. For this strategy to be effective, the instructor must provide clear objectives with specific instructions. Brookfield[24] identified themes characterizing critical thinking. One of those themes related to critical thinkers is the use of imagination and exploration of alternatives. Teamwork provides ample opportunity to spark imagination and creativity for the situation presented. Typically, group discussion leads to the identification of many alternatives; the group then evaluates and selects the needed interventions. This type of teaching/learning strategy promotes a second theme identified by Brookfield, namely the importance of context in critical thinking. No nursing situation is identical to another. Students must be able to assess each situation and to implement the required interventions. According to Linderman and McAthie,[25] when knowledge guides practice, it takes into consideration all other information gained through complementary means.

2. ***Reflective Journals:*** Students' use of journals is an important tool to encourage reflection on an experience and to evaluate one's performance and/or responses to the experience. Reflection provides an opportunity to weigh, consider, and choose.[26] Use of a reflective journal encourages students to think about their experiences and to examine the components as well as the overall experience. Students must see the need to examine their actions and determine areas that need improvements or changes. To be effective, instructors must provide specific guidelines on what information to include in the journal. For example, the student first describes the patient care situation. Next, students provide an analysis of significant events in the delivery of patient care and an exploration of feelings, reactions, and responses. In the last phase of journal writing, students "examine the outcomes of the reflective process."[27(p.1)] After this examination, students often identify changes to be made in future experiences.

3. ***Problem-Based Learning:*** This teaching/learning strategy focuses primarily on "process." A small student group works on a case study with the assistance of a faculty facilitator. This strategy links theory with clinical situations and encourages reasoning in a realistic situation using collabora-

tion and negotiation within the group. See Chapter 7 for more information on this strategy.

4. ***Questioning:*** Using questioning to reinforce learning is an excellent tool in the development of critical thinking. The use of questioning as a teaching tool can be traced back to Socrates in ancient Greece. Socratic questioning examines basic concepts or points, explores deeper into these concepts, and attends to problem areas of one's thinking.[28] Types of questions used in this teaching/learning strategy include clarification questions, probing questions, differing perspective questions, and consequence questions.[29]

## *Identification*

At this level, students become more "active" learning partners. Students identify with the experience at an emotional and personal level. As the experience becomes a part of the students, they desire to share the experience with others. As previously noted, teaching/learning strategies such as writing, case studies, and CAI continue to be important learning tools in the category of identification. With each of these strategies, there needs to be increasing complexity with more variables.

Additional teaching/learning strategies at the identification level should focus on organizing and applying concepts. Instructors play an important role at this level because they serve as a resource and moderator in students' use of information.[30] Other teaching/learning strategies for the identification category include:

1. ***Defensive Testing:*** Students at this level need to be challenged more on why they select one option over another. They need to recognize that nursing care is based on principles and knowing which principle matches a specific situation. Use of this strategy requires reflection, in other words "go beneath the surface structure of the situation, to reveal the underlying assumptions."[31(p.343)]

2. ***Debates and Critiques:*** Having students critique an article or other type of work provides a means of reinforcing the six critical thinking abilities identified by Linderman and McAthie.[32] These abilities include identifying possibilities/innovations, formulating and analyzing arguments, constructing meaning, using knowledge as context, negotiating, and critically reflecting on one's thoughts and actions. Seeking information and analyzing its meaning move students beyond basic concepts and challenge traditional use of these concepts. The strategy of debating is effective to developing critical thinking because it prepares students "to doubt, to challenge what is held to be true."[33(p.104)] If a student is required to debate the issue of abortion, he or she will formulate in-depth critical thinking about the purpose of abortion, its impact on a woman, and how society views access to this intervention. With debates and critiques, students "learn content, develop reasoning capabilities, and extend their ethical concepts."[34(p.30)]

3. *Problem-Based Learning:* With this teaching/learning strategy, students actively participate in problem solving. Discussion focuses on the problems presented in the case study and the identification of knowledge from previous experience with the identified problem(s).

## Skill

Now that students have developed an "attitude" of inquiry and the "knowledge" base needed, they need an opportunity to develop and apply knowledge in real-life situations. In nursing, these real-life situations are found in clinical settings. According to Adams and Hamm,[35] knowledge is beneficial only to the degree that it can be used to produce new knowledge.

The learning lab typically is located at the school of nursing and provides a tremendous opportunity for simulated learning. Although the learning lab traditionally has been used for learning of psychomotor skills, it offers students a safe, controlled environment to develop critical thinking. As students' nursing knowledge increases over the span of the curriculum, instructors can simulate or create situations in the learning lab that promote student exploration into the various options available for nursing care (without injury to the patient). In this nonthreatening environment, students are provided the opportunity to question, explore, and experiment. Students can apply reasoning skills without the constraints of limited time. See Chapter 22 for more discussion of the use of simulations to promote student learning.

The clinical setting is identified as any setting where students provide nursing care to "real" patients. Today, clinical settings range from in-hospital units to homeless clinics in the community. In these clinical settings, learning opportunities to develop critical thinking abound. The challenge of all clinical instructors is to construct clinical experiences that maximize student learning. The clinical setting requires students to be familiar with their patients' health problems, medications, procedures, and lab data. Using their knowledge of the textbook patient, students are challenged to develop skills in critical thinking in their efforts to implement appropriate care for an actual patient.

Care of patients in real-life situations reinforces that critical thinking is "contextual." Although the textbook lists specific interventions for patients with pneumonia, students must recognize the care needed for *that* patient at *that* time. Using a variety of mental processes, such as reasoning, prioritizing, judging, and inferring, students are able to select needed interventions. As knowledge and clinical skills develop, students' skills in critical thinking increase.

There is no "best" style for instruction in the clinical setting; however, several points should be considered to increase the effectiveness of the clinical experience.

1. Questioning by the instructor is an important part of the clinical experience. This process encourages students to "think" about the options available and

to select an intervention appropriate to *that* patient. A good technique to use when questioning students is asking the student to "talk aloud" while answering the instructor's questions.[36] Using this technique assists instructors in evaluating students' processing skills. Did they use appropriate reasoning skills? Was there a logical correlation between data and problem identification? Was the nursing process used appropriately, with logical sequencing of data—problem—goals—strategies or interventions—evaluation—follow-up with changes? Was there effective prioritization for that patient?

2. Students should be encouraged to "test" their thinking. Many health care alternatives are available today, and students need to explore what is best for their patients. The clinical setting provides the instructor with the opportunity to teach students on a one-on-one basis. Instructors need to seek every occasion when students perform correctly to verbally praise the student. Although clinical training is stressful and challenging, students need and deserve positive reinforcement of effective problem solving using critical thinking.

3. Instructors need to "empower" students to think critically. Students who feel a sense of empowerment take responsibility for the process of problem solving.

4. Instructors must see the importance and impact of role modeling. Using the teaching/learning strategy of modeling includes "leading the student through thoughts and experiences to one's own conclusions."[37(p.331)]

5. Written work related to clinical experiences is an important component in developing critical thinking. Students have the opportunity to take "textbook" patients and to select suitable interventions for their patients. The exercise of individualizing nursing care reinforces the contextuality of critical thinking and the need to explore all available options for patient care.

Kurfiss[38] discussed the elements of what she called *cognitive apprenticeship*, which include modeling or demonstration, coaching or assisting, guiding with gradual removal of the guidance, articulating or reasoning, reflecting or comparing, and exploring goals and options. All of these elements can be accomplished with clinical experiences. Clinical experiences expose students to the dynamic world of health care and practice with multiple concepts. Whether collecting data and relating their role to the patient's condition or developing an argument on why one intervention is better than another, students are developing skills in critical thinking. See Chapters 21 and 25 for more discussion of clinical instruction.

## EVALUATION OF CRITICAL THINKING

In the early 1990s, the National League for Nursing[39] revised its criteria for accreditation and incorporated the need for evaluation of critical thinking in undergraduate nursing programs. Since that time, nursing education has explored, pondered, and discussed how critical thinking should be evaluated. At the heart of evaluating critical thinking is nursing education's definition of critical thinking. How critical thinking is defined influences how it is evaluated.

In examination of nursing literature, several articles identify pertinent issues with tools for testing critical thinking inventories[40-44]; however, evaluation of critical thinking is an important component of nursing education. Teaching and evaluation clearly go hand-in-hand. Nursing education must identify and/or develop tools for evaluating critical thinking that reflect the individual program's definition and philosophy. With the use of multiple means of evaluation, nursing education gains a better understanding of teaching critical thinking and the impact of this instruction on student learning. Students should see evaluation as a learning tool; it is a positive means for determining the need for further learning, further clarification, and/or further directions by instructors.

## CONCLUSION

Nursing education's challenge to produce a nurse who can think critically has never been greater. Changing health care, increased acuity of patients, and a dynamic culture offer a tremendous challenge for nurses. Nursing education must attune itself to the task of reexamining the concept of critical thinking. This reexamination includes evaluation of all components of the teaching/learning process—curriculum, teaching/learning strategies, and evaluation measures. With the development of an effective curriculum, nursing education must create an attitude of inquiry in its students, develop the knowledge base needed, and provide ample opportunities for students to use their knowledge. Using a taxonomy such as the Steinaker and Bell[45] model provides an excellent framework to approach the development of critical thinking skills. In selecting approaches to develop critical thinking skills, nursing faculty can assure their students that as health care workers of tomorrow they will possess the necessary skills needed to deliver safe and competent nursing care.

---

### NOTES

1. J. Dewey, *How We Think: A Restatement of the Relation of Reflective Thinking to the Educative Process* (Chicago: Regnery, 1933).

2. F. Watson and E.M. Glaser, *Watson-Glaser Critical Thinking Appraisal* (Dallas: Psychological Corporation, 1980).

3. R.H. Ennis, A Logical Basis for Measuring Critical Thinking Skills, *Educational Leadership* 43, no. 2 (1985):44–48.

4. R.W. Paul, *Critical Thinking: What Every Person Needs To Know To Survive in a Rapidly Changing World* (Pohnert Park, CA: Center for Critical Thinking, 1993).

5. Paul, *Critical Thinking*, 20–23.

6. American Philosophical Association, *Critical Thinking: A Statement of Expert Consensus for Purposes of Educational Assessment and Instruction. The Delphi Report: Committee on Pre-College Philosophy* (ERIC Document Reproduction Service No. ED 315-423, 1990).

7. American Philosophical Association, *Critical Thinking*, 3.

8. N. Facione and P.A. Facione, Externalizing the Critical Thinking in Knowledge Development and Clinical Judgement, *Nursing Outlook* 44, no. 3 (1996):129–136.

9. N. Facione, P.A. Facione, and C.A. Sanchez, Critical Thinking Dispositions as a Measure of Competent Clinical Judgment: The Development of the California Critical Thinking Disposition Inventory, *Journal of Nursing Education* 33, no. 8 (1994):345–350.

10. *The California Critical Thinking Disposition Inventory (CCTDI) Test Administration Manual* (Millbrae, CA: The California Academic Press, 1994).

11. *The California Critical Thinking Disposition Inventory (CCTDI) Test Administration Manual*, 3.

12. E.L. Bandman and D. Bandman, *Critical Thinking in Nursing* (Norwalk, CT: Appleton & Lange, 1995).

13. Bandman and Bandman, *Critical Thinking*, 4.

14. R. Alfaro-LeFevre, *Critical Thinking in Nursing: A Practical Approach* (Philadelphia: W.B. Saunders, 1999), 8.

15. Alfaro-LeFevre, *Critical Thinking in Nursing*, 9.

16. Watson and Glaser, *Watson-Glaser Critical Thinking Appraisal*.

17. E.L. Klaassens, Improving Teaching for Thinking, *Nurse Educator* 13, no. 6 (1988):15–19.

18. N.W. Steinaker and M.R. Bell, *The Experiential Taxonomy: A New Approach to Teaching and Learning* (New York: Academic Press, 1979).

19. E.F. Pond, M.J. Bradshaw, and S.L. Turner, Teaching Strategies for Critical Thinking, *Nurse Educator* 16, no. 6 (1991):18–22.

20. C. Linderman and M. McAthie, *Fundamentals of Contemporary Nursing Practice* (Philadelphia: W.B. Saunders, 1999).

21. Pond, Bradshaw, and Turner, Teaching Strategies.

22. C.B. Olson, *Thinking/Writing: Fostering Critical Thinking Through Writing* (New York: Harper Collins, 1992).

23. Olson, *Thinking/Writing*, 23.

24. S. Brookfield, *Developing Critical Thinkers: Challenging Adults To Explore Alternative Ways of Thinking and Acting* (San Francisco: Jossey-Bass, 1987).

25. Linderman and McAthie, *Fundamentals*.

26. D.M. Adams and M.E. Hamm, *Cooperative Learning: Critical Thinking and Collaboration across the Curriculum* (Springfield, IL: Charles C Thomas, 1994).

27. M.M. Bratt, Reflective Journaling: Fostering Learning in Clinical Experiences, *Dean's Notes* 20, no. 1 (1998):1–3.

28. Paul, *Critical Thinking*.

29. M.H. Oermann, Evaluating Critical Thinking in Clinical Practice, *Nurse Educator* 22, no. 5 (1997):25–28.

30. Steinaker and Bell, *The Experiential Taxonomy*.

31. J.S. Ford and J. Profetto-McGrath, A Model for Critical Thinking Within the Context of Curriculum as Praxis, *Journal of Nursing Education* 33, no. 8 (1994):341–344.

32. Linderman and McAthie, *Fundamentals*.

33. F. Smith, *To Think* (New York: Teachers College Press, 1990), 104.

34. Adams and Hamm, *Cooperative Learning*, 30.

35. Adams and Hamm, *Cooperative Learning.*

36. S. Corcoran, S. Narayan, and H. Moreland, Thinking Aloud as a Strategy to Improve Clinical Decision Making, *Heart & Lung, The Journal of Critical Care* 17, no. 5 (1988):463–468.

37. D.E. Reilly and M.H. Oermann, *Clinical Teaching in Nursing Education* (New York: National League for Nursing, 1992), 331.

38. J.G. Kurfiss, *Critical Thinking: Theory, Research, Practice, and Possibilities* (College Station, TX: Association for the Study of Higher Education, 1988).

39. National League for Nursing, *Criteria and Guidelines for Evaluation of Baccalaureate Nursing Programs* (New York: National League for Nursing, 1991).

40. J.S. Hickman, A Critical Assessment of Critical Thinking in Nursing Education, *Holistic Nurse Practice* 7, no. 3 (1993):36–47.

41. D. Hartley and V. Aukamp, Critical Thinking Ability of Nurse Educators and Nursing Students, *Journal of Nursing Education* 33, no. 1 (1994):34–35.

42. C.J. Leppa, Standardized Measures of Critical Thinking: Experience with the California Critical Thinking Tests, *Nurse Educator* 22, no. 5 (1997):29–33.

43. B.C. Vaughan-Wrobel, P. O'Sullivan, and L. Smith, Evaluating Critical Thinking Skills of Baccalaureate Nursing Students, *Journal of Nursing Education* 36, no. 10 (1997):485–488.

44. B.L. Adams, Nursing Education for Critical Thinking: An Integrative Review, *Journal of Nursing Education* 38, no. 3 (1999):111–119.

45. Steinaker and Bell, *The Experiential Taxonomy.*

# CHAPTER 4

# Creativity

*Carol Picard*

Creativity is an elemental process, and the natural order of the universe according to Bohm, the Nobel prize–winning physicist.[1] In persons, creativity is the ability to make connections and to perceive patterns of relationship in novel ways. The artist Corita Kent said "To create is to relate."[2] Creativity is about imagining possibilities. It takes the shape of reflection on one's experience in the world, grounded in unique responses of engaging with the whole. Teilard de Chardin identified the human capacity for reflection and creative expression as its contribution to evolution—the noosphere, or thinking layer of the world.[3] Creativity can be expressed in a variety of modes and is a critical aspect of science and art. Kent believed that learning exercises that encourage the ability to connect and see new relationships foster a creative response to living.[4] To be in a creative state of mind, one must have an attitude of interest, which is wholehearted and total. Energy is not expended on protecting the self; instead, energy is released and free for the creative, imaginative process.[5]

Cultural blocks or conditions may prevent creativity from being expressed. Bohm described the need for openness, acknowledging barriers to the creative process in human beings. Society, as well as educational institutions, tends to "conformist, imitative and mechanical states of mind" that do not disturb the established order.[6] Nursing faculty face the challenge to prepare nurses who are competent and creative as beginning practitioners. The amount of content required to be competent can sometimes overshadow the process of becoming a reflective and creative practitioner. Watson cautions that the current nursing education often values the powerful prevailing medical discourse, choosing to emphasize data and content over experience and reflection.[7] She faults the technical and instrumental focus in the current health care environment as contributing to the lack of time devoted to the ontology of competence in nursing education and practice. Both Benner et al. and Watson critique teaching strategies in nursing education, which value critical thinking devoid of emotion.[8,9] The challenge is to foster creative responses to nursing situations that are grounded in nursing knowledge. Cultivating openness and self-awareness can support this goal.

Students model and respond to what they perceive is valued. Faculty may not be comfortable with an attitude of openness when curricula are content-driven instead of process-oriented. Process is an important element in cultivating critical thinking, which is essentially a creative process at its best. Nurses use creativity to sense patterns in clinical situations. Benner et al. challenge the use of standardized protocols and guidelines in nursing education and practice rather than including a more creative approach to appreciating the full complexity of clinical situations.[10]

The variety of innovative methods included in this text are examples of creativity in nursing education. Fostering creativity enhances the potential for knowledge development in the discipline because no two students are alike, and their ways of exploring phenomena of concern to nursing will also be unique.

## THEORETICAL RATIONALE

The goal of creative strategies in nursing education is to foster openness and a creative attitude in students. Creative strategies present opportunities for students to increase their awareness, which is a process of self-discovery. Watson recommended that nurses develop an awareness of self-in-relation, which is an essential component of transpersonal caring-healing, and the essence of postmodern nursing.[11] Watson encourages nurses to reflect on energy, consciousness, and caring as the basis for practice. Newman's theory of health as expanding consciousness describes the uniqueness of each person's pattern of consciousness.[12] This author believes that expanding consciousness is supported by creative activities. By mindfully reflecting on one's own pattern of response and engagement with others and the environment, consciousness expands. What better way to appreciate nursing theory than to live it. Newman encourages nurses to embody theory, melding theory and practice in a praxis approach to caring in the human health experience. Her theory is not something so much to apply, as it is to become. The teacher establishes a mindful presence to foster openness in students as a mirror or model for what students can later do with patients and families.

A creative approach is one requiring alertness and sensitivity. Although establishing a knowledge base can sometimes require habitual processes of thinking such as rote learning and memorization of facts, such activity can become a barrier to mindfulness. Calling students' attention to their capacity for heightening awareness can support energy available to creative responses to situations. The artist Alex Grey wrote that the creative process has six stages.[13] The first is formulation, where the subject or problem is discovered. The person then does research on this subject, saturating him or herself with knowledge about it. The next stage is to allow one's unconscious to sit with all of this knowledge and develop a response. How one responds is the inspiration, an internal process that is then translated into an outer form or activity, the creative act. The last stage of the creative process is to share it with others and get feedback.

Using resources and methods that are not typical for the nursing student can enhance the creative process because these methods are antidotes to ordinary habits of mind. Techniques involving several senses, such as the orange exercise that follows, or the use of poetry or film as artistic expressions of concepts and situations in the classroom example, can heighten focus on the subject at hand.

## CONDITIONS

Two important conditions support creative strategies. The first is safety. Because creative strategies foster openness, students may feel vulnerable as a result. Students must have confidence that the teacher is going to create a safe place for any risk taking of sharing ideas or feelings. As part of this creation of safe space, students must feel free to pass on any part of an activity. This freedom allows students to feel empowered and able to choose. Secondly, the teacher sets the tone of respect for the contributions of all participants. Because some activities, such as those described as follows, might cause a student to feel uncomfortable, the tone of respect is also the expectation of the teacher for the attitude of the whole group.

Creative activities can be part of a wide variety of teaching situations. The teacher is limited only by his or her own imagination. The goal is to cultivate an open, wholehearted spirit of inquiry. This creative act is teaching at its best. In preparing a lecture, ask yourself: How will students understand this new knowledge? How does it come alive? This is the teacher's creative process. In planning a lecture, sift through multiple sources on the topic, both from within and without the discipline. Let students know that it is assumed they have read some sources and will come together in dialogue. The goal is to make the material come alive so the student can engage with it.

## TYPES OF LEARNERS

These strategies can be used with both graduate and undergraduate students, and have been used in continuing education programs by the author.

## USING THE METHOD

In preparing for a lecture/discussion on caring for patients with mood disorders, the knowledge needed to care for a depressed person includes not only DSM-IV diagnostic criteria, etiological theories, and standard nursing care interventions but also an appreciation of the lived experience of depression. To invite the students to reflect on this state, I start the class with a poem by Sharon Olds entitled "Summer Solstice, New York City."[14] The poem depicts a suicidal person on a rooftop and those who rescue him. Other poetry on illness and disability and by nurses and other health care professionals is available in anthologies.[15,16] Weaving the poetic knowledge with the clinical descriptions and personal stories of patients, as well as inviting students to share their own knowledge of how depression is experienced, begin to color the class.

Frequently, students have cared for a person with depression in their clinical setting that week and illustrate with their new experiences. Others draw on experiences with close friends, relatives, or sometimes personal experiences that they choose to share. I have also brought former patients and other expert nurses to the classroom to share their experiences. When discussing the value of electroconvulsive therapy (ECT), I use a patient-education videotape on the topic, which takes the students to the bedside while the treatment is occurring. Because the treatment is still perceived by much of the lay public as something to be feared, I also show them why older people may have a great deal of anxiety. Many younger students have never seen the film *One Flew Over the Cuckoo's Nest*.[17] Using excerpts from the film helps them to appreciate an American iconic image of ECT, which their patients may remember. Class is over only when students reflect on the whole of the learning and consider what all of this means to their practice.

## Student's Creative Process in Smaller Group Situations: "Ode to an Orange"

This exercise can be part of a self-awareness activity, clinical seminar, or introduction to nursing course.

Needed: One orange for each student and the teacher. The activity can take place in a conference room, classroom, or any convenient space. Time allotment is one hour, including a breakout period of 15 minutes for small group activity.

This exercise makes use of a simple resource, fresh oranges, to gently invite the students to engage in and become aware of the creative process. Explain to the students that this is an exercise in awareness, where they are invited to be playful. There are no correct answers to this activity, only the ones they identify. The following are the stages of the creative process using the orange as a vehicle for the activity.

**Stage 1:** *Discovery of the subject.* Pass one orange to each student and invite the students to get to know their oranges. They can examine the fruit for all of its markings, mindfully concentrating on as much of the whole of the fruit as they can take in. When they are ready, collect all the fruit in one bag.

**Stage 2:** *Saturation.* Invite the students to now find their own orange. In the author's experience, this process is quick, and the students are somewhat surprised how easily they can identify their own orange. Invite the students to begin peeling the orange slowly, and to place the sections in front of them. The variability in how this process is done also allows for reflection on the uniqueness of each person in the room. For example, some people peel in one long spiral, whereas others are orderly about how they manage the skin pieces. Invite them to take in the scent of their orange and then to slowly eat one section, noticing the pieces of pulp for texture and taste. Invite descriptions of how the orange tastes. Students are then invited to share sections with each other and to compare the taste of each. The degree of variation can be striking within the same bag of oranges.

**Stage 3 and Stage 4:** *Incubation and Inspiration.* Invite the students to break into groups of three or four. The instruction is to create an "ode to orange" or a tribute to orange. Students may choose to create a song, essay, poem, picture, or other tribute to orange. They are invited to bring everything they know about orange to the task. Frequently, students brainstorm together using paper and collaborate on what their expression will be.

**Stage 5:** *Translation.* Student groups create an "ode."

**Stage 6:** *Integration.* The small groups perform their odes for each other and discuss the process as a whole. There is tremendous variability in how the ode is presented. Students have sung odes, written thoughtful reflections on the beauty of the fruit, danced, and crafted poems on the many dimensions of orange: color, variations in nature, and holiday associations, to name a few. The teacher encourages students to reflect on how they ordinarily explore new knowledge. Invite the students to consider how the exercise might apply to other dimensions of their student role. An example would be getting to know the patient: In what ways are there similarities and differences in patient needs? What are the assumptions we make based on a cursory review of information? When do nurses need to ask more in-depth questions? What is enough information?

Having to work in a group and take a risk to both create and perform their "odes" are often topics students want to explore. There is an opportunity to discuss one's private and public self, role in group collaboration, and the experience of creating something. Although the exercise is prescriptive in structure, it provides students with an opportunity to explore something in a more mindful manner. The teacher can end with some general thoughts on the creative process and invite the students to make links to clinical practice.

# EXAMPLE
# The Backpack Project

*Christine Bridges*

Clinical educators constantly seek to develop challenging learning experiences that have real-life relevance for students while meeting the requirements of a particular course. An added challenge is to make the experience meaningful and relevant for the clinical agency. The Backpack Project meets the needs of both the students and the agency and is a creative, scholarly, pragmatic, and fun course assignment. The project was originally developed in a school health setting, but it is easily applied to other populations and clinical areas.

School nurses, health educators, and others who work with children in schools recognize that the family is a critical partner in promoting children's health. More and more, however, the demands of busy lives make it difficult for parents to be part of the school day or to participate in evening programs. The Backpack Project was conceived as a way to establish a health communication link between the home and the school. This section describes the Backpack Project, identifies the learning objectives for graduate students in a community health nursing course, and provides an example of a backpack that has been developed.

The Backpack Project was preceded by an initial assessment of the community, which identified five health-related areas that parents wanted more information about for themselves and their children: exercise and fitness; health promotion and disease prevention; growth and development; nutrition; and mental health. The assessment also revealed that, although parents were eager for information, they were unable or unwilling to come to school-sponsored meetings, programs, or workshops. An outreach intervention was needed, and the Backpack Project was born. A list of backpacks that have been developed to date and the target age for each program is presented in Exhibit 4–1.

Thematic backpacks were developed around the five health-related areas that had been identified. Each is keyed to a specific topic. For example, "Healthy Snacks," "Stranger Danger," and "Sports Safety" are topics that have been addressed. A backpack contains a variety of resources and is borrowed from the school, like a library book, for a two-week period. Guidelines direct the development of a backpack's content and ensure that each backpack includes:

- didactic information
- individual activities

**Exhibit 4–1** Thematic Backpacks

| Health-Related Theme | Topic | Intended Grade Level |
|---|---|---|
| *I. Nutrition* | General Nutrition | K–2 |
| | Healthy Snacks | K–2 |
| | | |
| *II. Mental Health* | Stranger Danger | K–4 |
| | Self-Esteem | K–3 |
| | Self-Esteem | 4–6 |
| | Death and Dying | K–4 |
| | Loss | 4–6 |
| | It's Not Your Fault | 4–6+ |
| | Bully Prevention | 4–6+ |
| | Relaxation/Stress Management | 3–6 |
| | Depression/Suicide | 7–9 |
| | Multiple Intelligences | all+ staff |
| | | |
| *III. Exercise* | Your Body and How It Works | K–4 |
| | Sports Safety | 5–8 + coaches |
| | | |
| *IV. Health Promotion/ Disease Prevention* | Heart Smart | K–3 |
| | Asthma | K–4 |
| | Diabetes | K–4 |
| | Head Lice | 3–5 |
| | Germs | 3–5 |
| | Over-the-Counter Meds | 9–12 |
| | | |
| *V. Growth and Development* | Teen Concerns/Health Resources | 7–9+ |
| | Substance Abuse Prevention | 7–9+ |

- interactive family activities
- participatory, hands-on activities
- a bibliotherapy component
- resources

The guidelines, together with the students' learning objectives, provide a framework for determining what to include and how to present the material. Learning objectives focus on providing students with an opportunity to:

- build their clinical knowledge base in a selected area
- broaden their theoretical repertoire
- expand their teaching skills
- critically evaluate health resource materials

As clinical instructors, we seek to have students build their clinical knowledge and develop a broad repertoire of theories and models, which helps them to assess and plan for their clients. Additionally, students need to be able to find, critique, and evaluate available resources or adapt and develop materials if none are available as they hone their teaching skills. Creating a thematic backpack allows students to synthesize these three strands—theory, clinical knowledge, and resources—into a comprehensive and effective health education tool.

Whether the backpack's focus is diabetes or drug use prevention, nutrition or self-esteem, students must have a strong knowledge base of the clinical area of interest as a starting point. This requirement means reviewing the literature for the most current information and research. Only by having a thorough grounding in the clinical area will students be able to convey this knowledge to their clients in a meaningful way.

Appropriate models or theoretical frameworks underlie each backpack. For this population—school-aged children and their families—two theoretical orientations were especially helpful. Developmental theories were used to select the content area and to determine an appropriate level for the materials. For example, the young teen's need for autonomy and independence, the importance of peers, and the physiological changes of early adolescence helped shape decisions about the content focus of backpacks targeted to this age group. "Teen Concerns/Health Resources" and "Substance Abuse Prevention" backpacks were developed for children in grades seven through nine.

Consideration of cognitive, social, and emotional development help determine the level of content for the intended audience. For example, two self-esteem backpacks were developed. One was for young children in Grades K–3. The kinds of activities it contains are different from those developed for a self-esteem backpack for children in grades 4–6. Differences in levels of sophistication create an opportunity for graduate students to broaden the range of intervention strategies they bring to their practice. Planning and developing the intervention strategies, in turn, enhance and increase the students' teaching skills.

A second theoretical orientation that addresses the styles and needs of learners, Gardner's Theory of Multiple Intelligences,[18,19] provides the graduate students with a framework for developing interventions that move beyond simply presenting information with the hope that clients will act on it. Gardner is an educator who prefers to think not about how smart people are, but rather about how people are smart. He maintains that society has traditionally recognized and valued only two kinds of intelligences: linguistic and logical-mathematical (IQ tests, SATs, etc.). His theory of multiple intelligences proposes that we are smart in at least seven different ways and all have equal claim to priority. We don't all learn in the same way, and Gardner seeks to identify an individual's strengths and build on them. His work offers valuable insights into how people learn and how we might accommodate health education materials and approaches to the styles and strengths of the learners.

An example of a backpack itself best illustrates how clinical and theoretical knowledges are applied through creative nursing interventions. By way of example, the "Heart Smart" backpack will be described (see Exhibit 4–2). It was developed as one of the Health Promotion/Disease Prevention series for children in grades kindergarten through three.

Backpacks also contain a comprehensive list of resource materials, which includes books, relevant agencies and organizations, and Web sites. Each backpack is unique. The "Heart Smart" backpack includes an "Add-a-Recipe" binder, which invites every family to contribute its own favorite heart-healthy recipe. A backpack on death and dying has a Memory Book, and families are encouraged to fill a page with memories of a loved one who has died. Each backpack reflects the individuality and creativity of the nursing students who create them. The richness of this assignment lies in the fact that although the guidelines and objectives remain constant, no two projects are alike. The students are able to draw on their own intelligences and discover previously unknown talents and strengths.

---

**Exhibit 4–2** Heart Smart Backpack

| **Didactic Information** | Bibliotherapy: "The Magic School Bus inside |
|---|---|
| *Verbal-Linguistic Intelligence* | the Human Body" |
| *People learn best through* | Bibliotherapy: "Looking into My Body" |
| *reading, hearing, and* | Children and the Need for Physical Activity: |
| *seeing words.* | Fact Sheet |
| | Physical Activity and Cardiovascular Health: |
| | Fact Sheet |
| | Health and Fitness: You and Your Heart |
| | American Heart Association Position Paper: |
| | Exercise and Children |
| | American Heart Association Position Paper: |
| | Cigarette Smoking and Children |
| | What You Should Know about 22 Ways to a |
| | Healthier Heart |
| | Basic Food Groups |
| | Bibliotherapy: "The Golden Treasure" |
| | Bibliotherapy: "Gregory the Terrible Eater" |
| | Bibliotherapy: "Cloudy with a Chance of |
| | Meatballs" |

*continues*

**Exhibit 4–2 continued**

**Individual Activities**
*Intrapersonal Intelligence*
*People learn best through*
*    working alone, self-paced*
*    projects, and reflection.*
*Logical-Mathematical*
*    Intelligence*
*People learn best through*
*    questioning, reasoning,*
*    and working with patterns*
*    and relationships.*

Food Memory Game
First Heart Attack Risk Test
Activity Worksheets:
    Heart Message
    Build a Healthy Heart
    Good Advice Picture Puzzle
    Say "No" to Smoking
    Follow the Blood
    Count Your Heartbeats
    What's in Foods?
    Making Healthful Choices
    Activity Checkup
    What Foods Do You Need?

**Interactive Family**
**    Activities**
*Interpersonal Intelligence*
*People learn best through*
*    sharing and comparing*
*    experiences and relating*
*    to others.*
*Visual/Spatial Intelligence*
*People learn best through*
*    working with pictures,*
*    visualizing, and drawing.*

Video: "I Am Wonderfully Made"
The Healthy Body Cookbook
Quick and Easy Cookbook
Recipe: Good-for-Your-Heart Pretzels
Activity Worksheets:
    Fruits and Vegetables
    Activities for the Heart
    Family Fun
Add-a-Recipe Binder
Heart Smart Jeopardy Game

**Participatory, Hands-on**
**    Activities**
*Bodily-Kinesthetic*
*    Intelligence*
*People learn best through*
*    moving, touching, and*
*    processing knowledge*
*    through activities.*
*Musical-Rhythmic*
*    Intelligence*
*People learn best through*
*    rhythm, melody, singing,*
*    and listening to music.*

Food Pyramid Bingo
Food Charades
Be Like the Animals: Poems and Activities
    about Keeping Our Hearts Healthy
"My Pump" Song and Audiotape
"My Heart Is a Pump" Sponge and Water
    Activity
"My Pulse" Song and Audiotape
"My Pulse" Pulse Spots Activity and Stickers
"Flub-Dub" Song and Audiotape
"Heartbeats" Stethoscope Activity
"The Size of My Heart" Activity

## NOTES

1. D. Bohm, *On Creativity* (New York: Routledge, 1998).
2. C. Kent, *Learning by Heart: Teaching To Free the Creative Spirit* (New York: Bantam, 1992), 5.
3. P. Teilhard de Chardin, *The Phenomenon of Man* (New York: Harper & Row, 1959).
4. Kent, *Learning by Heart.*
5. Bohm, *On Creativity.*
6. Bohm, *On Creativity*, 16.
7. J. Watson, *Postmodern Nursing and Beyond* (New York: Churchill Livingstone, 1999).
8. P. Benner, C. Tanner, and C. Chesla, *Expertise in Nursing Practice* (New York: Springer, 1996).
9. Watson, *Postmodern Nursing and Beyond.*
10. Benner, Tanner, and Chesla, *Expertise in Nursing Practice.*
11. Watson, *Postmodern Nursing and Beyond.*
12. M. Newman, *Health as Expanding Consciousness* (Sudbury, MA: Jones & Bartlett, 1994).
13. A. Grey, *The Mission of Art* (Boston: Shambalala, 1998).
14. S. Olds, *The Gold Cell* (New York: Alfred Knopf, 1987).
15. C. Davis and J. Schaefer, eds., *Between the Heartbeats* (Iowa City: University of Iowa Press, 1995).
16. A. Belli and J. Coulehan, eds., *Blood & Bone* (Iowa City: University of Iowa Press, 1998).
17. M. Forman, *One Flew Over the Cuckoo's Nest* (Los Angeles: Warner Home Video, 1975).
18. H. Gardner, *Frames of Mind* (New York: Basic Books, 1983).
19. H. Gardner, *Multiple Intelligences: The Theory in Practice* (New York: Basic Books, 1993).

## SUGGESTED READING

Bryner, A., and D. Markova. 1996. *An unused intelligence.* Berkeley, CA: Conari Press.

Diaz, A. 1992. *Freeing the creative spirit.* San Francisco: Harper.

Gelb, M. 1998. *How to think like Leonardo daVinci.* New York: Delacorte.

Kent, C. 1992. *Learning by heart: Teaching to free the creative spirit.* New York: Bantam.

Richards, M.C. 1989. *Centering.* Middletown, CT: Wesleyan.

Root-Bernstein, R., and M. Root-Bernstein. 1999. *Sparks of genius.* Boston: Houghton Mifflin.

# CHAPTER 5

# Humor in the Classroom: Facilitating the Learning Process

*Sandra M. Hillman*

## DEFINITION AND PURPOSE

One of the most important functions of humor is to create a positive learning environment. Throughout history humor has been accepted as an important tool for the teacher in college classrooms. Most students can recall a learning experience they will never forget because it was presented in a humorous way. The effective educator symbolizes the world in a manner that is creative and insightful. This ominous responsibility requires the teacher to have many communicative strategies that can be meaningful for all students. Of all the communicative strategies that educators utilize, the use of humor is most promising but in many instances least understood.

Some of the benefits of humor in education include the improvement of problem solving, both interpersonally and in group settings; putting the educator and the participants at ease; and the promotion of expression and exchange of ideas. Robinson believes that what is learned with laughter is learned well.[1] Hizar and Bower found that humor and laughter increasingly presented as an approach that can assist in meeting specific goals and objectives.[2]

Sensitivity to humor can be taught to professors who are interested in creating a classroom community that is not afraid to take a reflective look at itself. Humor can be used in a variety of situations to display many different feelings and thoughts. The beauty of humor is that in order for it to be effective, it must be shared. Humor should be used by educators to facilitate and enhance the learning experience.

Humor is the recognition and verbal or written expression of that which is funny, ludicrous, or amusing. It connotes kindliness, a genial quality. Wit, on the other hand, denotes intelligence. Witty remarks reflect a quick ability to perceive and respond to incongruities and are designed to be entertaining or amusing. Sharpness, cleverness, spontaneity, or sarcasm may characterize wit. Wit is a form

54

of humor that has adaptive functions and can be potentially harmful or hostile. Laughter is the physical expression of what is humorous. It has bodily properties such as sounds, facial gestures, and usually involuntary muscle movements.[3]

There are three traditionally acknowledged theories of humor: superiority, incongruity, and relief.[4] From philosophical and psychological viewpoints, these theories have attempted to explain the complex phenomenon of humor.

Superiority theory dates back to Plato and Aristotle, who identified laughter as a form of derision, an expression of superiority over others.[5] Laughter was considered harmful to a person's character and incompatible with living a good life. As a type of humor, Lefcourt and associates found that students who had an internal locus of control preferred superiority humor.[6] This finding was related to the self-assuredness of these students, who could laugh at themselves when a prank was played on them. Here superiority was viewed as a person's ability to rise above one's own situation to laugh at oneself. Superiority theory also involves the therapeutic technique of distancing. The coping function of humor is exemplified through provision of distance between the person and the immediate situation.[7] The implication is that the person can become greater and more significant than the problem and can view the situation objectively. This type of superiority humor is not derisive. Perhaps variety in the forms of this theory of humor has made the generation of research problematic.

Incongruity theory emphasizes a cognitive side of laughter. According to this theory, laughter or amusement occur as an intellectual reaction to something unexpected, illogical, or inappropriate in some way.[8] Incongruity has been used extensively in children's humor. Research indicates that the recognition of incongruity occurs at about four months of age. In Sweden, this theory was validated by testing college students' emotional reactions to weights of different divergence from a range of expectancy.[9] Indeed, laughter resulted.

The relief theory of humor incorporates a physiological viewpoint in which laughter is seen as a venting of nervous energy. Freud supported this theory of humor. He believed that psychic energy is used in humorous situations and, as it becomes overabundant, is released as laughter, a physical process. Relief theory explains that laughter occurs because of the release of preexisting energy and the release of energy built up by the humorous situation itself. Freud felt that the pleasure experienced in humor was derived from psychic release and that humor served healthy and adaptive functions.[10]

Research to support and test these proposed theories has increased over the last 40 years. Although these theories represent philosophical views, they are relevant to the understanding and application of humor in the classroom environment.

Humor can assist the educator in bridging the gap between professor and students. As a stimulation of mental function, humor is used in adult education processes to facilitate the learner's receptivity to the information presented and his or her willingness to explore new ideas. The implementation of humor through the use of games, simulations, role-play case studies, and other related activities are all applications of the principles of adult learning.

Just as humor aids in the retention of concepts learned, it also stimulates creativity and critical thinking. The psychological function of humor allows for the expression of feelings, such as empathy and anger, in a constructive, witty manner. Because the affective domain strongly influences the learner's willingness to apply knowledge and skills in daily work, educators should strive to use strategies such as cooperative games that address this learning domain.

Games use an interactive process that facilitates acquisition and application of cognitive, affective, and psychomotor knowledge. When dealing with sensitive issues such as bioethics and cultural differences, the use of humor in simulation games and role-play can foster an openness and willingness to examine other viewpoints. Looking at the comical side of situations in which personal value conflicts frequently arise may lessen the learner's sense of threat when the game is conducted in an informal atmosphere.[11]

Despite the recognition of the importance of humor, nursing educators have made little attempt to consciously or deliberately use humor in the educational setting. The planned use of humor in the educational process as content in the curriculum and as a learning tool remains an uncommon occurrence. Unfortunately, the educational process has long been associated with formal discourse. Educators speak about the serious, apathetic student. Regardless of how good an educator is at presenting, content alone is not necessarily going to keep everyone's attention and interest for the entire presentation. Using humor in the classroom enhances the learning process and fosters the student-teacher relationship, and can become the vehicle for developing the student's ability to relate in a warm and friendly way to others.

Four interrelated aspects should be considered in the area of education and humor. The first is enhancing the learning process itself through humor. Second is using humor to facilitate the process of socialization. Third is teaching the concept of humor as a communication and intervention tool. Fourth is modeling the use of humor as a vehicle for facilitating the other three.

Higher education is currently faced with an entirely new goal for survival—adaptation to change through learning. The concepts of creativity and change are closely related to each other and to humor and education. Cultivating our sense of humor requires that we learn to thrive on change.

## THEORETICAL RATIONALE

Extensive research by Ziv demonstrated that humor does improve learning in schoolchildren and that it is positively correlated with creativity.[12] A humorous approach stimulates divergent thinking, the creation of new ideas, and new ways of looking at situations.

Laughter has a liberating effect on the flow of ideas. Studies have shown that the open, humorous teacher in the classroom is more effective in creating an atmosphere that is conducive to better academic work. Higher humor that is relevant to what is being taught—not sarcasm or ridicule, but humor that invites everyone to share in those defects common to all humans—improves learning. Ziv also found that humor may be a better indicator of leadership IQ.[13]

Zillman and Bryant (1983) demonstrated the positive effects of humor in learning.[14] They found that humor used with college-age students must be relevant to the subject being taught. Unrelated humor used by the professor detracts from the student-teacher rapport and has detrimental effects on the acquisition of information. On the other hand, the involvement of relevant humor that is well integrated into the educational message may lead to superior retention of the information and is likely to make the learning experience more enjoyable as well as enhance the student-teacher rapport. Fry points out that some of the physiological results of laughter include the stimulation of the production of adrenaline in the brain, which increases alertness and memory, thereby enhancing the learning process.[15]

Humor must be a component of any learning theory. Instead of a relationship to one particular theory of learning, humor and laughter contribute to all of those necessary principles of learning regardless of the theory: enjoyment; creativity; interest; motivation; a relaxed, open, warm environment; a positive student-teacher relationship; and decreased tension and anxiety. Probably, humor most closely aligns itself with the humanistic approach to education. Building a positive self-image, identifying the self-actualized person, and finding meaning in one's life are the goals of the humanistic movement. Maslow, who pioneered this movement, defined the self-actualized human as having a philosophical, non-hostile sense of humor.[16] Humor and laughter can produce a momentary experience related to self-actualization in terms of creating new and innovative perspectives.

This approach enables the educator not only to take him or herself lightly but also to use a sense of humor to remind others of their vulnerability. Maslow defines humor and laughter as education in a palatable form. To be real and genuine is one of the most important qualities of a teacher who facilitates learning. Having a sense of humor is an aspect of being real. Eble states that laughter creates the very air in which learning thrives.[17] Laughter is the physical expression of what is funny and forces a physical giving that relaxes for a moment the inner self. Such giving is necessary to prepare the self for learning. Eble suggests that parents consider laughter even before love because laughter keeps love from smothering, and if we laugh we are bound to love.

## CONDITIONS

Humor can be used in a variety of ways in the classroom. The use of humor to facilitate the learning process by creating an open, trusting environment that puts students at ease and prepares them to relax, be themselves, and experience new concepts and ideas is one condition for the use of humor. In addition, faculty can use humorous examples or present concepts humorously to help students comprehend and retain lecture material.

Another use for higher humor is to help socialize the student by releasing strain and tension. The use of humor in education is a mechanism that does not destroy one's self-image but provides a way to criticize, show mistakes, and express values, yet save face for students and imply caring in so doing.

Robinson (1995) points out that when relating humorous experiences, the educator may indicate mistakes that he or she has made as well.[18] This process can help students, who usually have unrealistic expectations of their own performances, to take themselves less seriously and enjoy the learning process.

With any teaching strategy, the effective use of humor needs to be learned and refined. Before using humor in teaching situations, educators may want to assess their sense of humor using a humor profile such as the one developed by White and Lewis.[19] The score obtained on the humor profile reflects the degree to which educators could improve their abilities to use humor as a teaching strategy. Completion of a humor profile may provide insight into an educator's ability to lightheartedly accept and tolerate him or herself and others and a willingness to transgress from conformity to innovation in instruction.

Once educators have assessed their sense of humor in teaching, the next step is to make a commitment to explore ways to include humor in the educational content. Learning and humor can be effectively integrated with the use of icebreakers, jokes, games, and fun activities. Observing others who use similar techniques is often helpful. Humorous material should be collected by listening and talking with colleagues and by writing down humorous anecdotes.

## TYPES OF LEARNERS

Humor is appropriate for both undergraduate and graduate students, provided it is relevant to the content being taught. College students respond well to the use of relevant humor in the learning process, both on ground and in distance learning online courses. The use of humor in the form of game playing or joke telling makes learning fun and enhances retention and application of content. What is taught in an atmosphere of fun and open, honest interaction is learned well.

## RESOURCES

Humor can be used in all settings; however, if games, cooperative play, or magic techniques are chosen, tiered lecture halls inhibit the students from relating in the game format. Special equipment can be used depending on the objectives and type of humor implemented. The use of humor to facilitate learning can require no additional resources if the educator chooses to tell anecdotal stories of his or her own experiences. If games are chosen to facilitate learning, then various props and video/audio equipment may be required. The object is to use whatever equipment is necessary to integrate the humor activity into the educational process.

## USING THE METHOD

Using humor in the learning process can take several forms. Some faculty may feel most comfortable using spontaneous storytelling by relating their own experiences to enhance the learning process. Jokes, anecdotal situations, and humorous exercises may be used to establish a sense of trust and to increase the learner's receptivity to information and participation during content presentations. Educators who have never used, or are not comfortable using, spontaneous humor in the classroom might choose to use predeveloped exercises or games. It is important to ensure that the participants do not become so involved in the chosen activity that they miss the point of the educational content. White and Lewis recommend that if this approach is taken, the educator should select the game/exercise after the learning objective has been set.[20] Before using a game or exercise, it is recommended that a pilot test be done at least once with a group not involved with the immediate presentation. This test will help to determine the effectiveness of the game in meeting the preconceived objectives. Faculty must realize that what works for some people does not necessarily work for others.

Games may have different outcomes each time they are used. Like different types of teaching, these structured games/exercises must be evaluated for their effectiveness. An educator's primary responsibility is to ensure clarity and precision of information. If the teacher can keep animated by providing entertainment value, receptivity of the participants to the game or exercise will be enhanced.

Facilitators must debrief all of the exercises and games carried out during educational sessions. Debriefing puts the participants back together when the game has finished and allows the educator and participants to experience their feelings and outcomes of the game. Kroehnert found that incorporating play through the use of games in the classroom is not only fun for both the educator and the participants but also greatly enhances the learning process.[21]

In stressing the significance of using critical thinking skills when confronted with a problematic situation, Bornemeier describes an exercise that requires both creativity and analytic ability.[22] The students are given the task of removing an object from a tall cylinder, using any resource at their disposal, without tipping the cylinder. It is common for many participants to identify elaborate, time-consuming solutions. At the end of a specified time, the less obvious but most effective solution is demonstrated. As water is poured from the educator's water pitcher into the cylinder, the object rises to the top. Most of the students laugh and acknowledge the foolishness of their efforts and their inability to identify the most simple, efficient, and creative solution to the problem. Becoming actively involved, with each phase requiring critical thinking skills, is more beneficial than merely listening to an explanation of the concept. In the end, the learning process is more explorative and imaginative.

With the recent development of online distance learning, methods to infuse humor into the virtual classroom to promote a positive learning environment have begun to emerge. One example is the following:

### *You Know You're Becoming a Computer Junkie When . . .*

1. You wake up at 3 AM to go to the bathroom and stop to check your e-mail on the way back to bed.
2. You get a tattoo that reads: "This body best viewed with Netscape Navigator 3.0 or higher."
3. You name your children Eudora, Mozillia, and Dotcom.
4. You turn off your modem and get this awful, empty feeling, like you just pulled the plug on a loved one.
5. You spend half of the plane trip with your laptop on your lap . . . and your child in the overhead compartment.
6. You decide to stay in college for an additional year or two, just for the free Internet access.
7. You laugh at people with 28,800-baud modems.
8. You start using smileys in your snail mail.
9. Your hard drive crashes. You haven't logged in for two hours. You start to twitch. You pick up the phone and manually dial your ISP's access number. You try to hum to communicate with the modem—and you succeed.
10. You find yourself typing "com" after every period when using a word processor.com
11. All of your friends have an @ in their names.
12. Your cat has its own home page.
13. You check your mail. It says "no new messages." So you check it again.
14. You move into a new house and decide to Netscape before you landscape.
15. You start tilting your head sideways to smile. :-)

## POTENTIAL PROBLEMS

Educators must be completely honest and open with their participants. This includes not using hidden agendas, not misleading students, and not setting anyone up. In addition, it is important that participants are not deceived or their efforts used for personal gain. Humor in the classroom setting is undesirable if a student is the target of the humor. It is important to note that the genders react to humor in significantly different ways. When a game is chosen for the classroom and an assessment of its potential effects is made, the educator should consider the following:

- Does the game encourage the players to "laugh with" as opposed to "laugh at" one another?
- Is it cooperative in nature?
- Does the game take positive action?
- Is the game inclusive in nature?
- Do the participants feel more connected with the other members of the class as a result of playing the game?
- Does the game provide opportunities for the players to be imaginative and spontaneous as well as provide room for recreation?
- Can the participant's goals and standards be met?
- Is it challenging?
- Does it facilitate the content being taught?

It is evident that humor can be a valuable tool for the educator. Humor promotes the creation of a positive learning environment for students. In addition, the implementation of games, role-play, and simulations helps to create a sense of community in and outside the classroom. Faculty have a responsibility to identify creative ways to incorporate humor into their learning laboratory, which complement their unique teaching styles. Ultimately, humor in the classroom creates the climate in which learning thrives!

---

## NOTES

1. V. Robinson, *Humor and the Health Professions,* 2nd ed. (Thorofare, NJ: Slack Inc., 1995).
2. H. Hizar and M. Bower, The Dynamics of Laughter, *Archives of Psychiatric Nursing* 6 (1992):132–137.
3. M. Brody, The Meaning of Laughter, *The Psychoanalytic Quarterly* 19 (1950):192–201.
4. J. Morreall, *The Philosophy of Laughter and Humor* (Albany, NY: State University of New York, 1987).
5. J. Morreall, *Taking Laughter Seriously* (Albany, NY: State University of New York, 1983).
6. H. Lefcourt, C. Sidoni, and C. Sidoni, Locus of Control and the Expression of Humor, *Journal of Personality* 42, no. 1 (1974):130–140.
7. J. Simon, Therapeutic Humor: Who's Fooling Who? *Journal of Psychosocial Nursing and Mental Health Services* 26, no. 4 (1988):8–12.
8. Morreall, *Taking Laughter Seriously.*
9. Nerhardt, Humor and Inclination To Laugh: Emotional Reactions to Stimuli of Different Divergence from a Range of Expectancy, *Scandinavian Journal of Psychology* 11 (1970):185–195.
10. H. Williams, Humor and Healing: Therapeutic Effects in Geriatrics, *Gerontion* 1, no. 3 (1986):14–17.
11. L. White and D. Lewis, Humor: A Teaching Strategy To Promote Learning, *Journal of Nursing Staff Development* 6 (1990):60–64.
12. A. Ziv, Using Humor To Develop Creative Thinking, in *Humor and the Health Professions*, 2nd ed., ed. V. Robinson (Thorofare, NJ: Slack Inc., 1990), 114.

13. Ibid.

14. D. Zillman and J. Bryant, *Uses and Effects of Humor in Educational Ventures* (New York: McGraw-Hill, 1983).

15. W. Fry, Humor, Physiology and the Aging Process, in *Humor and the Health Professions,* 2nd ed., ed. V. Robinson (Thorofare, NJ: Slack Inc., 1990), 114.

16. A. Maslow, *Motivations and Personality* (New York: Harper Row, 1970).

17. K. Eble, *A Perfect Education* (New York: McGraw-Hill, 1966), 45.

18. Robinson, *Humor and the Health Professions.*

19. White and Lewis, Humor.

20. Ibid.

21. G. Kroehnert, *100 Training Games* (New York: McGraw-Hill, 1991).

22. W. Bornemeier, Sphincter Protecting Hemorrhoidectomy, in *Humor and the Health Professions,* 2nd ed., ed V. Robinson (Thorofare, NJ: Slack Inc., 1990), 121–122.

---

**SUGGESTED READING**

Loomans, D., and K. Kolberg. 1993. *The laughing classroom.* Tiburon, CA: H.J. Kramer, Inc.

Robinson, V. 1995. *Humor and the health professions.* 2nd ed. Thorofare, NJ: Slack Inc.

# PART II

## Teaching in Structured Settings

Part II presents concept-based topics that are applicable in a myriad of situations, regardless of the level of the learner, the topic, or the class size. The universal concepts evident in each chapter include the importance of planning and preparation on the part of the teacher, the manner in which information is conveyed, and the importance of active student involvement and responsibility for learning.

The principles presented in Part I, the Introduction section, are seen in the chapters in this section. Application of teaching and learning theories and planned activities directed toward critical thinking are apparent. Educators can use creative innovations with time-honored strategies, such as lecture, to bring a refreshing approach to teaching.

# CHAPTER 6

# Lecture Is Not a
# Four-Letter Word!

*Barbara C. Woodring*

## INTRODUCTION

> What all the great teachers appear to have in common is love of their
> subject, an obvious satisfaction in arousing this love in their students,
> and an ability to convince them that what they are being taught is deadly
> serious.[1]

The authors of the various chapters in this text provide an introduction to several creative and innovative teaching strategies that are currently in use in higher
education. During the evolution and development of these newer strategies, the
lecture has been relegated to the status of a second-class citizen—at least that is
how it appears in the literature. It has become trendy to "lecture bash," to describe
our colleagues who openly espouse the use of lecture techniques as old-fashioned
and out of step with educational trends. To many educators, the term *lecture* has
been added to their list of unspeakable four-letter words. But, a lecture is only a
means to an end—intrinsically, it is neither good nor bad; its success depends on
how it is delivered.

In practice, however, the lecture format is alive and well regardless of the negative overtones that may be attributed by some people. The lecture remains the
most frequently utilized teaching method in the repertoire of post-secondary educators.[2] In this chapter, the reasons for the long-term popularity of this teaching
strategy, how to improve its utilization, and how to become a better lecturer are
explored.

## DEFINITION AND PURPOSES

By definition, the lecture is one method of presenting information to an audience. Prior to the invention of the printing press, when only scholars had access to
handwritten information sources, the lecture was the primary means of transmit-

ting knowledge. Learners would gather around the master-teacher and take notes related to what was said. The lecture remained the common mode of disseminating information until printed resources and technological advancements became more affordable.

It would appear that when students were able to purchase their own textbooks and computers, methods of presenting information would have changed. Interestingly, change has occurred slowly. Today, with textbooks, computers, and study guides galore, the lecture remains a commonly used technique. It is suggested that there are two major reasons for this longevity: (1) most current educators learned via the lecture, and it is well known that individuals teach as they were taught unless they make a specific effort to alter their approaches; and (2) the lecture is the safest and easiest teaching method, allowing the educator the most control within the classroom. Some of the common advantages and disadvantages of using the lecture method are listed in Table 6–1. Whatever the rationale, positive outcomes can still be achieved by using the lecture, especially when the lecture and lecturer are well prepared.

## THEORETICAL RATIONALE

Few lecturers take time to contemplate the theoretical basis of this practice, but the lack of a theoretical or organizational framework may be one reason that learners perceive some lecturers to be disorganized and/or difficult to follow. The teacher may derive a basis for lecturing from a variety of philosophical and theoretical processes. Three common approaches are communication, cognitive learning, and pedagogical/andragogical theories. The theories supporting effective communications should be common knowledge to nurses; therefore, they are not discussed here. Nurse educators should also have an understanding of cognitive learning theory because it is the underpinning of developmental concepts found in many nursing courses. Pedagogical/andragogical theories are not as well understood and are addressed briefly.

Over the past few decades, graduate nursing education has focused on advanced nursing practice (clinical specialization and nurse practitioners) rather than on educational processes. This change has resulted in limited numbers of younger nursing faculty members who have strong backgrounds in curricular design and learning theory. Pedagogy, a portion of learning theory, loosely refers to educating the chronologically or experiential young or immature. A major tenet of pedagogy lies within the fact that someone external to the learner decides who, what, when, where, and how information will be taught; the learner becomes a passive recipient of knowledge. Historically, nursing content and practice have been taught from a framework based on the medical model; pedagogical principles have worked well. Within the pedagogical context, the lecture strategy establishes the teacher as the one in command, the authority from whom answers come. This

**Table 6–1** Advantages and Disadvantages of Using Lectures As a Teaching Strategy

## ADVANTAGES

+ permits maximum teacher control
+ presents minimal treats to students or teacher
+ able to enliven facts and ideas that seem tedious in text
+ able to clarify issues relating to confusing/intricate points
+ teacher knows what has been taught
+ lecture material can become basis of publication
+ students are provided with a common core of content
+ able to accommodate larger numbers of listeners
+ cost-effective student:teacher ratio 2-200+:1
+ economy of time: teacher can present content in much less time than to elicit from student

+ teacher controls the pace of presentation
+ reward for teacher who becomes known as an expert in specific area/ topic
+ encourages and allows deductive reasoning
+ enthusiasm (role model) of teacher motivates students to participate and learn more
+ can add the newest information on a moment's notice
+ permits auditory learners to receive succinct information quickly
+ enables integration of pro and con aspects of topic
+ teacher can model kind of thinking desired for student
+ lecture produces better immediate recall of information

## DISADVANTAGES

− attempt to cover too much material in given time
− an easy teaching method, but a far less effective learning strategy
− 80% of lecture information forgotten one day later and 80% of remainder fades in one month
− presumes that all students are learning at the same pace
− not suited to higher levels of learning
− classes tend to be too large for personalized instruction
− creates passive learners
− provides little feedback to learners
− student attention wavers in less than 30 minutes

− teacher attempts to teach all that he or she has learned in a lifetime about a subject in one hour
− inhibits development of inductive reasoning
− poorly delivered lecture acts as a disincentive for learning
− viewed by students as a complete learning experience; think lecturer presents all they need to know
− affective learning seldom occurs
− if lecture is not written out, information may not be delivered accurately—if it is written out, why not just allow students to read

Source: Adapted from Woodring, B. Lecture Is Not a Four-Letter Word. *Innovative Teaching Strategies in Nursing (2nd)*, p. 359, 1994, Aspen Publishers, Inc.

approach may provide a rationale for lecturing being viewed as "traditional" and out of step with innovation and creativity in the academic process.

In recent years, both the age and experiential backgrounds of "traditional" college students have shifted, causing scholars to question the appropriateness of the previously used pedagogical methods. In response, educators such as Knowles,[3] Kidd,[4] and Cross[5] introduced and refined the concept of andragogy. The principles previously utilized in teaching the young (pedagogy) were adapted and applied to "mature" learners (andragogy).

Those educators who ascribe to andragogical theory treat the learner as an adult who brings a variety of rich, valuable experiences to every learning situation. The who, what, when, and where of learning emanate from within the learner. Table 6–2 illustrates the comparison of andragogy and pedagogy within the educational process. The information included in Table 6–2 emphasizes that the teacher must know as much as possible about both the learners and the topic before deciding on a specific teaching strategy. When a lecture is used in the andragogical context, it is often accompanied by other adjuncts, such as lecture-discussion (which will be discussed following), to allow the input of the adult learner.

## TYPES OF LEARNERS

A lecture can be used effectively with learners who represent a variety of developmental and cognitive levels. In fact, that adaptability is one of the most positive aspects of this method—a teacher may, at a moment's notice, alter the depth, sophistication, and level of the material being presented. These alterations can be made based on the needs, interests, and/or responses of the learners. The assumption is made that the lecturer has a sufficient command of the subject matter, as well as the presence of mind and flexibility, to alter the content and teaching plan (these assumptions may not be accurate with novice educators, or when material is being presented the first time).

Combining the lecture with pedagogical approaches to teaching/learning is especially useful in basic and/or beginning courses in a sequence, as well as in orientation to new clinical areas or agencies. Novice learners of any age tend to prefer the structure of pedagogy, rather then andragogy; however, the more mature and secure teachers and learners become, the more they enjoy the flexibility and challenge of integrating andragogical concepts into the lecture format.

## TYPES OF LECTURES

Lectures survive because like bullfights and "Masterpiece Theater" they satisfy the need for dramatic spectacle and offer an interpersonal arena in which important psychological needs are met.[6]

**Table 6–2** Comparison of Characteristics: Andragogy vs. Pedagogy

| Characteristic | Pedagogy | Andragogy |
|---|---|---|
| Concept of learner | • Dependent<br>• Passive learner<br>• Needs someone outside self to make decisions about what, when, and how to learn | • Independent/autonomous<br>• Self-directed<br>• Wants to participate in decisions related to own learning<br>• Students will increase effort if rewarded rather than punished |
| Role of learner's experiences | • Past experiences given little attention<br>• Narrow, focused interest<br>• Focuses on imitation | • Wide range of experience, not just in nursing, which impacts life/learning<br>• Broad interests—likes to share previous experience with others<br>• Focus on originality |
| Readiness to learn | • Determined by someone else (society, teachers)<br>• Focus on what is needed to survive and achieve<br>• Tends to respond impulsively | • Usually in the educational process because they have chosen to be<br>• Wants to assist in setting the learning agenda<br>• Tends to respond rationally |
| Orientation of teaching/ learning | • Looks to teacher to identify what should be learned and then to provide the information and process to learn it<br>• Focuses on particulars, concerned with the superficial aspects of learning (grades, due dates)<br>• Needs clarity/specificity<br>• Evaluation of learning done by the teacher or society (grades, certificates) | • Teachers are facilitators, providing resources and supports for self-directed learners<br>• Evaluation is done jointly by teacher, learner, and sometimes by peers<br>• Likes challenging, independent assignments that are reality-based<br>• Tolerates ambiguity |

*Source:* Adapted from Woodring, B. Lecture Is Not a Four-Letter Word. *Innovative Teaching Strategies in Nursing (2nd),* p. 360, 1994, Aspen Publishers, Inc.

A lecturer may vary his or her approach from a presentation that is formal to a much less formal monologue. Lowman[7] has described three types of lectures: formal, expository, and provocative. The *formal lecture* is sometimes referred to as an oral essay. In the formal setting, the lecturer delivers a well-organized, tightly constructed, highly polished presentation. The information provided primarily supports a specific point and usually is backed by theory and research. The presentation may be written and read to the audience. Preparation of a formal lecture is time consuming; therefore, this method probably would not be used for every class period during a school term. It may, however, be appropriate to tie things together either at the beginning and/or end of a course. One of the major problems with a formal lecture is that it ignores the interactive dimension and sometimes fails to motivate students.

A variation on the formal lecture is *lecture-recitation.* This process is integrated into the formal lecture: the lecturer stops and asks a student to respond to a particular point or idea by reading/presenting materials he or she had prepared. An example of this approach may be a formal lecture related to the pathophysiology of sickle cell anemia (SCA), followed by a student-presented case study about a patient with SCA.

The *expository lecture* is considered the most typical type of lecture. It is much less elaborate than the formal oral essay. Although the lecturer does most of the talking, questions from students are occasionally entertained.

In the *provocative lecture,* the instructor still does most of the talking, but he or she often provokes students' thoughts and challenges their knowledge and values with questions. This type of lecture allows for numerous variations on the theme and is becoming more popular in today's college classrooms. Included in this category are *lecture-practice,* where the instructor uses props to illustrate or demonstrate the subject and may include lecture-computer link and video integration; *lecture-discussion,* where the instructor speaks for 10 to 15 minutes and then stimulates student discussion around key points presented (the lecturer acts only to clarify and integrate student comments); *punctuated lecture,* when the presenter asks the students to write down their reflections on lecture points and submit them; and *lecture-lab,* where the lecture is followed by students conducting experiments, interviews, observations, and so forth during the class period. This lecture method may involve various types of interactive learning activities, where the lecture technique does not stand alone.

Keep in mind that a lecture, in and of itself, is not a bad or inappropriate approach to teaching. It may be the most effective method when dealing with certain groups; however, like any strategy, it is most effective when not used as the singular, exclusive technique. Eble, in *The Craft of Teaching,*[8] suggested that the lecture should be thought of as a discourse—a talk or conversation—not an authoritative speech. As a discourse, the lecture can be viewed as a planned portion of the art or craft of teaching. As such, lecturing becomes a learnable skill that improves with practice.

## USING THE METHOD

When presenting an oral essay, or formal lecture, preparation must begin well in advance of the presentation date. Planning, organization, and written preparation are essential and time consuming. Less formal forms of lecture may take less time, but their preparation should not be procrastinated either. If the lecture is one in a sequence (or within a course), the best time to begin the final preparation of a lecture is at the completion of the preceding one. Significant ideas that need to be reemphasized are still fresh in the presenter's mind, as are the questions that were raised, or should have been raised, by the students. The lecturer can recall the presentation strategies that worked with this group of participants, and those that did not. Changes that might have made the lecture more effective can be identified. Most lecturers, however, do not heed this advice, and lecture preparation is often relegated to a brief time immediately prior to the presentation. In order to present an effective lecture, the speaker must invest time preparing for several crucial time segments: the first five minutes, the main portion or body of the lecture, and the last five minutes.

## Lecture Introduction (First Five Minutes)

During the first five minutes of the lecture, two significant things occur: (1) the speaker outlines the objectives, outcomes, and expectations held for the participants, and (2) the audience decides whether to trust the speaker to produce what was promised (objectives) and whether to invest energy in following the presentation.

"There is too much material to be covered within the time allocated, but I'll do the best I can." From a teacher's point of view, this statement is always true, but it should never be said to an audience. If a lecturer opens with such a statement, the listener has already been conditioned to expect a less than topnotch presentation. The participant asks himself or herself, "Why should I bother to listen if I can't possibly learn what I need in this hour?" Once this statement has been made, the lecturer will have difficulty regaining the full attention of the listener. So, no matter how tempting it may be to use, eliminate that statement from your repertoire.

Instead, begin by identifying what the learner should gain from this lecture: state the objectives in clear, interesting, pragmatic, and achievable terms. Then, make a solid connection with the listeners by using an example of how the lecture material can be (or has been) used in practice or life in general. Outline the key concepts that will be addressed, and use your expertise and clinical experience to provide some background and rationale for this lecture. The key points should be limited in number. Research on what is remembered following classes indicated that most students can absorb only three to four major points in a 50-minute lecture and four to five points in a 75-minute presentation.[7] Conclude the introduction by establishing an open atmosphere and describing the "rules of operation" (e.g., "feel free to ask questions at any time," "there will be time at the end of the lecture for questions"). An open atmosphere can be established by posing a question, making a bold statement, using a controversial quote, using humor, or using a visual aid or cartoon. The better one knows the audience, the easier and more successful this introduction becomes.

**Body of Lecture**

Like the human body, the lecture is divided into specific parts. Begin with the definitions of concepts or principles illustrated by pragmatic, personal examples. The speaker conveys the critical information the learner needs to know in the body of the lecture. It should be well organized, with smooth transitions between topics. The experienced presenter knows that a lecturer cannot carry the primary responsibility for conveying all information or imparting all skills. Readings or problem-solving assignments must be made to accomplish those goals, and students need to be appraised of this connection. The body of the lecture should contain (1) general themes that tie together as many other topics as possible, (2) topics that are difficult for students to understand, (3) sufficient depth and complexity to retain the learners' interest, and (4) testimonies and exhibits (statistics, analogies, etc.) to support main points.[9]

The speaker's presentation style is most evident during the body of the lecture. Tips and suggestions made in the Resources section of this chapter will enhance your presentation style.

**Lecture Conclusion (Last Five Minutes)**

The lecture needs a definite ending. Closing a notebook, running out of time, or dismissing the class is not an acceptable conclusion. An effective communicator knows that any interaction deserves closure; the lecture is not an exception. By focusing the learners' attention during the last five minutes of class, the lecturer is able to establish finality and make a link between what was taught and what the learners will be able to use in life or practice. A good conclusion ties the introduction and the body together in a manner similar to that of an abstract that precedes a well-written paper.

The objectives and outcome statements that were used as a portion of the introduction can be reiterated, assuming they have been accomplished. The conclusion should also contain a review of the key points or topics covered and allow time for elaborating, amplifying, and/or clarifying issues presented. The lecturer must resist the temptation to present new information during the conclusion. Offering suggestions related to the application and transfer of knowledge may be helpful to the participants. Using this approach allows the learner to quickly rethink the content, stimulate continued interest, and consider further action. The participants will leave the lecture hall feeling a sense of accomplishment because they can specify what has been learned. Thus, each lecture should be carefully planned and presented with an introduction (first five minutes), a well-organized body, and a conclusion (last five minutes).

**RESOURCES**

The major resource needed to utilize the lecture technique effectively is you, the lecturer. Presenting an informative and interesting lecture is a craft and a learnable skill. Because the speaker is the key element for this strategy, the following points are presented to help polish your presentation skills.

- *Conveying enthusiasm is the key element in presenting an effective lecture.* Enthusiasm is contagious and is demonstrated by facial expressions, excitement in the voice, gestures, and body language. A lack of enthusiasm on the part of the speaker is interpreted by the listener as a lack of self-confidence, lack of knowledge, a disinterest in the learner, and/or disinterest in the topic. If you do not have an effusive personality, practice adding a smile and small hand gestures to each lecture. Once these movements are comfortable, add other interactive methods.
- *Understand the content.* Even a written, formal lecture will not hide the insecurity of being unprepared or underprepared.
- *Use notes.* The use of notes is generally the option of the speaker; however, to avoid the distress of losing your train of thought or incorrectly presenting complex information, the use of some type of notes is highly recommended. For ease of handling, record the notes all on the same size paper or card (four-by-six- or five-by-seven-inch notecards or 8½-by-11-inch sheets of paper work well). Sequentially number each card/page; this task is a great asset should you drop or have a fan or air conditioner blow away your notecards. The depth and content of lecture notes should fit the lecturer's comfort level (use of anything from a skeletal outline to a full manuscript is acceptable). Notes should be written leaving white space that is easy for the eye to follow. This layout can be accomplished by typing or handwriting in a double-space format. Major points should be highlighted so the eye can easily pick up a cue when scanning a page. Although the use of notes is perfectly acceptable, the verbatim reading of notes is *not* acceptable. Rehearse your notes as long and as often as needed so the lecture will appear spontaneous and enthusiastic and will be completed within the given time frame.
- *Speak to an audience of 200 as if they were a single student.* Speak clearly and loudly enough to be heard in the back of the room. The use of a microphone may be necessary if you are presenting in a large room or auditorium. Always use the microphone if there is any doubt that your voice will not be heard in the last row. It is sometimes helpful to have a friend sit in the back and signal if your voice is not being heard during the presentation. The use of a small clip on the microphone is preferable to using a hand-held or stationary microphone because it allows the speaker to move away from the podium and frees one's hands to handle notes. If a microphone is to be used, the speaker should arrive in the assigned room early enough to try the equipment and to regulate microphone position and sound levels. If the lecture is being transmitted to multiple sites, as in distance/distributive education settings, be certain to test the sound levels at all sites prior to beginning the lecture.
- *Make eye contact.* Select a participant at each corner of the room with whom you plan to make eye contact. Slowly scan the audience until you have seen

each of the designated participants. Smile at familiar faces. Review informa-tion related to the process of group dynamics; that review may come in handy. Again, if the lecture is being transmitted to multiple sites, be certain to make eye contact via the monitors with participants in the distant sites. You may wish to make a concerted effort to look into each monitor as you visually scan the lecture hall.

- *Use creative movement.* Movements of the speaker's head and hands in ges-turing should appear natural, not forced. Be careful when standing behind a podium; do not grip the sides tightly with your hands or to lock your (shaky?) knees. This action produces a circulatory response that could cause the speaker to faint. Occasionally step away from the podium and toward the listeners, which conveys an attitude of warmth and acceptance. Avoid dis-tracting mannerisms such as pacing, wringing your hands, clearing your throat, or jamming your hands into pockets.

- *The use of a stage or podium places an automatic barrier between the speaker and the listeners.* This gulf needs to be bridged early and often dur-ing the lecture. Suggestions for bridging the gulf include: (1) use notecards rather than a manuscript because they are more portable and allow freedom to move away from the podium on occasion; (2) step out from behind the po-dium, especially if you are short in stature. The audience does not wish to see a "talking head"; (3) walk toward the listeners, which is interpreted as a sign of warmth and reaching out to the audience; (4) address the right half of the audience, the left half of the audience, and then the audience at each distant site (each monitor). Do not turn your back to either side of the audience or transmitting cameras; (5) call on at least one participant in the audience and at each distant site by name; (6) use hand gestures to accentuate words, but be careful not to overdo this action (this caution is especially important if the lecture is being transmitted to multiple sites because large hand gestures are more distracting when seen on a monitor than when viewed in person); and (7) if given the opportunity to be seated on a stage/platform, be aware of the eye level of the audience. Should speakers seated on a platform feel the need to cross their legs, they should cross them at the ankles.

- *Create a change of pace.* An astute lecturer constantly assesses the audience and reads participants' signals. Facial signals indicate agreement/disagree-ment with what has been said and may express understanding/misunder-standing of content. Another signal is given when listeners begin having side conversations or squirm in their seats. These signals call for intervention, response, or a change of pace by the speaker. The change of pace can be as simple as turning off the overhead projector (the sound and changing light pattern will cause the listener to refocus attention on the speaker, away from the visual); shifting the focus from the speaker to a handout; using a humor-ous example; altering the tone or inflection of your voice; requesting written or verbal feedback from participants; dividing into small groups for a brief discussion or taking a "stand and stretch" or a few-minutes' class break. Keep this rule of thumb in mind: an individual's optimal attention span is roughly one minute per year of age up to the approximate age of 45 (e.g., a five-year-old has a five-minute attention span; a 25-year-old, 25 minutes). Therefore, plan a change of pace or break according to the average age of your audience. "The mind can only absorb as much as the seat can endure" is a fairly valid guideline.

* *Distribute a skeletal outline only if it will help the learners to identify key points.* Emphasize principles and concepts. Do not copy charts, graphs, and materials that are found in the learners' texts. Handout information should supplement the lecture. The lecture should not be a rehash of basic information from the learners' textbook. If handouts are used, they should be clear and contain a limited amount of information so the learner is not overwhelmed. Handouts printed on colored paper stand out and are more likely to be read than those printed on white paper.

Several publications that may be of assistance in keeping the lecture process fresh are *The Teaching Professor*, a monthly newsletter from Magna Publications; *Change*, a monthly publication of the Association of Curriculum and Development; *The National Teaching & Learning Forum,* which is published bimonthly by Oryx Press; and the Sage Publications' *Survival Skills for Scholars* series.

## POTENTIAL PROBLEMS

Nothing is perfect. As with any method or technique, some problems exist with the use of the lecture as a teaching strategy. A key question to be answered is: "What makes lectures and lecturers unsuccessful?" Over the past decade, graduate nursing students have responded to that question, and each year student responses were consistent.[10] The most frequently repeated negative characteristics of lectures/lecturers focused on the person doing the presenting, *not* the method. Examples of these negatives and some suggestions for improvement are found in Table 6–3. The remainder of this section is devoted to dealing with negative perceptions, which are more generic than the characteristics in Table 6–3.

### Student Boredom

Educators today face challenges that our predecessors did not even dream about! How can one obtain and retain the attention of the "Nintendo generation"— a generation of learners who are accustomed to fast-paced, action-packed, colorized entertainment at the flick of a switch. To compensate for this situational dilemma and still utilize the lecture technique effectively, the teacher should ex-

**Table 6–3** The Perceived Negative Factors Related to Lecturing

| Negatives | Suggestions for Improvement |
|---|---|
| • Disorganized or hard to follow<br>• Lack of outline or outline too detailed | • Prepare and follow brief outline for each lecture |
| • Wears clothing that is distracting<br>• Lacks professional appearance | • Dress as a professional role-model. (If you don't care about wearing stripes and plaids together, enlist the help of a colleague whom you consider to be a professional.) |
| • Lack of facial expression<br>• Monotone voice (nervous, shaky voice)<br>• Lack of enthusiasm | • Audio- and/or videotape one of your lectures and analyze it and establish some goals for improvement; then view it with a friend or colleague to support your decisions for change. |
| • Won't take eyes off notes<br>• Reads the lecture material | • Practice your lecture in front of a mirror or videotape it.<br>• Practice until you know the main points by memory. Use only as many written notes as are absolutely essential. Write cues in the margin for yourself (smile-walk-relax!) |
| • Often sits behind podium to lecture (referred to as the "talking head" because that is all that students see!) | • Don't stand behind a podium unless you are six feet tall.<br>• Ask for a shorter, lower lectern or table. |
| • Uses no visual aids or visuals of poor quality | • Teachers tend to put too much information in small print on slides and overhead transparencies.<br>• Ask your librarian, media center, or learning center for assistance in preparing visuals. |
| • Lacks knowledge of educational principles<br>• Doesn't acknowledge that adult learners like to participate | • Review techniques for keeping adult learners engaged.<br>• See references by Cross, Kidd, and Knowles. |

*continues*

**Table 6–3** continued

| Negatives | Suggestions for Improvement |
| --- | --- |
| • Inconsiderate of learners' needs; doesn't give breaks | • Implement planned change-of-pace activities. |
| • Distracting habits or characteristics: pacing; staring out windows; playing with objects (paper clips, rubber bands, change); using nonwords (ah, um) and repetitious phrases (you know, like, well uh) | • Use a videotape of your lecture to identify repetitive habits.<br>• Repositioning hands or holding notecards may help the "nervous hands" problem.<br>• Make a list of alternate words that could be substituted for the frequently repeated pet phrases.<br>• Nonwords are a verbalization that allows your speech to catch up to what your brain is thinking. Becoming aware of the use of nonwords may or may not be all you need to eliminate them; when they occur, stop, take a deep breath, and then go on. |

Source: Reprinted from Woodring, B. Lecture Is Not a Four-Letter Word. *Innovative Teaching Strategies in Nursing (2nd)*, p. 369, 1994, Aspen Publishers, Inc.

periment with combining advanced technologies and the lecture in the classroom. Some examples are the in-class use of a textbook on disk with capabilities of adding supplementary information presented during the lecture; the use of a computer-linked electronic blackboard, which transmits data from the computer or electronic blackboard to the video screen in the classroom or to individual student desk/laptop monitors; and/or the integration of PowerPoint-type visual aids during the lecture. These electronic capabilities allow the lecturer to interject computer-generated charts, graphs, diagrams, student input, and up-to-the-minute research findings into the lecture. An additional possibility is the assignment of out-of-class computer-assisted instructional programs (such as ADAM or subject-disease-specific learning packages), communications packages (e.g., WebCT, WebCrossings), Web-based assignments, and so forth to complement the lecture.

**Institutional Blocks**

Physical, political, and situational blocks exist within every institution, any or all of which may contribute to dissatisfaction with any given instructional approach. The timing of a class offering cannot be overlooked. Traditionally, teachers have disliked teaching and students have disliked attending classes offered at 7 AM or 9 PM. No one likes getting up that early or staying in class that late! Classes taught immediately after meal time are considered "sleepers" because blood leaves the brain and moves to the gastrointestinal tract, making everyone sluggish. Classes taught late in the afternoon or early evening are bad because the students and teachers are tired. Try as one may, short of one-on-one teaching, the perfect time to hold a class will probably never be found. Speakers must make their presentations stimulating and motivating at any time of the day!

Another institutional barrier to be considered is the number of students proportional to the size of the classroom and the number of students in proportion to the number of faculty (student:faculty ratio). Lecturers are often placed in small, crowded classrooms with large numbers of students or large, cavernous classrooms with smaller numbers of students. Often, geographical relocation of desks/ tables could ease the space configuration and provide a more positive learning atmosphere. Figure 6–1 depicts some alternative seating arrangements that facilitate the presentation of lecture and enhance listener attention. The large student:faculty ratio will probably not be decreased in post-secondary education in the near future. It is seen as very cost effective to have one faculty member lecture to 100 to 300 or more students at a given time. The cost barrier will continue to impose restrictions that are exacerbated by the increase in distributed and multisite class sessions. This disproportionate student:faculty ratio will require lecturers to implement the tips list under the previous Resources section, as well as utilize technological support, teaching assistants for smaller group interactions, and other creative strategies to enhance student learning for large lecture sections.

## Negative Press

The faculty member who consistently lectures may be subjected to student-generated negative comments, such as "This class is so boring, all he does is lecture"; "It's awful, she reads to us right out of her book"; or "I can't learn to think critically if all she does is lecture!" In fairness, it is generally not the method but the teacher who is at fault if such comments are disseminated. Try to break this negative stereotype by acknowledging that the situation has existed in the past. In order to correct negative press, introduce at least one additional teaching method (e.g., discussion, video, question-and-answer, small group interaction, role-play) into each lecture session. This approach will increase student interaction and should increase student satisfaction. In addition, you will have gained the participants' respect because you have acknowledged their feelings and made an overt effort to respond to them.

## Knowledge Retention

The problem of retaining information gained from a lecture should be acknowledged and addressed. Although those educators who enjoy using the lecture

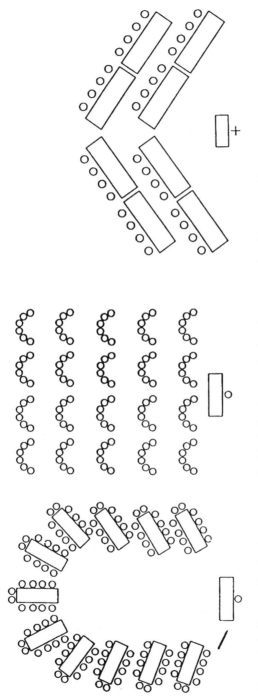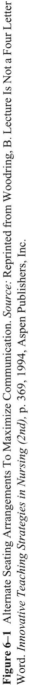

**Figure 6–1** Alternate Seating Arrangements To Maximize Communication. *Source:* Reprinted from Woodring, B. Lecture Is Not a Four Letter Word. *Innovative Teaching Strategies in Nursing (2nd),* p. 369, 1994, Aspen Publishers, Inc.

method hate to admit it, research has proven that 80 percent of information gained by lecture alone is not recalled by students one day later, and that 80 percent of the remainder fades in a month. Research has also shown, however, that the more a learner's senses (taste, touch, smell, sight, and hearing) are involved in the learning activity, the longer and the higher the volume of knowledge is retained.[11] Therefore, it would appear that if certain types of equipment were used to illustrate a point (touch, sight), a video clip was inserted into the midst of the lecture (sight, hearing), or any other active learning process were introduced, the student's knowledge retention would increase.

In recent years, the use of *punctuated lectures* has also been viewed as a method to increase retention of information. The punctuated lecture requires students and teachers to go through five steps: (1) Listen (to a portion of a lecture), (2) Stop, (3) Reflect (on what they were doing, thinking, feeling during that portion of the lecture), (4) Write (what they were doing, thinking, feeling during that portion of the lecture), and (5) Give (the written feedback to the lecturer).[12] This approach provides the lecturer and the students with an opportunity to become engaged with the learning process, as well as to self-monitor their in-class behaviors. In addition, Brookfield[13] suggests that students cannot read the lecturer's mind; that students cannot be expected to know what we expect, stand for, or wish them to value unless we make an explicit and vigorous effort to communicate. The reflective teacher, according to Brookfield, must build a continual case for learning, action, and practice instead of assuming that students see the self-evident value of what we are telling and asking of them. Utilizing these suggestions should enhance knowledge retention emanating from a lecture.

## EVALUATION

An evaluation of the lecture/lecturer must be completed in a timely manner. The most useful time is at the completion of the individual lecture. This task need not be laborious. Ask the listeners to respond to a few specific questions, and then allow them to provide additional comments in an anonymous format. This feedback is especially helpful for the novice lecturer. The evaluation process should aim to provide constructive criticism and comments for improvement. (The author utilizes this technique with graduate students. They may make any comments they wish; however, a negative comment cannot be made without offering a suggestion for its resolution.)

If this evaluation technique is used often, then the learners become accustomed to it. The process can be completed in five minutes or less. Often, teachers are so interested in assessing whether the course objectives have been met that they forget to evaluate the means by which they were met. Lecturers will not improve without suggested change, and suggested change can best be obtained via a planned evaluation tool/method. The evaluation of a lecture or lecturer should not occur in isolation; it must be viewed as a portion of an overall evaluation plan (see Chapter 29), and should be conducted only when there are plans for growth, follow-up, and change.

## CONCLUSION

Presenting an effective lecture is more than simply standing in front of a group and verbalizing information. The lecturer must consider the learners' needs, abilities, and learning styles; the cognitive and developmental levels of the learners; the stated objectives and desired outcomes of the class; and the individual objectives of the learners. The lecture should be divided into three major segments: introduction (five minutes), body, and conclusion (five minutes). Each section should be planned and presented in an organized manner, never "off the cuff." The prepared lecturer will be considerate, credible, and in control (not to be mistaken for rigidity).

Several factors enhance the presentation of a lecture, but none is more important than genuine enthusiasm. The lecture should not be considered a secondary teaching strategy. In many situations, it is the most appropriate methodology to be used. To elicit the best results, the lecture should be accompanied by at least one of the other effective strategies discussed in this text.

---

**NOTES**

1. J. Epstein, *Masters: Portraits of Great Teachers* (New York: Basic Books, 1981), *xiii.*

2. J. Davis, *Better Teaching, More Learning: Strategies for Success in Postsecondary Settings* (Phoenix, AZ: Oryx Press, 1993).

3. M. Knowles, *The Modern Practice of Adult Education: Androgogy versus Pedagogy* (New York: Association Press, 1970).

4. J.R. Kidd, *How Adults Learn* (New York: Association Press, 1973).

5. K.P. Cross, A Proposal To Improve Teaching, *AAHE Bulletin* (September 1986):9–15.

6. J. Lowman, *Mastering the Techniques of Teaching,* 2nd ed. (San Francisco: Jossey-Bass Publishers, 1995), 130.

7. J. Lowman, *Mastering the Techniques of Teaching.*

8. K. Eble, *The Craft of Teaching* (San Francisco: Jossey-Bass Publishers, 1982).

9. J. Lowman, *Mastering the Techniques of Teaching.*

10. B. Woodring, *Student Evaluation of Teaching Effectiveness* (unpublished manuscript, 1997).

11. K. Roberts and H. Thurston, Teaching Methodologies: Knowledge Acquisition and Retention, *Journal of Nursing Education* 23, no. 1 (1984):21–26.

12. K.P. Cross and M.H. Steadman, *Classroom Research: Implementing the Scholarship of Teaching* (San Francisco: Jossey-Bass Publishers, 1996).

13. S.D. Brookfield, *Becoming a Critically Reflective Teacher* (San Francisco: Jossey-Bass Publishers, 1995).

## SUGGESTED READING

Cramer, R. 1999. Large classes, intimate possibilities. *The National Teaching & Learning Forum* 8, no. 4:5–6.

Creed, T. 1997. PowerPoint, no! Cyberspace, yes. *The National Teaching & Learning Forum* 6, no. 3:5–7.

Desrochers, C. 1999. Multi-purpose lecture breaks. *The Teaching Professor* 13, no. 10:1–2.

Driver, R. 1999. Wither: The lecture. *The Teaching Professor* 13, no. 1:2.

Fenstermacher, G., and J. Soltis. 1998. *Approaches to teaching.* 3rd ed. New York: Teachers College Press.

King, A. 1994. Inquiry as a tool in critical thinking. In *Changing college classrooms,* ed. D.A. Halpern, 13–38. San Francisco: Jossey-Bass Publishers.

Loxterman, A. 1998. Student-centered lecturing. *The Teaching Professor* 12, no. 10:4.

Middendorf, J., and A. Kalish. 1996. The "change-up" in lectures, *The National Teaching & Learning Forum* 5, no. 2:1–4.

Mintz, E., and J. Yun, eds. 1999. *The complex world of teaching.* Cambridge, MA: Harvard Education Publishing Group.

Olmstead, J. 1999. The mid-lecture break: When less is more. *Journal of Chemical Education* 76, no. 4:525–527.

Powers, B. 1993. Instructor excellence: Mastering the delivery of training. San Francisco: Jossey-Bass Publishers.

Rhem, J. 1998. Humor in the classroom. *The National Teaching & Learning Forum* 7, no. 6:10–12.

The Carnegie Foundation. 1999. Scholarship is the 'big picture.' *The National Teaching & Learning Forum/Carnegie Chronicle,* May:7–9.

# CHAPTER 7

# Problem-Based Learning

*Gayle W. Bentley*

Problem-based learning is a teaching/learning strategy that is implemented within a small group setting with a faculty facilitator. This strategy centers around a realistic clinical case scenario, and students are active participants in the learning process. Their learning is self-directed and motivated by the need to understand and resolve the case scenario. Problem-based learning is a useful method in a profession where critical thinking, problem solving, and lifelong learning are essential to the practice.

This chapter presents definitions, theoretical rationales, and specific information on the implementation of problem-based learning into nursing education. Types of courses, conditions, and learners suited for this method are identified, as well as resources essential to the success of the problem-based learning strategy. The faculty and student roles are defined, and a clinical case scenario is presented for implementation in a nursing course. The advantages and potential problems inherent with this method are delineated within this chapter.

## DEFINITION AND PURPOSE

Problem-based learning is an innovative, student-driven learning strategy that challenges students to think critically. Within this framework, students develop skills in self-directed learning, critical thinking, self-evaluation, interpersonal communication, and the ability to retrieve, access, and use information.[1,2,3] A small group of students participates in an interactive process directed at understanding a staged but realistic sequence of a clinical case scenario. The identifying characteristic of problem-based learning is that the content needed to solve the problem is *not* presented to the students. This needed content and other information regarding the problem must be identified by the group, researched by the individual students, and then presented to the small group for discussion. The problems serve as the stimulus for learning, and the students make the knowledge relevant by putting it in the context of situations. The pursuit of information based on these real-life situations enables students to integrate and organize information for application to future clinical situations. The faculty serves as the small group facilitator, and resources are made available to assist the students. This strategy is not teacher centered, but student-learner centered.

## THEORETICAL RATIONALE

Problem-based learning in professional education has its origin in the medical disciplines in the mid-1960s. Over the past 30 years, this method of learning has spread to schools of health sciences, such as nursing, dentistry, pharmacy, and public health, and into schools of architecture, business, engineering, law, and many other professional fields. It appears especially relevant to those professions that have an applied practice component. According to authors in the field of problem-based learning, the increased adoption of problem-based learning in higher education is influenced by the perceived deficiencies in traditional professional education.[4] The challenges of information explosion in professional knowledge and the need to acquire skills for lifelong learning are the impetus for the implementation of problem-based learning in higher education. This method for learning is important in the education of professionals where skills in independent problem solving and self-motivation are essential to practice.[5]

Traditional teaching methods evolve from a subject-focused approach. Making an assumption that the learner knows little about the content, the faculty provides the learner with the information in a preselected arrangement. On the other hand, problem-based learning acknowledges the learners' prior knowledge and supports the learners to identify their own learning needs. Traditional teaching strategies, which tend to overload students with content, do not assist students in developing the competencies needed for practice. Without an understanding of the problem and application to a situation, students may do no more than commit the unassimilated data to short-term memory. Memorizing information does not assist them in handling the complex problems found in the health care environment. Students need to learn how to link learned facts, concepts, and principles with new knowledge in order to make the sound decisions required for dealing with the variety of problems they may encounter in practice.[6]

Problem-based learning is primarily a *process-driven* method for learning. The ultimate goal is not the solving of the problem. The process of group interaction, self-directional retrieval, and the utilization of information for reasoning within a clinical scenario is the goal. Students need to acquire skills to direct, analyze, and critique their reasoning skills as they work with realistic clinical situations. The process involves critiquing the adequacy of their own knowledge and directing their own learning.[7]

Problem-based learning can also can be *content-driven*. This learning strategy can serve as the vehicle to introduce new information or to integrate prior knowledge. The use of problem-based learning scenarios based on realistic clinical cases can complement any course-specific content. The goal is to integrate theory into practice and to facilitate application to clinical situations.

The problem-based learning strategy is designed to challenge learners to demonstrate effective reasoning and critical thinking skills. In addition, students learn to collaborate with others in shared decision making as they solve problems. The interactive strategy fosters teamwork and communication skill development.

Camp cites that, according to Savery and Duffy, problem-based learning is consistent with a constructivism view of human learning.[8] This principle includes a belief that understanding comes from interactions with one's environment, that cognitive conflict stimulates learning, and that knowledge evolves through social negotiation and evaluation of the viability of individual understanding. The strategies of problem-based learning support these principles.

## CONDITIONS

The type of course most suitable for implementation of the problem-based learning strategy is the clinical application course. The strategy facilitates the integration of theory into practice. The case scenario is the basis for the strategy and can be designed to match most course outcomes.

Problem-based learning occurs best in a small group setting that enables the students to interact and to collaborate in the clinical reasoning process. The ideal group would consist of five to seven students with one faculty facilitator. Each small group functions independently and at its own pace. It is recommended that these small groups meet for weekly group sessions that last approximately two hours. The group process is essential because participants bring with them life experiences and various levels of knowledge on the subjects.

## TYPES OF LEARNERS

As a practice discipline, health care professionals can benefit from the use of problem-based learning in order to simulate realistic clinical situations. Problem-based learning is appropriate for all types of learners and is especially appealing to the adult learner. Adult learners are motivated to focus on practical application of what is learned and wish to apply knowledge to immediate circumstances.[9] Problem-based learning is based on reality and the contextual nature of practice. Actively involving learners in the learning process is important for understanding and retention of information. The more mature students with strong communication skills and experience with group dynamics would initially be more comfortable with this method, but development of these skills is a goal of the problem-based learning strategy.

## RESOURCES

The most essential resource for implementation of problem-based learning is faculty facilitators for each of the small student groups. A faculty facilitator serves as a member of each small student group. Within each small group, the faculty facilitator acts to guide the group process in the development of cognitive skills and is responsible for the evaluation process. Continuity is established by ensuring that the faculty member remain with the same small group; however, a faculty member may facilitate more than one group.

A realistic clinical case scenario is the essential element for the use of problem-based learning. The faculty facilitator develops the case scenarios, which consist of a realistic clinical case that addresses course outcomes or curriculum goals. A faculty guide or a listing of learning concepts to accompany the cases is helpful for linking with course outcomes or for consistency of content material to be covered within each small group. Initially, faculty preparation time could be intensive as problem-based learning scenarios and faculty guides are developed.

Library resources, informational resources, and technology support are also needed for problem-based learning. Typically, student utilization of these resources increases with the implementation of problem-based learning as students are challenged to research answers to learning issues. Resources for information include faculty experts, consultants, texts, journals, and a computerized data retrieval system, as well as field and clinical experiences.

## ROLE OF FACULTY

In problem-based learning, faculty members are no longer the deliverer of facts and bodies of knowledge. The role of the faculty facilitator is clearly defined as not being the content information source. Ideally, the faculty facilitator would be an expert as a group facilitator and an expert in the case scenario content areas; however, the most essential skill is that of group facilitator. Faculty may express concern about not being an expert in the content area, but facilitating the student's learning in the clinical reasoning process is the most critical faculty skill necessary.

This more passive faculty role monitors the learning process and helps students to create a positive learning atmosphere. The faculty facilitator role guides, models, and coaches and fades in the group learning process.[10] The faculty facilitator may ask leading or open-ended questions to guide the group initially if needed, but the role is primarily to encourage critical reflection and to make suggestions only when necessary. The guidance should offer students insight into the types of questions they should be asking themselves as they approach the case scenario. The faculty facilitator needs to mentor good interpersonal skills for the group by establishing a climate that promotes the exchange of ideas and consensus of decisions. Encouraging students in their decision-making skills and in their collaborative efforts is another important responsibility of the facilitator. As the students become more adept in the process, the faculty facilitator deliberately and progressively fades from the group interactions, and students become independent. The desired outcome is that the faculty eventually becomes unnecessary to the group process.

The performance of the faculty facilitator in problem-based learning is crucial to the outcome. The faculty is responsible for outlining the goals of the sessions by identifying what is to be accomplished and how the process works. Because students naturally defer to the faculty in a teaching/learning situation, the faculty facilitator needs to clearly establish that role in the process and to remind students that their opinions are most important in this learning process.[11]

Although the student evaluation is done by both the faculty facilitator and the students, the faculty must guide this process. The faculty facilitator discusses the evaluation process with the students, including the philosophy of self- and peer evaluation and the application of the evaluation criteria. If the student is to assume responsibility for learning, then he or she needs to be able to assess his or her own ability to work with a problem accurately.[12] Students perform self- and peer evaluation in terms of group dynamics, contribution to learning, identification of learning issues, and the effectiveness of the resolution of the problem[13] (Exhibit 7–1). The facilitator gives students feedback regarding their self-evaluation and their evaluation of their peers.

The faculty facilitator evaluates each student's contribution to the process, his or her identification of learning needs, the accuracy and completeness of the information obtained, and the reasoning process. Because the evaluation process is both formative and summative, timely feedback from the faculty facilitator concerning group dynamics and the learning process should occur at the end of each session.

## APPLICATION OF THE PROBLEM-BASED LEARNING STRATEGY

An orientation for faculty facilitators and the students is important at the initiation of the problem-based learning strategy. This orientation defines goals and objectives as well as clarifies roles and responsibilities of the faculty and students in the group. In the first group session, the role definitions and process guidelines for problem-based learning are presented. Time is dedicated to each member's introduction and brief sharing of interests and backgrounds. Essential for the success of the problem-based learning process is an environment that fosters open communication. The faculty facilitator needs to model behavior conducive to group interaction to help establish such a learning environment.

Problem-based learning occurs in a sequence of steps, with Part 1 of the case scenario being introduced in the first session and subsequent parts being introduced at later sessions (Exhibit 7–2). Student learning results from the process of working toward the understanding of the clinical case. Students learn to search for information to help them understand aspects of the case and possible ways to resolve it. The learning is self-directed and motivated by the need to understand and resolve a clinical case scenario.

**Exhibit 7-1** Peer Evaluation

Please use the indicated scale to rate each of the 5 areas for each member of the group. Please include comments as needed.

5—Always    4—Almost always    3—Sometimes    2—Hardly ever    1—Never

| Group Member | Seeks and provides resources for an equal share of the tasks related to the case scenarios. | Active participant toward effective resolution of the case scenarios. | Assumes responsibility as a participant in group discussions and in the leadership of the group. | Works toward harmonious and productive group sessions. | Completes research and input in an appropriate and timely manner. | Average Score |
|---|---|---|---|---|---|---|
| | | | | | | |
| | | | | | | |
| | | | | | | |
| | | | | | | |
| | | | | | | |

Additional Comments:

Student Signature: _____

**Exhibit 7–2** Case Scenario for Problem-Based Learning

---

**Case Scenario: Mr. Cook**
**PART 1**

You are the Home Health Registered Nurse who has received a referral for a new client. Dr. Craig has referred Mr. Henry Cook, a 68-year-old Caucasian, to your home health care agency for daily wound management of an ulcer resulting from an injury to his left foot. Mr. Cook has Medicare Part A and Part B. Significant medical history includes diabetes mellitus, hypertension, and gout. His diabetes is being managed with an oral hypoglycemic agent and dietary restrictions (1800 calorie ADA). He developed bilateral peripheral neuropathy about seven years ago. His health is otherwise good, and he has previously been independent in all his activities of daily living, including driving his car. The physician has ordered daily wet-to-wet dressing changes for Mr. Cook's wound management.

Current Medications:
Chlorpropamide 100 mg po bid
Captopril 25 mg po bid
Allopurinol 300 mg po daily

During your first visit with Mr. Cook, you obtain the following assessment data: Mr. Cook is a retired salesman and recent widower who lives alone in a townhouse apartment. He has lived in this present neighborhood for 30 years and has an extensive network of friends and neighbors. His two children live out of state. He is 5' 9" and weighs 210 pounds. Although he quit smoking cigarettes 15 years ago, he occasionally chews tobacco. When you arrived for your visit, you found Mr. Cook in the kitchen soaking his injured foot in vinegar and tap water. Mr. Cook's response to your questions concerning this treatment for his ulcer was, "My neighbor had a sore like this on his heel and this cleared it right up." Mr. Cook developed an ulcer on the dorsal aspect of his left heel approximately one month ago when "something was stuck in my shoe and rubbed a hole in my heel." The ulcer is approximately the size of a quarter, with white purulent drainage. The surrounding area is swollen, erythematous, and painful to touch. Mr. Cook states that he has never been taught to check his blood sugar and manages his diabetes with the daily "sugar" pill and "not eating too many sweets." The results of your checking a random blood glucose reading were 188 mg/dl.

His vital signs were:
Temperature: 97°F
Pulse: 88/minute
Respirations: 20/minute
Blood Pressure: 170/90

You found Mr. Cook to be alert, oriented, and with obvious hearing difficulties. Mr. Cook ambulated awkwardly with the cane as he accompanied you to the door and mumbled, "Nothing has gone right since Emma died this spring!"

*continues*

**Exhibit 7–2** continued

**Case Scenario: Mr. Cook**
**PART 2**

You have been working with Mr. Cook for the past several weeks, focusing on wound care and enhancing his compliance with diabetes control. His wound is not improving; in fact, it appears to be increasing in size and depth. After a telephone consult, his physician orders hydrocolloid dressing changes BID.

Today's assessments reveal:
Temperature: 99°F
Pulse:- 66
Respiration:- 18
BP:- 166/94
Blood sugar: 244 (2 hours pp)

Mr. Cook has become more verbal about his wife's death just seven months ago. His neighbor stopped you on the sidewalk outside Mr. Cook's house and expressed his concern that Mr. Cook never goes out of the house anymore and is always sitting in the same kitchen chair alone in the dark. The neighbor states that his late wife had always managed the house cleaning, shopping, and meal preparation, and he worries that Mr. Cook is not eating right. Because the bedrooms are upstairs, he suspects that Mr. Cook is sleeping on the couch.

You have noticed a gradual weight loss in Mr. Cook and increasing clutter in the house. Your 24-hour diet recall reveals:

Breakfast: OJ 6 oz., scrambled eggs (2), toast (2 slices) with grape jam, bacon (2 strips), coffee (2 cups, black)
Lunch: Turkey, lettuce, and tomato sandwich with mayonnaise; potato chips; and ice tea (1 glass, unsweetened)
Dinner: Chicken Pot Pie (microwave), tea (2 glasses), and apple pie (1 slice)
Snacks: Peanuts (boiled, canned, 10 oz.), OJ (4 oz.), fruit cake (3 slices), banana (one small)

During this visit, you plan to prepare Mr. Cook for your absence next week because you will be attending an out-of-town nursing conference and another nurse will be making the daily home visits while you are gone.

**Case Scenario: Mr. Cook**
**PART 3**

It is six months later. Multiple wound care treatments were not successful, and Mr. Cook's ulcer progressively worsened. The ulcer had doubled in size, had yellow purulent drainage that had not responded to penicillin, and the edges were necrotic with bluish discoloration. Peripheral pulses on the edematous left foot were absent for weeks. His blood sugars were approximately 200 to 250.

*continues*

**Exhibit 7–2** continued

This nonhealing foot ulcer has resulted in a below-the-knee amputation of his left leg. The physician has requested that you arrange for his home health care following discharge. He is to be discharged from the hospital tomorrow after this four-day hospitalization. You will make a "day of discharge" visit to readmit him to your home health care caseload. The physician reports that Mr. Cook's suture line appears to be healing well, and a program to form his stump for prosthesis has been initiated by the physical therapy department. He had been out of bed minimally during the hospital stay. The physician requests the home health care nurse to visit Mr. Cook three times a week. His oldest daughter arranged a leave of absence from her family and employment to stay with Mr. Cook during the hospitalization and the first week at home.

**Case Scenario: Mr. Cook**
**PART 4**
Mr. Cook has continued to improve. You will be preparing Mr. Cook for discharge from home health over the next few weeks. He is making progress with his ambulation and accepting the prosthetic positively. He reports occasional episodes of phantom pain. His medications for control of his diabetes remain the same, although his blood glucose consistently remains elevated above 180 mg/dl.

The results of his last laboratory tests are:

Hemoglobin 14 g/dl
Hematocrit 48 g/dl
WBC 4500/mm$^3$
Na 136 meq/L
K 3.6 meq/L
BUN 20 mg/dl
Creatinine 1.8 mg/dl
Glucose 210 mg/dl
Hemoglobin A1C- 18 %
Uric Acid 7.0 mg/dl

On your visit last Friday, Mr. Cook and his neighbor were planning the transportation for Mr. Cook's return to church. Mr. Cook's grandson and his family have made plans to move to Mr. Cook's neighborhood and to assume responsibility for much of his care. You told Mr. Cook that you would reduce your visits to once per week for three weeks, and then discharge him from the service after the fourth and final visit.

*Source:* Reprinted with permission from G.W. Bentley and K.E. Nugent, Problem-Based Learning in a Home Health Course. *Nursing Connections,* Vol. 9, No. 4, pp. 29–39.

A copy of the first part of the sequenced clinical case scenario is provided to each group member by the faculty facilitator. At the beginning of each session, students choose from among themselves a reader and a scribe or recorder. The recorder keeps a record of the group discussions or responses using the following headings: Analysis of the Problem, Potential Nursing Diagnoses, Student Learning Issues, and Informational Resources[14] (Exhibit 7–3).

The reader reads aloud as the group goes over each sentence of the case, line by line, and decides what facts are known about this case. This information is recorded under "Analysis of the Problem." Using the facts obtained from the case, the group then generates appropriate diagnoses. Each response is recorded.

As the group members continue to analyze the information presented in the case, they identify the limitations of their knowledge. Information recorded is linked as "What Is Known" and "What Is Unknown." Unknown information becomes the knowledge needed to better understand and to pursue further the clinical problem. This unknown information becomes the student learning issues and

---

**Exhibit 7–3**  Example of Problem-Based Learning Group Recordings: Mr. Cook Part 1

**Analysis of the Problem** (What Is Known)
Elderly male, recent widow
Lives alone in townhouse apartment
Has private physician and Medicare (part A&B)
Two children live out of state; close neighbors/friends
Recent foot ulcer requiring daily wet-to-wet dressings
Medical History:
  NIDDM: does not self-monitor blood sugars, diet "avoids sweets"
  Random BS: 188mg/dl, daily medication
  Hypertension: BP 170/90, daily medication
  Gout: daily medication
  Neuropathy: bilateral peripheral
Overweight    Height: 5'9" Weight: 210 pounds
Prior independent in ADLs: uses cane, awkward
Owns/drives car
Chews tobacco occasionally; quit smoking cigarettes 15 years ago
Hearing impairment
Wife died last spring

**Potential Nursing Diagnoses**
Impaired skin integrity
Knowledge deficit concerning diabetes management
Knowledge deficit concerning wound care
Potential for falls related to foot ulcer and need for use of cane
Adjustment to recent death of wife (r/t loss, role function, lifestyle changes)
Alterations in nutrition
Impaired hearing

*continues*

**Exhibit 7–3** continued

**Student Learning Issues** (What Is Unknown)
What are the types/classifications of ulcers and treatments?
How to accurately document wound management and healing progress?
What effect does neuropathy have on wounds/healing?
What are the benefits/harm of vinegar and tap water on ulcer?
For each medication, what are indications and precautions, especially for elderly?
What are the nutritional needs/requirements for Mr. Cook? His IBW?
How to assess the environment and client's safety with ADLs?
How to assess the client's knowledge level/deficits to begin teaching plans?
What is significance of his blood glucose 188mg/dl? Is "tight" control recommended?

**Informational Resources**
Textbooks, Internet, Journals/Articles; Personnel/Experts in the Field/Community (i.e., Home Health Nurses, Physicians, Counselors, Physical Therapists, Social Workers, Health Department, Mental Health Facilities, Counseling Services)

*Source:* Reprinted with permission from G.W. Bentley and K.E. Nugent, Problem-Based Learning in a Home Health Course, *Nursing Connections,* Vol. 9, No. 4, pp. 29–39.

is recorded under the appropriate heading. Students are encouraged to identify areas in which more information/learning is needed to analyze the case. The group then identifies resources needed to meet the identified learning needs; sources typically include those found in the library, on the Internet, and from expert persons in the content area and persons within community agencies. The identified resources are recorded under "Informational Resources," with the name of the student who is responsible for finding the information. Students are expected to consult a variety of available resources to uncover these learning needs. Optimally, students choose the learning issues of personal interest, and then it becomes recognized as an individual learning issue. At the end of the session, the group breaks, typically for a week. Each student has responsibility for researching the selected learning issue(s) and then begins the retrieval process. The goal of this learning strategy is an active, student-driven process, with students taking responsibility for their own learning.

The next session begins with each student sharing the information that he or she researched. Each student begins by identifying the resources he or she utilized to retrieve the needed information and often presents referenced notes or handouts for the group. This process gives the students opportunities to develop their communication and presentation skills. The group critiques the resources for accuracy, applies the new knowledge, and then reassesses prior knowledge and thinking related to the case. After students have presented and discussed all new information, a consensus is reached concerning a summative status of the clinical case management.

Before continuing with Part 2 of the case scenario, the group must agree that all learning issues were covered. The negotiation and collaboration within the small group is an invaluable part of the problem-based learning experience. Students are then given the second part of the case and the process continues. The case concludes when the final part is presented and the students reach conclusions concerning the analysis of the problem, management of the case, and resolution of student learning issues.[15] For each case scenario, a faculty facilitator guide or a list of the course learning concepts can be consulted to assist in focusing students on key aspects of the situation related to course outcomes (Exhibit 7–4). These faculty facilitator guides or lists of the case scenario learning concepts also assist with the continuity among groups if the process is content driven and specific course content areas are to be covered within each group.

---

**Exhibit 7–4**  Learning Concepts and Facilitator Guides for Case Scenario: Mr. Cook

**Case Scenario Learning Concepts**
- Home Health Care
  Services, referral, eligibility, and admission requirements
  Impact of health care delivery system and policy on services
- Diabetes Mellitus
  Management with medications, diet, and exercise
  Nursing role as care provider, educator, and advocate
  Complications and special considerations for elderly
- Wound Management
  Types of wounds and treatment options
  Documentation of wound care and status
  Home remedies
- Gout: monitoring and treatment
- Nursing care for a patient with an amputation
- Health promotion and levels of prevention
- Community resources and barriers for aging population
- Teaching/learning strategies in special populations
- The nurses' role in working with human loss and grief
- Developing trust in the nurse-patient relationship

**FACILITATOR'S GUIDE**
**Case Scenario: Mr. Cook**
**PART 1**
1.  What criteria qualify Mr. Cook for this referral to home health care?
2.  What is gout? How is it diagnosed? How is it treated?

*continues*

**Exhibit 7–4** continued

3.  Medications: What are *three* types of oral hypoglycemic agents (compare mechanisms of action, drug interactions, nursing implications)? Are the dosages of the medications high? Low? What are the medications' indications? Nursing implications?
4.  When checking a blood glucose, which is better: random or fasting? Why? What drugs and external forces influence a high or low blood sugar? What are nursing actions and teaching for clients who continue to have *high* blood sugars?
5.  What type of wound care would be appropriate for this type of ulcer? Why? How would you monitor the client's response to the wound care treatment? How would you document the ulcer and circulatory status of the foot?
6.  What are common complications in the elderly diabetic? What is the Diabetes Control and Complications Trial (DCCT) study? What is the latest research concerning recommendations for Type II diabetes management?
7.  How would you respond to Mr. Cook's response about using vinegar and tap water in the wound management? Would you use a sterile or clean dressing change technique? Why?
8.  What level of prevention would you anticipate practicing: primary, secondary, or tertiary? How and why?
9.  What factors should be considered when teaching this client? Describe techniques that could be used to enhance the client's learning.
10. How do you see motivation, compliance, and health beliefs affecting this case?
11. What would you expect in the process of normal grief and loss?

**FACILITATOR'S GUIDE**
**Case Scenario: Mr. Cook**
**PART 2**
1.  What role adaptations are required of Mr. Cook? What is the nurse's role in assisting Mr. Cook with his grief and loss?
2.  What community resources are available to Mr. Cook in regards to his diabetes? His hypertension? His foot care? What are the potential barriers to his involvement with these resources?
3.  What is neuropathy? What is the difference in etiology of the neuropathy? Signs and symptoms? Medical management?
4.  What is the purpose of a hydrocolloidal dressing? What signs would indicate a positive response to this wound management? What are three methods of wound debridement?
5.  How would you address the concerns about Mr. Cook's nutritional status? What are his caloric needs? Ideal weight? Evaluate the 24-hour diet recall. Is he following an 1,800 cal ADA?
6.  What lab tests reflect data concerning nutritional status? What are potential reasons for his weight loss? Psychological? Physical?
7.  Create two menus for an 1,800 calorie ADA diet (breakfast, lunch, dinner, and snacks). Make one menu feasible for a *low-income* budget.

*continues*

**Exhibit 7–4** continued

8. How would you prepare for a week's absence from your clients? Prepare for termination of a relationship? How would you maintain continuity of care?

**FACILITATOR'S GUIDE**
**Case Scenario: Mr. Cook**
**PART 3**
1. What is the proper way to culture a wound? Penicillin is effective against what organisms? What are several implications to remember about the use of penicillin?
2. What health care needs do you anticipate for Mr. Cook after surgery? What are your most important assessments?
3. What are the greatest dangers to the elderly amputee after surgery?
4. What equipment would you anticipate him needing? Where would he get the equipment? What financial costs are involved and what are his resources? What will Medicare cover?
5. How would you communicate with other members of the health care team in the overall management for Mr. Cook?
6. What do you see as the role of the home health nurse in discharge of this client from the hospital?
7. How soon after the amputation should rehabilitation begin? What are the types of leg prosthesis and their pros/cons? What are the guidelines concerning care of the stump? What teaching is indicated?
8. What are the risks and the benefits of providing a wheelchair for the elderly amputee? What home safety issues are involved in his care?
9. What is the anticipated reaction and adjustment that may occur in response to a loss such as this amputation?
10. Compare the rehabilitation of a young adult with that of this elderly client. What are the similarities and differences?
11. What are the latest medical advances concerning prevention of amputation in ambulatory clients?

**FACILITATOR'S GUIDE**
**Case Scenario: Mr. Cook**
**PART 4**
1. What health promotion and lifestyle change issues are pertinent for Mr. Cook? What would you like to see and evaluate prior to discharge? Why?
2. What is phantom pain? Will the pain eventually go away by itself? Would you expect a younger or older person to be more likely to experience prolonged phantom pain?
3. What concerns do you have associated with his lab values, his diabetes control, and his medications? What are the reasons for his elevated blood sugar? What is the relationship of K+ to glucose? Why is creatinine a better indicator than BUN?

*continues*

**Exhibit 7–4** continued

Uric Acid is a byproduct of what? Purpose of prescribing A1C? WBC? What DIFF do you look for to indicate you can fight infection?

4. What community resources are available to Mr. Cook at this time? What resources might be needed if his condition had left him unable to live alone? What financial commitments would be indicated for these options?

5. What aspects of the process of aging need special attention?

6. How does Healthy People 2010 address the needs of this population? What are the risks for this aggregate population? What costs are associated with falls in the elderly?

7. What potential responses could this client have in response to discharge from the services? Review issues related to preparation for termination of the nurse-client relationship.

*Source:* Reprinted with permission from G.W. Bentley and K.E. Nugent, Problem-Based Learning in a Home Health Course, *Nursing Connections,* Vol. 9, No. 4, pp. 29–39.

At the conclusion of each session, approximately 10 minutes should be dedicated to an evaluative discussion among the group. This discussion should include constructive evaluation of the faculty facilitator role performance and the performance of each student. The students are evaluated in terms of reasoning and problem-solving skills, self-directed learning, and support of the group process. Specific feedback from each student concerning what was most helpful and what seemed to hinder the learning process is expected in order to assist the students in gaining confidence and skills needed for the process of lifelong learning. The formal individual student evaluation should occur at midpoints and at the conclusion of the problem-based learning course.

Problem-based learning can be integrated into the clinical component of courses in a variety of ways. The clinical faculty's utilization of the format "what is known" and "what is unknown" verbally on the clinical units can help to stimulate the student's thinking abilities and problem-solving skills in the actual clinical settings. Students would continue to think in terms of "why" in providing care. The faculty may choose to utilize this format for the identification of learning needs or clinical preparation needs when making clinical assignments. Students could gather information on their assigned clinical patient and complete an individual preparation for their clinical assignment based on identification of the "known" and "unknown." This process would lead the student's identification of their learning issues needed to prepare for the clinical experience.

## ADVANTAGES OF PROBLEM-BASED LEARNING

1. Development of self-directed, lifelong learners
2. Integration of knowledge and building on prior knowledge
3. Application to future experiences

4. Development of critical thinking abilities
5. Realistic and highly motivating for students

In problem-based learning, students are the active participants in searching, assessing, organizing, and sharing information. Evidence suggests that problem-based learning students retain knowledge longer than students taught conventionally and that these students are better able to transfer concepts to new problems.[16] In addition, problem-based learning promotes critical thinking in students, thus fostering their critical reasoning through the synthesis of information. The small group setting promotes collaboration, interpersonal communication, and peer evaluation. These skills are essential for practice in collaborative health care.

This strategy has the potential to strengthen the clinical component of courses by integrating dyadic information into a reality-based case scenario. Utilizing problem-based learning, the students explore the physical, mental, and social issues interwoven into the patient's primary problem. These clinical situations may not otherwise be experienced by students, so problem-based learning expands opportunities to encounter clinical situations within a group setting.

An advantage of problem-based learning is the increased student motivation based on interest in the real-life situation. The real-life situations are intriguing for students and can be linked easily with future recall, which is invaluable for future professional life and practice. Students assume responsibility for the learning process. Experiences that foster lifelong learning and self-directed learning prepare students to practice in a changing and complex health care delivery system.

**POTENTIAL PROBLEMS**

1. Student motivation
2. Faculty role adjustment
3. Institution and program commitment and resource allocation

Although students participating in problem-based learning are most often reported as being highly motivated,[17] potential problems with student motivation do exist. Self-study is a large part of the student's time, and some students may need assistance with maintaining the motivation that is needed with this independence. Students who have been prepared by secondary schools as passive learners may have difficulty adjusting. Often, students are subject/course bound in their personal traditional study habits. In problem-based learning, the faculty facilitator, as well as peers, helps keep students on track as group processes evolve. Some groups may need guidance with group dynamics and level of responsibility in the learning process.

The faculty comfort level in this new role is essential. Relinquishing control and leadership of the group may be problematic for some faculty who serve as faculty facilitators. The faculty who are often quick to give answers and turn sessions into lectures defeat the purpose of the problem-based learning precept. Some faculty as well as students may have difficulty with the role in which faculty change from "expert" to mentor and students are regarded as colleagues who are novices. The atmosphere is more casual, and faculty must be approachable. The faculty need to be educated on the role definition for problem-based learning and to develop an attitude that is appropriate to the faculty facilitator role to maximize student learning.

The culture of teaching and learning for any institution needs to be considered prior to implementing problem-based learning in the curriculum. A commitment to this goal and philosophy of learning is needed from the administration in order to have the support and resources for implementation. This commitment to the problem-based learning method requires consideration of the faculty resources needed to be successful. Administrative planning for the number of faculty and the faculty time commitment for the small group implementation of this strategy is essential.

## CONCLUSION

Problem-based learning is a student-centered process of working toward the understanding and resolution of a problem. It is unique in that it stresses the development of problem-solving skills. A clinical case scenario based on lived experiences can provide an opportunity for students to reason through the clinical problems effectively. This strategy is useful in learning new information as well as in building on prior knowledge as students progressively take responsibility for their learning. The faculty facilitator is responsible for mentoring the desired outcomes of collaboration, shared decision making, and skills of group dynamics. The group work fosters collaboration and teamwork, which are essential skills for practice in the changing health care environment.

---

# EXAMPLE
# Problem-Based Learning
# The use of the exemplar family as the basis for learning health promotion and illness/injury prevention

*Veronica Kane*

Problem-based learning (PBL) was the teaching method of choice for a family nurse practitioner course in health promotion and illness/injury prevention (HP/IIP). The uniqueness of PBL is that all learning stems from the problems themselves. PBL deliberately utilizes the ill-structured as the foundation for learning because these constructs mirror those encountered in the real world.[18] From this starting point, the student first identifies the problem(s), specifies what is known and what is hypothesized about the problem, and determines the directions to be taken to further understand the problem and to develop a solution for it.[19] The exploration might range from anatomic relationships to pathophysiological mechanisms to psychosocial theories to any relevant area of study.

In developing the course, there were several priority objectives. The format of the class needed to provide the students with the opportunity to operationalize the principles of health promotion/illness-injury prevention, while facilitating the development of the clinical reasoning process. Another core objective of the course was the integration of the family system into all levels of the health care. A final critical objective was to support and develop collaborative learning in the students. In order to meet the objectives, the scenario of a multigenerational family was developed (see Exhibit 7–A). This family provided the lens through which HP/IIP principles were studied. The cumulative data in the exemplar family scenario were designed for exploration of gender, lifespan, cultural, interpersonal, and public health arenas.

---

**Exhibit 7–A** Portrait of the Exemplar Family

> The members of the exemplar family are all clients in your family practice clinic. Some information that you will need to know to care for them is as follows.
>
> **Father:** JACK is a 42-year-old self-employed contractor. He started the business with an old military buddy after retirement (retired Army NCO) three-and-a-half years ago. His business is going well. Six months ago, he was awarded a contract to renovate several old buildings as part of a district revitalization plan. He was married before, but his first wife died in a car accident seven years ago. He has two children from that marriage, Alan, 15 years old, and Christina, 12 years old, who live with him. Jack admits to drinking several beers an evening to unwind and dipping Copenhagen snuff. He smoked until he turned 30 and stopped because of his daughter's respiratory problems at the recommendation of the primary care provider. At that time, he took up chewing tobacco. He has been married for five years to Marta, and together they have one child with another one on the way. Neither child was planned, but they are not unwelcome. Jack's medical history is unremarkable except for some nonspecific low back pain that he has been followed for occasionally, recent suspicion of hyperlipidemia (his wife had him check it at the mall), and a nagging, persistent cough for the past two

continues

**Exhibit 7–A** continued

months. Growth parameters: 71 inches tall, 180 lbs.; this reflects a recent weight loss of 10 lbs., which he attributes to the increased activity at work lately. He is not sure what immunizations he has had, but definitely none since he left the military.

**Mother:** MARTA (nee Guitterez) is a 36-year-old lab technician at a local hospital's blood bank and has been married to Jack for the past five years. She has a child from her previous marriage, and her ex-husband remains involved with his daughter despite a two-hour drive for visitations. This daughter, Abigail, is eight years old. Marta's mother lives nearby and is very involved with the family. Marta comes from a very traditional Mexican family (her grandparents emigrated). Marta has just determined by home pregnancy test that she is pregnant. Her health history is noncontributory. G2P1, with no complication during her first pregnancy. She does not drink alcohol at this time. Immunizations: Dt was three years ago, does not remember when she had OPV; HEP-B 1-3, completed two years ago, HEP-A 1 was received eight months ago. She had chickenpox when she was five years old. Growth parameters: 65 inches, 120 lbs.

**Children:**

ALAN is a 15-year-old high school sophomore. He is the eldest child of Jack's first marriage. He was a very positive, outgoing child before his mother's death, but he has become withdrawn, moody, and inconsistent in his academic performance. Jack thinks that Alan is just being a teenager, but stepmother Marta is concerned and maybe feels a little guilty that the introduction of so many changes in the family over the past few years may be taking a toll on Alan. Alan does go out with friends on weekends, and Marta suspects that the boys are drinking, but Jack just says that "boys will be boys." Alan is not involved in sports, although he likes to shoot hoops with his friends. He spends a lot of time playing the saxophone and Nintendo 64.

Alan has demonstrated normal growth and development. His only hospitalization was following the car crash in which his mother died. He suffered a femur fracture and mild concussion, but he has no physical sequelae from that event. His general health has been excellent, with no more than an occasional cold or strep throat in his history. Immunizations received to date include: DPT 1-5, OPV 1-3, MMR-1. Last TB test was 1990, negative.

CHRISTINA is a 12-year-old in seventh grade and is a child of Jack's first marriage. She is a quiet but pleasant child, who the teachers have always enjoyed having in class. She competes in gymnastics and is active in Girl Scouts. She gets along well with other children and has many friends with whom she is frequently on the phone or meeting at the mall. She gets harassed a lot by Alan, but she has developed a good relationship with Abigail, her stepsister. She has just completed the Red Cross babysitting course and now gets paid for watching her younger brother, Andy, for short periods.

*continues*

**Exhibit 7–A** continued

Christina has a negative health history, except for asthma. She was hospitalized several times for this condition as a young child, but in recent years she is well controlled on inhaled medication and occasional nebulizer use for exacerbations. She uses her inhalers to prevent exacerbations associated with exercise, and her asthma has not interfered with her gymnastics. Fall and spring are her most difficult seasons, and during these times she minimizes outdoor sports and activity. She is Tanner stage III, with some breast development and pubic hair, but no growth spurt or menarche. Growth parameters: height 40%, weight 35%. Immunization status: DPT 1-5, OPV 1-4, MMR-1, last TB test was 1994, negative.

ABIGAIL, 8 years old, is in the third grade. Abby was adopted by Marta and her first husband after being in foster care with them for six months. She is multiracial, Korean and African-American, and her adoptive father is African-American. She enjoys her visits with her dad (every other weekend, and alternating holidays) and speaks with him often on the phone. She enjoys her stepsister, Christina, but she complains that Alan always tries to annoy her. In school, she has several good friends but is not involved in anything extracurricular. Just this year, she started piano lessons and is really having fun with that. She also likes to watch her stepsister's gymnastics, but she does not believe that she could ever be as good at it, so she doesn't want to join.

Abigail was diagnosed last year with Attention Deficit with Hyperactivity Disorder and has demonstrated an improvement in school behavior and performance since starting on Ritalin. Her growth parameters reveal a height percentage of 40%, but a weight percentage of 75%, a marked increase over the last two years. There are no other health problems. Immunization status: DPT 1-5, OPV 1-4, MMR 1-2, HIP 1-3, HEP-B 1-2, last TB test was 1995, negative. She had chickenpox when she was 20 months old.

ANDREW is 17 months old. Andy spends 40 or more hours per week in a neighborhood daycare. He has no identifiable words yet, but he points and grunts to make his needs known. He started walking last month and is still pretty unstable. Marta thinks that he is into the terrible twos early because he has recently escalated his temper tantrums and oppositional behavior. His dietary habits have become very "selective" and sporadic. He loves milk and is still on the bottle by day and night. Andy has been in good health except for colds and ear infections. His immunizations to date are: HEPB 1-2, DPT 1-2, OPV 1-2, HIB 1-2. Growth parameters: height 50%, weight 25%.

**Grandparents:**

ROSA, 70 years old, mother of Marta, has been widowed for 20 years. She is an RN, who is employed part-time at a local AIDS hospice. She is active in the Seniors Quilt Group and as a Mall Walker. She is very involved with her grandchildren, teaching them stories from Mexican folklore, songs in Spanish, and cooking Mexican foods for them. She has lived in the same house for

*continues*

**Exhibit 7–A** continued

35 years and gets help maintaining it from her two sons. Rosa is on no medications but has not come for a check-up in two-and-a-half years. She is coming in now because her daughter convinced her that she should. She has experienced some gastric burning over the past few months and has self-medicated with antacids with intermittent relief. She has also noticed that when she lifts a patient at work or sneezes or laughs, she wets herself. This is becoming at times embarrassing because she thinks others can tell that she is wetting, so she usually wears sanitary pads when she goes out of the house.

ELLIOTT, 74 years old, father of Jack. His first wife died 10 years ago. He remarried the following year to the woman who lived in the next door apartment and had been a good friend for years, Marion. He loves his grandkids and sees them often. He is a retired professor of English. He and Marion have been busy socially with a bridge group and travel yearly on cruises or bus tours. Elliott has poorly controlled hypertension, non-insulin-dependent diabetes, glaucoma, and arthritis in his knees. Medications include Precose, Diabinase, Tenormin, Lasix, Naprosyn, Tylenol, and Timolol. Lately, he has noticed that his vision is getting dimmer, he is more forgetful, and he feels like he is getting weaker. His wife confides that he has gotten more forgetful some evenings; once he even forgot how to play bridge in the middle of a game.

MARION, 62 years old, stepmother of Jack, wife of Elliott. Marion teaches elementary school and is well-liked by the faculty and students alike. She is very active in the community, but she worries that she will need to stay closer to home to watch Elliott if he becomes more forgetful. She has a twin sister in Florida, but they seldom see each other since Elliott's retirement because of financial concerns. Marion is in good health. She treats her high cholesterol with various herbs and vitamins from the health food store. She has been on Oscal and Prempro since menopause began six years ago.

New skills must be acquired for this new role. The facilitator need not be the content expert as in the traditional classroom, but he or she does need to be well versed in the acquisition, evaluation, and application of information. Knowing the right answer is of secondary importance to asking the pertinent question that leads the student toward discovery. The facilitator assists the students' development by guiding the learning of group skills, lifelong learning skills, and self-assessment skills. If interruptions of the collaborative process are too frequent or inappropriate, then the power base for learning will shift from the students back to the faculty member. The interruptions impact on the students as if they have been doing something wrong. The shift in power base undermines the self-directed learning that is at the heart of PBL. Students need to access a variety of literature, community, consumer industry, regulatory, and professional resources throughout their careers, and they must learn to critically appraise the information that they find. The facilitator's job is not to provide the answers, but rather to design problems and tutor students as the students assume full responsibility for learning.

The students were provided with a list of HP/IIP issues (see Exhibit 7–B) to serve as a starting point for the discussion of each family member. The

---

**Exhibit 7–B** Health Promotion/Illness-Injury Prevention Issues

Consider the following areas when analyzing this family. This list is not inclusive. Additional areas of analysis are welcomed and encouraged.

1. Health promotion: theorists, history of movement, goals, client education
2. Role of the family (adoption, blended issues, dynamics)
3. Role of nutritional status (growth and maturation, impact on future illness, assessment, weight management, food refusal behaviors, feeding aberrations)
4. Role of exercise/fitness (sports participation, effects on bone, heart, circulation, psychological status; indications, contraindication: motivation: risks, benefits)
5. Role of psychological status (cognitive function, depression, anxiety, stress, suicide)
6. Role of environment (occupational risks, heavy metals, day care exposures, rural vs. urban, safety, injury prevention)
7. Role of age (growth and development, impact of developmental level, needs, assessments: aging: menopause, skin examination)
8. Role of pregnancy (norms, management, impact, risks)
9. Role of health maintenance (screenings, immunizations (discuss diseases), benefits, schedules, anticipatory guidance, health promoting activities)
10. Role of lifestyle (homosexuality, sexual activity, indigent)
11. Role of alternative health care practices (folk medicine, chiropractic, cranial manipulation, acupuncture, Christian Scientist, humor/impact of outlook on disease)
12. Role of substance use and abuse (tobacco, alcohol, recreational drugs, over reliance vs. addiction)
13. Role of sensory input (impairments, impact of socialization, development, precautions)
14. Role of biostatistics and epidemiology
15. Role of finances
16. Role of culture/spirituality
17. Role of disease prevention
18. Role of interactions (polypharmacy, OTC misuse, substances and pharmaceuticals)
19. Role of ethics
20. Role of chemoprophylaxis

list is not exhaustive, and students are encouraged to explore additional relevant areas. In the initial class, students were oriented to the continuum of health promotion and family systems theory. They also were instructed in the process of PBL. The expectations for participation and the self-directed learning goals were clarified.

Instead of being topic-driven, class sessions focused on individual family members, as well as how each member impacted or was affected by the other members and events. This reflects the approach taken in clinical practice, where one does not focus a narrow beam on a specific diagnosis, but rather investigates multiple layers of information in assessing patient concerns and needs in order to develop a plan of care.

## TYPICAL CLASS

In preparation for class, the students familiarized themselves with the family profile, focusing on each member in turn and considering each of the HP/IIP issues in that relationship. Using a brainstorming technique, all known data were extrapolated and listed on the board. Next, the discussion of "what we think we know from the data given" was listed. At this point, the students made some preliminary hypotheses. These could take the form of positives, negatives, or risk factors that were perceived at this point; describe pathophysiology; or refer to deficits in the database.

In the next phase, students identified their learning needs and developed strategies for obtaining needed information. Learning resources were identified, and the students distributed study assignments within the group. During the following class, all new information was shared, and hypotheses were refined. When it was agreed that all aspects of HP/IIP care for the individual had been exhausted, the focus then switched to another member of the exemplar family.

The faculty member's involvement was primarily to reflect questions and thoughts back to the students or to provide some guidance if the students were at an impasse. Guidance typically took the form of asking questions to nudge the students along.

## EVALUATION

As predicted by prior studies, the student reaction to learning through this format was mixed. Many students expressed anxiety that they were not learning the *facts* that were necessary for them to pass their RN board examinations. They mourned the absence of lecture and expressed resentment that they had to "teach themselves." By the time they concluded their second problem-based course, they were efficient, effective, self-directed learners, but they emotionally relied heavily on the presence of the faculty member. In the third and final PBL course, the students established themselves as colleagues, collaborating on cases, sharing resources, and challenging presented information. Their perception was that transition to the work force was smoother than their counterparts from other programs.

**NOTES**

1. H.S. Barrow, A taxonomy of problem-based learning methods, *Medical Education* 20 (1986):481–486.

2. H.S. Barrow, *The Tutorial Process* (Springfield, IL: Southern Illinois University of Medicine, 1988).

3. A. Doring, A. Bramwell-Vital, and B. Bingham, Staff Comfort/Discomfort with Problem-Based Learning. A Preliminary Study, *Nurse Education Today* 15, no. 4 (1995):263–266.

4. D. Boud and G. Feletti, *The Challenge of Problem-Based Learning* (New York: St. Martin's Press, 1991).

5. Barrow, *The Tutorial Process*.

6. R. Tornyay and M. Thompson, *Strategies for Teaching Nursing* (New York: John Wiley & Sons, 1987).

7. Barrow, *The Tutorial Process*.

8. G. Camp, Problem-Based Learning: A Paradigm Shift or Passing Fad? *Medical Education Online* 1 (1996):2.

9. M. Knowles, *The Modern Practice of Adult Education: From Pedagogy to Andragogy* (New York: Cambridge University Press, 1980).

10. Barrow, *The Tutorial Process*.

11. G.W. Bentley and K.E. Nugent, Problem-Based Learning in a Home Health Course, *Nursing Connections* 9, no 4 (1997):29–39.

12. Barrow, *The Tutorial Process*.

13. Bentley and Nugent, Problem-Based Learning, 29–39.

14. Bentley and Nugent, Problem-Based Learning.

15. Bentley and Nugent, Problem-Based Learning.

16. Camp, Paradigm Shift.

17. Camp, Paradigm Shift.

18. S.L. Finkle and L.L. Torp, Introductory Documents (available from the Center for Problem-Based Learning, Illinois Math and Science Academy, 1500 West Sullivan Road, Aurora, IL 60506-1000), 1995.

19. T.H. Click and E.G. Armstrong, Crafting Cases for Problem-Based Learning: Experience in a Neuroscience Course, *Medical Education* 30 (1996).

# CHAPTER 8

# Reflective Practice

*Hollie T. Noveletsky-Rosenthal*

## DEFINITION AND PURPOSES

Reflective practice is the process of examining one's own nursing practice in order to uncover those factors that one brings to nurse-patient or nurse-colleague interactions that either hinder or enhance one's ability to interact therapeutically. Johns[1] refers to reflective practice as the process of exposing the contradictions in practice. In exposing the contradictions, the nurse must first come to understand what he or she defines as ideal practice. Then the nurse examines the multiplicity of factors within the clinical interaction that either hindered or enhanced the nurse's ability to achieve ideal practice. Johns developed a model of Structured Reflection to aid nurses in identifying and understanding the complexities of factors within clinical interactions so that they may develop and access their own tacit knowledge.

Benner[2] identifies expert nurses as those nurses who are able to immediately grasp the whole of a situation. The expert nurse is able to understand the multiplicity of factors at play within a given situation. In order for a nurse to develop this expert knowledge, he or she must first develop and access his or her own tacit knowledge. The process of reflection gives access to the tacit knowledge gained in clinical practice. Boud, Keogh, and Walker[3] outline three stages in the process of reflection. In the first stage, one identifies and describes a significant event or interaction. In the second stage, one evaluates the event or interaction in order to identify factors that either hindered or enhanced one's learning. In the third stage, one integrates the knowledge gained with his or her past experiences in order to access one's own tacit knowledge. Thus, the reflective process allows nurses the ability to uncover knowledge embedded in clinical experience.

Schon[4] described two types of reflection. The first is reflection in action, and the second is reflection on action. Reflection in action is the process of analyzing or thinking about one's actions while carrying out the action. Reflection on action is the process of retrospective analysis of one's action. For the novice nurse, reflection in action is difficult. As a novice, the nurse is still trying to gain theoretical knowledge and mastery of psychomotor skills. At this level, reflection in action is mainly focused on applying appropriate theoretical knowledge within a given clinical situation; however, reflection on action provides the novice nurse with the opportunity for retrospective analysis of clinical situations in order to gain a deeper understanding of the multiplicity of factors involved within the clinical situation. This deeper understanding allows the novice nurse to begin to develop his or her own tacit knowledge for clinical practice and to identify ways to bring his or her practice closer to a defined ideal practice level.

## THEORETICAL RATIONALE

According to Habermas, there are three types of knowledge: empirical, interpretive, and critical. Taylor[5] equates Habermas' typology of knowledge with technical, practical, and emancipatory knowledge, respectively. Empirical or technical knowledge is generated through scientific inquiry and allows for the description, prediction, and control of phenomena. Interpretive or practical knowledge is knowledge that is relative and context dependent. Interpretive knowledge is generated through new insight that may allow for evolution or change in perception. Critical or emancipatory knowledge is also knowledge that is relative and context dependent; however, critical knowledge is generated with the specific intent to bring about change. Taylor[6] states that "reflection creates interpretive knowledge for generating meaning and change through raised awareness" and critical knowledge for intentional change that enables the nurse to move his or her practice closer to ideal practice.

## CONDITIONS

Reflective practice as a teaching method requires the development of a safe environment for disclosure. Therefore, reflective practice is appropriate for small group seminars or one-on-one conferencing. Group members need to be encouraged to participate fully and to work toward the development of a safe and respectful environment that allows for disclosure and free discourse.

In addition, students need to develop an understanding of the process of reflection. Foundational readings on Johns' model of Structured Reflection are necessary to establish a framework from which to process clinical interactions.[7] The facilitator is essential to the process of reflection. The facilitator encourages the students to move beyond superficial examination of interactions toward a level of critical reflection in order to develop their own tacit knowledge. Johns developed reflective cues and eight framing perspectives to assist the students in examining the interaction from multiple perspectives in order to gain a fuller understanding of the complex dynamics of the interaction. The reflective cues center on the five types of knowledge: aesthetics, personal, ethics, empirics, and reflexivity. These reflective cues take the form of questions that facilitate the student in examining the interaction from different perspectives. The framing perspectives provide different angles from which to examine the interaction in order to gain a deeper understanding of the dynamics. These framing perspectives include framing the development of effectiveness, philosophical framing, role framing, theoretical framing, parallel pattern framing, problem framing, reality perspective framing, and temporal framing.

## TYPES OF LEARNERS

Because reflective practice is an evolving process, there are no standardized prerequisites or outcome measures. Growth is measured individually. Therefore, reflective practice is appropriate for all levels and types of students, including undergraduate, graduate, and doctoral students. Because the focus of the reflection is on clinical interactions, however, all participants should be concurrently in a clinical placement.

In addition, reflective practice is an effective method of staff development. In staff development, a novice nurse would be paired with an expert nurse or would participate in a weekly seminar where the focus of the experience was to critically reflect on significant clinical interactions. This method would provide the novice with a safe environment within which to develop his or her own tacit knowledge.

## RESOURCES

The seminar facilitator is an important resource. The facilitator needs to be expert in both theoretical and clinical knowledge and should be competent in the process of reflection. The facilitator does not necessarily need to have expert knowledge within a specific clinical area, however. The role of facilitator is to assist the student in the reflective process through the use of Johns' reflective cues.

The setting of the seminar needs to provide a sense of privacy so that safe disclosure can occur. In addition, the room should be arranged so that all group members are facing one another in order to help foster a sense of group and equality.

## USING THE METHOD

Seminar groups should meet weekly for approximately two hours per session. Seminar expectations are reviewed during the first class. Expectations include: (1) each student is expected to participate in the group discussion, and (2) each student is expected to work toward the development of a safe and respectful environment that allows for disclosure and free discourse. In addition, each student is to keep a weekly reflective journal. At least one entry per week will examine a clinical encounter with a patient, family, or colleague that the student wishes to further understand. Students are instructed to write a narrative describing the experience. Then, using Johns' model of Structured Reflection and the reflective cues, students are encouraged to examine those factors that the student brings and those factors that the other brings to the interaction that either hinder or enhance the student's ability to interact therapeutically. The facilitator reviews the journals on a weekly basis, and written feedback is provided regarding the students' insights.

Each student is expected to share three journal entries with the group over the course of the seminar. The student presents the narrative of the interaction and his or her reflective thoughts on the nature of the interaction. This presentation provides a starting point for group reflection on the dynamics of the interaction. This process affords each student the opportunity to gain knowledge vicariously and to facilitate each other's learning.

At the completion of the seminar course, students are instructed to reflect back on the course by reviewing their weekly journal entries. Students are instructed to write a final reflective paper that examines their own process and product of the seminar experience. This exercise allows the students to realize their growth and the usefulness of reflective practice within their professional lives. The final reflective paper also provides the facilitator with an individualized measure of each student's development.

## POTENTIAL PROBLEMS

The most significant potential problem associated with reflective practice as a teaching method is related to the development of a safe environment for disclosure. If the seminar group is unable to bond together in a cohesive, supportive group, individuals will not feel safe to disclose personal feelings and reflections. Group discussion will be stifled. Addressing this issue with the group may help to raise individuals' awareness of the group's dynamics. Because individuals within the group will be at various levels of self-knowing, however, raising the individuals' awareness may not bring them collectively to a point of enough awareness to develop a sense of group cohesiveness. If the group is not able to develop a sense of cohesiveness, then the reflective process will have to be carried out mainly through the use of the reflective journals.

Another potential problem is students who have difficulty expressing themselves publicly. Despite the development of a safe environment, some students are reluctant to openly express their personal reflections. Again, the reflective journals provide a safe avenue for exploration of both the clinical interactions and the students' inability to reflect within the group setting. Reflective discourse between the student and seminar facilitator can occur through the reflective journals. This discourse increases the facilitator's awareness of the individual's needs while assisting the student to reflect on both clinical interactions and his or her personal growth potential.

Finally, the process of facilitating a seminar group using the teaching method of reflective practice requires a high level of personal commitment among the group members. As the group evolves over time, the group members develop a stronger sense of cohesiveness and commitment to the group. The facilitator, as a member of the group, also develops a strong sense of cohesiveness and commitment. As a result, termination of the group becomes difficult. Some time must be devoted to preparing the group for termination. One strategy to assist in termination is that of identifying alternate methods of continued group cohesiveness. For example, an Internet list serve can be developed as a means to continue the group after termination. In addition, the facilitator needs time to reflect back on the experience in order to process the loss of the group before starting another group. If this process of reflection is not performed, then a sense of loss may interfere with the ability to adequately facilitate the subsequent group.

## CONCLUSION

Johns' model of Structured Reflection provides a useful framework for examining clinical interactions. The structure of the model assists the students in sorting out multiple, competing factors that impact their daily practice while acknowledging the constraints of reality. This model allows the students to critically reflect without assuming unwarranted blame or guilt. One student noted:

Through the development of reflective thinking in practice, I was reminded of the meaning and value of being truly present. Although it is my habit to examine situations in a reflective way, I realize that it was previously with the motive of fault-finding, usually my own, as if when things went wrong that was proof that I was somehow not good enough, did not measure up, was not able for the task at hand. This semester, reflective practice took on new meaning. Rather than searching for fault and using that as an excuse to give up, I could search for a reason, an explanation, and use it as a springboard to improve . . . Repeatedly asking the questions, "What do I bring to the table?" and "How does my presence change things?" made me realize that there is always an answer to those questions. The assumptions underlying the questions are that I do bring something to the table, and my presence does change things. To be aware of those questions makes it possible to change the answers if need be. It makes the answers purposeful rather than inadvertent.[8]

This statement underscores the role of reflection in the development of interpretive and critical knowledge. Students then use this knowledge to change their practice to more closely approximate ideal practice. Through the process of reflective practice, students are able to develop tacit knowledge embedded in clinical practice and to begin the journey from novice to expert nurse.

## NOTES

1. C. Johns and D. Freshwater, eds., *Transforming Nursing Through Reflective Practice* (Malden, MA: Blackwell Science, 1998).

2. P. Benner, *From Novice to Expert* (Menlo, CA: Addison-Wesley, 1984).

3. D. Boud, R. Keogh, and D. Walker, *Reflection: Turning Experience into Learning* (London: Kogan Page, 1985).

4. D.A. Schon, *The Reflective Practitioner: How Professionals Think in Action* (New York: Basic Books, 1983).

5. B. Taylor, Locating a Phenomenological Perspective of Reflective Nursing and Midwifery Practice by Contrasting Interpretive and Critical Reflection. In *Transforming Nursing Through Reflective Practice,* eds. C. Johns and D. Freshwater (Malden, MA: Blackwell Science, 1998), 134–150.

6. Ibid., 138.

7. Johns and Freshwater, *Transforming Nursing.*

8. H.T. Noveletsky-Rosenthal and K. Solomon, *The Use of Johns' Model of Structured Reflection in Graduate Nursing Education* (Cambridge, England: Paper presented at the meeting of the Fifth Reflective Practice Conference, June 1999).

## SUGGESTED READING

Hallet, C.E. 1997. Learning through reflection in the community: The relevance of Schon's theories of coaching to nursing education. *International Journal of Nursing Studies* 34, no. 2:103–110.

Johns, C. 1997. Reflective practice and clinical supervision—Part 1: The reflective turn. *European Nurse* 2, no. 2:87–97.

Johns, C. 1997. Reflective practice and clinical supervision—Part II: Guiding learning through reflection to structure the supervision 'space.' *European Nurse* 2, no. 3:192–204.

Johns, C., and D. Freshwater, eds. 1998. *Transforming nursing through reflective practice.* Malden, MA: Blackwell Science.

Marland, G., and W. McSherry. 1997. The reflective diary: An aid to practice-based learning. *Nursing Standard* 12, no. 13-5:49–52.

Riley-Doucet, C., and S. Wilson. 1997. A three-step method of self-reflection using reflective journal writing. *Journal of Advanced Nursing* 25, no. 5:964–968.

Wong, F.K., D. Kember, L.Y. Chung, and L. Yan. 1995. Assessing the level of student reflection from reflective journals. *Journal of Advanced Nursing* 22, no. 1:48–57.

# CHAPTER 9

# Teaching Sensitive Subjects

*Elaine W. Young*

## DEFINITION AND PURPOSES

Sensitive subjects are intricately entwined in cultural values and, by their very nature, are heavily laden with attitudes and feelings. These values are basic to one's identity as a member of a culture, and as such, individuals often hold personal values as "truths." When people believe that their values are truths, they are reluctant to question the validity of these values; however, the questioning of one's values leads to critical thinking and ultimately to a reformation or change of personal basic concepts. This change is crucial to the education process and, therefore, imperative for all nursing students.

Further, it is important to consider that although general agreement exists that holistic care is integral to nursing practice,[1,2,3] the literature reveals that nurses avoid certain "sensitive" areas related to patient care.[4,5] These sensitive areas are often associated with our culture's traditional values.[6] For example, in the past, the health care system used to (1) dictate how a person "should" die and provided few choices; (2) avoid addressing the possibility of closet drinking, professional substance abuse, or that young people were using street drugs; (3) consider that only young and heterosexual people were sexual; and (4) consider it the "right" of families to use violence in order to control its members. Through research and practice, such traditionally held values have since been found to be harmful to the health of individuals and, therefore, were in need of change. These areas, and more, continue to be avoided by nurses in the clinical arena.

To be effective practitioners, however, nurses must continually confront unhealthy traditional values that are intrinsic to our culture. Such confrontation in the clinical arena is likely to cause patients discomfort, but nurses must address this possible discomfort.[7] Nurses need to know how to address these sensitive subjects in the lives of their patients. But first, nursing students need to confront their own unhealthy values. Thus, affective education is important for all nursing students to help empower them to effect patient change.

## THEORETICAL RATIONALE

The objectives of affective education call for the provision of accurate, relevant information to assist students with exploring personal values, behaviors, and attitudes. Such teaching incorporates the behavioral, cognitive, and affective domains of knowledge and promotes critical thinking on the part of the student. A process of critically questioning both self and the world in which one exists allows the student to be an active developer and not just a passive receiver of knowledge.[8] The examination of one's self and environment serves as the motivation for the change of values. A student may, indeed, discover uncomfortable feelings when considering a patient's sexuality. Teachers then need to provide these students with a classroom milieu in which they can develop skills in communication and self-exploration. Opportunities for communication with classmates and teacher help students to discover the various perspectives that make the familiar strange and the strange familiar.[9] As students encounter patients in need, they will discover a variety of values that will at first seem strange. The nurse must assess such values for their effect on health behaviors. The nurse is better able to assess the patient's values if his or her own values are clear.

Traditionally held values are often found to interfere with healthy behaviors, for example, the belief that women should be subservient to men. The sense of traditionally held values for the sake of tradition begins to crumble when students are provided with information as well as an opportunity to safely express negative feelings associated with such tradition. The student then begins to adopt personal values that are more satisfying and healthful. The goal of learning and teaching affectively is less the acquisition of facts than the development of greater self-knowledge and understanding.[10] The atmosphere of the classroom must be one of trust because the students must be willing to share emerging thoughts and feelings and be comfortable to reflect on these thoughts as they share with other class members for possible criticism.[11] People feel most vulnerable sharing embryonic thoughts because they are difficult to defend in the face of questioning from others. But the embryonic stage of thought development is often the best time to evaluate and build neoteric thoughts.[12] The teacher must be aware of this vulnerability and provide a safe atmosphere.

The classroom is the environment in which such critical thinking begins. The wise student takes new thoughts, opinions, and feelings to other areas of his or her life and tests them on family and friends to help gain further insights. "Theoretical, empirical, and experiential evidence all indicate that the cognitive, affective, and behavioral domains work in consort to affect one's behavior and that dealing with any domain in isolation significantly reduces the impact of the learning experience."[13] Such multidimensional holistic learning experiences are important for any educational setting. Nursing curriculum and clinical experiences provide the student with an array of opportunities in which further values clarification can take place. The teacher, however, will find it difficult to evaluate affective learning in the classroom because value change often only begins in the classroom and continues through later experiences.

## CONDITIONS

If an educator is to teach sensitive topics, then he or she must understand the need to teach about values without preaching or taking sides. A teacher cannot *tell* students what to value—only promote self-exploration. Thus, the teacher must be well-educated to teach affective education so that his or her personal values do not impede a student's educational progress. The teacher's values must be supportive of health values because such support helps to clarify conflicts. When a student's values conflict with health values, the teacher needs to help the student understand how a personally held value may conflict with good health care. Such a conflict can become an obstacle to learning. "We construct our own model of truth in negotiation and struggle with our ancestors, who bequeathed us theirs."[14] Educators need to understand that the real obstacle to learning about values is often cultural and not intellectual, and the student may need to change "traditional truths."

The teacher must also know how to pose the right questions and guide the student to deep, thoughtful responses. The teacher's task is to help students transform cultural values that are harmful into more helpful values. In such a trusting, comfortable classroom, the student learns through the example of the teacher how to confront unhealthy values. Student nurses need to build a culture that values health if they are going to help their patients promote better health. Because values are tied to cognition, the teacher can help the students think for themselves in order to develop more healthful values.[15] Values can and do change over time. If students and professor agree from the outset that basic health values are important, then students are able to change those values that inhibit health care and promotion. The same process is true for patients. The student learns that giving information only is not an effective means to change patients' behaviors. But the changing of unhealthy values to healthful values is the start of long-term healthful behavior change.

## TYPES OF LEARNERS

The education about values, or sensitive subjects, is part of the total education experience known as *affective education*. Affective education differs from purely cognitive learning in that it requires the students to become reflective and introspective of their own lives. The students become the basis of knowledge. Cognitive learning is mostly the accumulation and understanding of facts and rarely is concerned with the individual student's feelings or attitudes. Without self-understanding of values, it is most difficult to effectively help others understand that values may hinder healthy behaviors. Thus, the clinical arena remains bereft of values clarification because of the lack of proper time and courses that address affective education. Nursing educators must establish clearly that "sensitive" subjects are critical to the holistic care and prevention strategies of patients, and they must require that all nursing students study these subjects.

Student and teacher must begin with a basic agreement on health values. Examples of basic health values are that people have the right to (1) obtain health care, (2) decide for themselves what course their health shall take, (3) refuse care, (4) be respected by health care workers, and (5) be protected from communicable diseases.[16] As agreeable as these values may seem, other values may interfere with these basic health values, respectively: (1) only the wealthy deserve health care and people "should" work harder to earn money, (2) only physicians and nurses know enough to make sound medical decisions to determine the course of care, (3) a physician will tell a person what care he or she must receive, (4) health care workers have the right to refuse to care for certain groups of people, and (5) children may not be responsible enough to learn about certain communicable diseases such as AIDS. Thus, health values can clearly be in conflict by well-meaning, thoughtful people. The teacher must encourage the learner to analyze, evaluate, and synthesize in order to operate at a higher level of abstraction to build a strong concept of health. Beyond accepting a set of health values, the student must then be guided to learn how personal cultural values may conflict with these health values.

## RESOURCES

The classroom is best arranged so students may face each other and discuss issues with their classmates. At least two hours is needed because handouts with facts take time to discuss, but students' experiences and feelings take more time for analysis.

## USING THE METHOD

The following method demonstrates the changing of negative feelings and attitudes toward homosexuality. The need for changing these negative feelings is based on the health value that patients deserve health care free of discrimination. Negative feelings associated with homosexuality may be the cause for neglect or insensitivity on the part of the nurse in the care of a gay person. To provide holistic care requires that the nurse holds no prejudices against people. Homosexuality, in our culture, is a sensitive subject that many people do not know how to handle and often become confused by their negative feelings. Even our federal governmental officials are not clear about homosexuality, but most nurses probably would agree that they "shouldn't" be prejudiced, and intellectually they may "try" to be more accepting. It has been shown, however, that some nurses do hold prejudices against homosexual people.[17] Thus, it is possible for student nurses to hold the value that homosexuality is wrong, sinful, and responsible for a variety of negative feelings such as disgust, pity, and repulsion.[18] Such feelings would definitely interfere with holistic care of gay people.

Because students intellectually know that their negative feelings are not conducive to caring, they are often reluctant to share such negative feelings in a group. In order to change unwanted feelings, it is best for the student to first recognize such feelings and then to share them in a safe environment. An effective means for people to recognize and share negative feelings in a group is to ask them to write their feelings and share them anonymously. Thus, they avoid being embarrassed by publicly owning such feelings. Experience using this method (as listed in Exhibit 9–1) has revealed that students often confuse feelings with thoughts. Unless a careful explanation and discussion of feelings is carried out, students will make such responses as "I think homosexuality is wrong or sinful" without revealing the feelings associated with that thought.

The second question of "why" gives the student the opportunity to examine the cognitive reasons for their feelings. A common dialogue reveals that students feel "disgust" when they hear the word, with the reason that homosexuality is against their religious beliefs. Class discussion will probe further along the lines of, "do you feel the same disgust when you hear the term non-married sex or unwed mother?" Both behaviors are against many religions, but students will often reflect and state that these terms do not evoke the same negative feelings, and the students will then become confused. Such confusion is the beginning of change because the

---

**Exhibit 9–1** Affective Teaching Method

1. Provide each student with a slip of paper. (Everyone should have a similar piece so that individual slips cannot be identified with an individual student.)
2. Define and discuss the meaning of a feeling in preparation for the activity.
3. Ask students to write the first feeling or feelings felt when they hear the word "homosexuality."
4. Then ask them to write *why* they think they feel the way they do.
5. The final question is "Do you want to change your feelings?"
6. Collect the slips in a bag and pass the bag so that each student withdraws another student's slip.
7. The class then reads aloud the feelings expressed by members of the class and discusses the results.

students must gain insight to understand why they are able to feel no negative feelings for one breach of religious belief and not the other.

There are a variety of reasons that people hold negative feelings toward homosexuality, such as that homosexual men act feminine or their sexual behaviors are "unnatural." Cognitively, it is important to point out that generalizing sex role behaviors may hinder full development of individuals, and future critical thinking exercises can lead to the analysis of traditional sex roles as well. There is no agreed-upon definition of "natural" because most human sexual behaviors are learned and, again, in-depth discussion of this reason is needed to understand the underpinning of this feeling of "disgust." Much knowledge regarding homosexuality, and sexuality in general, is important to discuss. At each point, the teacher must consider the students' feelings as well.

The third question of wanting to change negative feelings is crucial. If the students have no desire to change, then there is little chance that they would go through the effort to gain insight. The teacher then would have to refocus the discussion to the basic value of people deserving unprejudiced care. The teacher then helps the student to see that negative feelings associated with homosexuality carry evidence of prejudice. Although they are helpful, history, statistics, and personal disclosure clearly do little to address the basic values of the students in the class. Students' feelings and attitudes regarding such information guide the students to change.

A common belief is that if a person has negative feelings toward a group of people, then the "professional" is able to keep such feelings to him or herself and not let them interfere with patient care. Because feelings and attitudes are insidious, it is next to impossible to keep feelings to one's self. Negative feelings are expressed through avoidance, facial expressions, and outright abusive behavior.[19] Thus, truly effective affective education *changes* negative feelings rather than attempting to hide or ignore them.

## POTENTIAL PROBLEMS

Because personal values will become evident, discussions often become heated. Time may need to be taken to review communication skills and behaviors and to allow further time for processing. Time in future classes may also be needed because students often think of further points to be considered and discussed. This method of addressing negative feelings is useful for a variety of sensitive topic areas. Often, nursing students know how they "should" feel regarding sensitive areas, but they rarely are given the opportunity to openly express these feelings in a safe environment in order to analyze themselves and begin the changing process. Students are at first surprised that the class, as a whole, holds so many negative feelings associated with homosexuality (or any of the other sensitive subjects). As the discussions proceed, though, they are often relieved to be able to openly discuss negative feelings that have long "bothered" them personally. Self-analysis and values clarification can be an enlightening experience!

## NOTES

1. M. Attree et al., Students' Evaluation of the Process of Conducting a Patient Assessment, *Nurse Education Today* 14 (1994):372–379.

2. J. Waterhouse and M. Metcalfe, Attitudes Towards Nurses Discussing Sexual Concerns with Patients, *Journal of Advanced Nursing* 16 (1991):1048–1054.

3. E.W. Young, Patients' Plea: Tell Us About Our Sexuality, *Journal of Sex Education and Therapy* 10, no. 2 (1984):53–56.

4. C.L. Coyle and E.W. Young, Affective Sexuality Education in Graduate Nurse Practitioner Programs in the United States, *Journal of Sex Education and Therapy* 23 (1998):62–69.

5. E.W. Young, Sexual Needs of Psychiatric Clients, *Journal of Psychosocial Nursing* 25 (1987):30–32.

6. C.L. Brown, Ethics and Health Policy—Introduction, *Image: Journal of Nursing Scholarship* 31 (1999):253.

7. C.L. Brown, Ethics and Health Policy.

8. W.H. Shubert, *Curriculum: Perspective, Paradigm, and Possibility* (New York: Macmillan, 1986).

9. M. Greene, *Landscapes of Learning* (New York: Teachers College Press, 1978).

10. P.B. Koch, Integrating Cognitive, Affective, and Behavioral Approaches into Learning Experiences for Sexuality Education, in *Sexuality and the Curriculum: The Politics and Practices of Sexuality Education*, ed. J.T. Sears (New York: Teachers College Press, 1992), 256.

11. W.E. Doll, Teaching a Post-Modern Curriculum, in *Teaching and Thinking about Curriculum: Critical Inquiries*, eds. J.T. Sears and J.D. Marshall (New York: Teachers College Press, 1990).

12. P.C. Scales, The Centrality of Health Education to Developing Young Adolescents' Critical Thinking, *Journal of Health Education* (Supplement), November/December.

13. P.B. Koch, Integrating Cognitive, Affective. and Behavioral Approaches.

14. E. Beverly and R.W. Fox, Liberals Must Confront the Conservative Argument: Teaching Humanities Means Teaching about Values, *The Chronicle of Higher Education* (November 1, 1989):A52.

15. K.J. Winkler, Experts on Moral Development Find Common Ground under Fire from Critics of America's Schools, *The Chronicle of Higher Education* (October 26, 1988):4A, 8A.

16. The White House Domestic Policy Council, *The President's Health Security Plan: The Clinton Blueprint* (New York: Random House, 1993).

17. E.W. Young, Nurses' Attitudes toward Homosexuality: Analysis of Change in AIDS Workshop, *Journal of Continuing Education in Nursing* 19, no. 1 (1988).

18. Ibid.

19. Ibid.

## RESOURCES

Following are organizations that would be helpful for current information in sensitive subjects:

**American Association of Sex Educators,**
  **Counselors, and Therapists (AASECT)**
P.O. Box 238
Mount Vernon, IA 52314-0238
Phone 319/895-6203
www.aasect.org

**Knowledge Exchange Network (KEN)**
ken@mentalhealth.org

**Sex Information and Education Council of**
  **the U.S. (SIECUS)**
130 West 42nd Street, Suite 350
New York, NY 10036-7802
212/819-9770
www.siecus.org

**The Jason Foundation, Inc.**
116 Maple Row Blvd., Suite C
Hendersonville, TN 37075
www.jasnfoundation/office.htm

**Human Rights Education Associates**
P.O. Box 382396
Cambridge, MA 02238
617/661-0278

# PART III

## Simulation and Imagination

The teaching-learning strategies presented in Part III promote the use of imagination as a way of encouraging students to stretch their thinking and explore their understanding of concepts in different ways. Effective learning requires active participation. When students use their imagination to play a role, take an opposing viewpoint to their held view, or learn to express themselves in new and different ways, they become involved in their learning. The role of nursing faculty is a facilitating one, helping students to interact with each other to bring out other possibilities, to reinforce learning objectives and help students develop insight into the translation of classroom to clinical.

Clinical experience is a mainstay of nursing education. However, it is more and more difficult to find student clinical experiences in today's managed care world, when providers are under the gun to reduce patient length of stay, and restrict the time and amount of ambulatory care visits. The requirement for increased provider productivity does not allow time for teaching. In addition, the informed health care consumers of today may or may not be willing to allow neophyte students to practice their skills. Simulation allows students to gain experiences that may not be available in the immediate clinical area, but will be part of their practice in the real world of health care.

Students can be encouraged to use stimulation and imagination to learn how to adapt their clinical knowledge to the practical world. Simulation and imagination techniques encourage students to avoid being locked in to one solution to a problem, and provide an opportunity to learn to develop different approaches to the problems they face.

# CHAPTER 10

# Role-Play

*Arlene J. Lowenstein*

## DEFINITION AND PURPOSES

Role-play is a dramatic technique that encourages participants to improvise be-haviors that illustrate expected actions of persons involved in defined situations. A scenario is outlined and character roles are assigned. The drama is usually unscripted, relying on spontaneous interplay among characters to provide material about reactions and behaviors for students to analyze following the presentation. Those class members not assigned character roles participate as observers and contribute to the analysis.

Part of the category of simulation, role-play allows participants to explore why people behave as they do. Participants can test behaviors and decisions in an envi-ronment that allows experimentation without risk. The scenario and behaviors of the actors are analyzed and discussed to provide opportunity to clarify feelings, increase observational skills, provide rationale for potential behaviors, and antici-pate reactions to decisions. New behaviors can be suggested and tried in response to the analysis.

Role-play is used to enable students to practice interacting with others in certain roles and to afford them an opportunity to experience other people's reactions to actions they have taken. The scenario provides a background for the problem and outlines the constraints that may apply. Defining the important characteristics of the major players establishes role expectations and provides a framework for be-haviors and actions to be elicited. The postplay discussion provides opportunity for analysis and new strategy formation.

Although it is a dramatic technique, the focus is on the actions of the characters and not on acting ability. An actor plays to the audience; the role-player plays to the characters in the scenario. The audience also has a role, that of observing the interplay among characters and analyzing the dynamics occurring. The instructor's role is that of facilitator rather than director. The impetus for the analysis and discussion belongs with the learners. The instructor's role is more passive, clarifying and gently guiding.

Role-play is a particularly effective means for developing decision-making and problem-solving skills.[1] Through role-play the learner can identify the systematic steps in the process of making judgments and decisions. The problem-solving process—identification of the problem, data collection and evaluation of possible outcomes, exploration of alternatives, and arrival at a decision to be implemented—can be analyzed in the context of the role-play situation. The scenario can include reactions to the implementation of the decision as well as the evaluation and reformulation process.[2,3]

Role-play provides immediate feedback to learners regarding their success in using interpersonal skills as well as decision-making and problem-solving skills. At the same time, role-play offers learners an opportunity to become actively involved in the learning experience but in a nonthreatening environment.

## THEORETICAL RATIONALE

Role-play developed in response to the need to effect attitudinal changes in psychotherapy and counseling.[4] Psychodrama, a forerunner of role-play, was developed by Moreno as a psychotherapy technique. Moreno brought psychodrama to the United States in 1925 and continued to develop it during the 1940s and 1950s.[5] In psychodrama, players may be required to recite specific lines or answer specific questions and may represent themselves, whereas in role-play players are encouraged to express their thoughts and feelings spontaneously, as if they were the persons whose roles they are playing.[6]

Psychodrama provided a foundation for further development of role-play as an educational technique. Corsini and other psychotherapists and group dynamicists began using role-play to assist patients to clarify people's behavior toward each other.[7] Further development led to the use of role-play in sensitivity training, a technique that became popular in the 1970s. Human relations and sensitivity training events share a common educational strategy. The learners in the group are encouraged to become involved in examining their thought patterns, perceptions, feelings, and inadequacies. The training events are also designed to encourage each learner with the support of fellow learners to invent and experiment with different patterns of functioning.[8] Role-play can be used to meet those educational objectives and is often used in human relations and sensitivity training but has many other uses as well. DeNeve and Hepner, in a study comparing role-play to traditional lectures, found that students believed that the use of role-play was stimulating and valuable in comparison to the traditional lecture method, their learning increased, and they remembered what they had learned.[9]

## CONDITIONS

Role-playing is a versatile technique that can be used in a wide variety of situations. One set of learning objectives might be role-play dealing with the practice of skills and techniques, whereas another different group of objectives would use role-play to deal with changes in understanding, feelings, and attitudes. Van Ments points out that role-play is conducted differently for these two sets of learning objectives.[10] The role-play used for the practice of skills may be planned with the emphasis on outcome and overcoming problems. The second type of objective may be best met with an emphasis on the problems and relationships. This method explores why certain behaviors are exhibited and requires expertise from the instructor in dealing with emotions and human behavior. The teacher is responsible for helping the students to avoid the negative effects that could come from the exploration of their feelings and behaviors.

## PLANNING AND MODIFYING

Teachers who are new to the technique need to plan before class, but they should monitor the needs of the group as the experience progresses and be able to modify those plans if necessary. The situation developed should be familiar enough so that learners can understand the roles and their potential responses, but it should not have too direct a relationship to students' own personal problems.[11] It may also be effective to use two or more presentations of the same situation with different students in the roles if the objective is to point out different responses or solutions to a given problem. When that method is used, the instructor may choose to keep those students involved in the second presentation away from viewing the first presentation, to avoid biasing their reactions. The same role-play scenario can be used throughout the semester to allow students to react to changing events within the same scenario.[12]

Role-play strategy qualifies as an adult-learning approach because it presents a real-life situation and tries to stimulate the involvement of the student. It has special value because it uses peer evaluation and involves active participation.

## TYPES OF LEARNERS

Role-play is appropriate for undergraduate and graduate students. It is especially effective in staff development programs because of its association with reality. It is used effectively to reach affective outcomes. Role-play can be simple or complex, depending on the learning objectives. Regardless of the simplicity of the play itself, it is important to allow adequate time for planning, preparing the students for the experience, and postplay discussion and analysis. The actual role-play may be as brief as 5 minutes, although 10 to 20 minutes is more common. Van Ments suggests that the technique be broken into three sections: briefing, running, and debriefing. Equal amounts of time may be spent for each session for simple objectives, or a ratio of 1:2:3, with most time spent on the debriefing or analysis, for more complex learning objectives.[13]

## RESOURCES

Role-play can be used in most settings, although tiered lecture rooms may inhibit the ability of the players to relate to each other and to the observing students. In that setting, the theatricality of the technique is likely to be emphasized over the needed behavioral focus.[14]

Special equipment or props may be simple or not used at all, again depending on the objectives. An instructor may choose to use video or audio taping. This can be especially helpful to review portions of the action during the debriefing and analysis section. Reviewing tapes may also be helpful for participating students who, because of their roles, were not in the room to hear and see some of the interaction that occurred in other role-plays.

Outside resources are not usually needed for most role-play situations, although additional instructors, trained observers, or specific experts may appropriately be used to meet certain objectives. The technique is best for small groups of students so that those not involved in the character parts can be actively involved in observing and discussing the action in the debriefing or analyzing portion. Van Ments finds role-play increasingly unsatisfactory as a technique in groups with more than 20 to 25 students, although there may be exceptions, depending on objectives and strategies for involving the audience.[15]

## USING THE METHOD

Planning is crucial to effective use of role-play as a learning technique. It may be helpful to pilot the exercise before running it in the class situation to allow the instructor to anticipate potential problems and evaluate if the learning objectives can be met. Discussing critical elements of the role-play with colleagues can be useful if full-scale piloting is not feasible. A small amount of time going through the plans with someone else may prevent a critical element from going wrong and disrupting the exercise.[16]

Selecting a scenario and deciding on character roles is an important part of planning. McKeachie cautions that situations involving morals or subjects of high emotional significance, such as sexual taboos, are apt to be traumatic to some students.[17] He has found that the most interesting situations, and those revealing the greatest differences in responses, are those involving some choice or conflict of motives. Student input into planning can also be effective.

To implement the role-play, the scenario and characters need to be described briefly but with enough information to elicit responses that will meet the learning objectives. Allowing students in the character roles to have a few minutes to warm up and relate to the roles they will be playing is often helpful. Spontaneity should be encouraged, so it is preferable to avoid a script, other than bare outlines of the action. Observing students absolutely must be briefed on their role. Enough time must be allotted for discussion and analysis of the action. This debriefing also allows for evaluation of the success in meeting the learning objectives.

In addition to the development of learning objectives and planning, the instructor is responsible for setting the stage for the role-play, monitoring the action, and leading the analysis. Students need a clear understanding of the objectives, the scenario, the characters they are to play, the importance of the role of the observers, and the analysis as a vital part of the process. On occasion, the instructor may take a character role, but usually character roles are given to students.

When planning a role-play session, the instructor needs to be concerned with the amount of time students may be excluded from the room while waiting for their turn to participate. This issue is especially important when two or more presentations of the same situation are to be used, or the role-play has characters who should not be exposed to the dialogue that occurs before they appear in their roles. It is important to avoid the need for the excluded students to roam the corridors with nothing to do for long periods.

In some instances, it may be appropriate to have students switch roles during the role-play. This technique can be useful if the group is large and more students need to be involved in the action. This approach also may provide students with an opportunity to see and feel different reactions to similar situations. Another example of when to use this technique might be when the objective is to learn how to conduct a group. Students may benefit by playing group member and switching to leader or vice versa during the exercise.

The instructor needs to encourage students to respond to interactions in the role-play in a spontaneous, natural manner, avoiding melodrama and inappropriate laughing or silliness. Effective use of role-play focuses on student participation and interaction. The instructor, as facilitator, channels the discussion to meet the learning objectives but avoids monopolizing the play or discussion. The instructor must also be able to monitor and control the depth of emotional responses to the situation or interplay as needed, terminating the play when the objective has been met or the emotional climate calls for intervention.

Students need to understand the importance of playing the character roles in ways in which they believe those characters would act in a real-life situation. Students who act as observers must be strongly encouraged to present their observations and contribute to the discussion and analysis. Students can also take part in the development of role-play scenarios, identifying their learning objectives, issues, and problems they feel need to be explored, and scenarios that may provide that exploration.

## POTENTIAL PROBLEMS

Van Ments refers to the "hidden agenda"[18] and warns that stereotyping may occur as roles are presented, often reflecting the expectations and values of the students or the teacher. This stereotyping may lead to unanticipated learning that can reinforce prejudices and preconceptions. Instructors need to be aware of this possibility and avoid writing in stereotypes. They should describe only functions, powers, and constraints of the role described. Roles should be rotated to avoid overidentification of one student with a specific role. In the debriefing session, the students are invited to question and challenge assumptions.

Students may not always make a distinction between an actor and a role.[19] Criticism of the student playing the role must be avoided, while allowing for critique of the behavior of the role character. The instructor must be aware of the emotional tones involved in the role-play and channel the emotions into activities that will lead to successful attainment of the learning objectives.

Planning and learning objectives should determine the course of the role-play. Students may take the role-play in an unexpected direction, possibly because they have a need to explore another issue or problem. If it is not appropriate to revise the learning objectives to accommodate student needs, then the play can be terminated. In that case, the postplay discussion can be used to assist students in recognizing why the technique was not effective. Students should advise how to improve the role-play or develop a different teaching strategy. Repeating a scenario with the same or different characters can sometimes afford a more in-depth examination and add to the experience.

The instructor and students need to be aware that this is not a professional drama. Although at times it may be appropriate to change actors if the role-play does not seem to be going well, it is important not to blame the students. In most cases, the teaching strategy needs changing, rather than the actors. Role-play can be an effective and creative strategy to provide active student participation to meet specific learning objectives.

---

# EXAMPLE
## Understanding Patient Adherence

*Inge Corless, Donna Gallagher, Ronald Borans, Elizabeth Crary, Sara E. Dolan, and Sarah Kressy*

The apparent success of highly active antiretroviral therapy (HAART) for the treatment of HIV/AIDS demonstrated by a falling mortality rate was soon tempered by the challenge of maintaining a complex drug regimen.

The complexity of the initial HAART drug regimens was not only due to the large number of pills to be taken and their frequency, but also because of significant requirements of either food or fasting when taking these regimens.

Too often, health professionals prescribe these "miracle" regimens without the required education that is necessary to support the patient. Consequently, patients often take these medications at the wrong times, with the wrong foods, or not at all.

As part of an HIV course, students received a great deal of information about HAART: how it's prescribed, approximate combinations, side effects, and so forth. Additionally, as a learning exercise, students were given selected "HAART" regimens to which they were to adhere for one week. Students were given the frequency of dosings (but not the quantity) and were asked to adhere to the regimen with substitute candies, which they were given. Students were also asked to maintain a diary. As will be noted, students included in their diaries some symptoms that they knew might occur with their specific regimen.

### Student 1

Nelfinavir (Viracept): 750 mg tid with food

(PI) side effects: diarrhea, fat redistribution, increased triglycerides/cholesterol, hyperglycemia with insulin-resistant type II diabetes mellitus

**Day 1:** Today is my start day. I did not have to work today, but I worked all night. I took my first dose around 6 AM with food—not a full meal because working nights I really don't have the appetite for a full meal. I was so tired that I slept through my afternoon dose and was able to take my evening dose around 6 PM.

**Day 2:** I worked today 7:00 AM to 7:00 PM. Because my meal schedule was a bit more normal today, I was able to take all of my doses, although at different times. I wasn't able to eat lunch until 2:30 PM. Working as a nurse, I could see how it would be difficult to take my pills in front of my peers. I definitely would go into the bathroom to take them. I didn't have dinner until after 8:30 PM because I got home around 8:00 PM, so my time schedule was off again.

**Day 3:** Had clinical today from 9:00 AM to 5:30 PM. Was able to take pills as scheduled: 8 AM, 12 noon, 6 PM—because day schedule was more regimented. Would definitely take pills in bathroom at lunch to avoid questions.

**Day 4:** Worked 11 PM to 7 AM. Took pills in AM with minimal food. Once again slept through 12 noon dose. Took PM pills around 7 PM with dinner. Working the night shift makes taking pills *very* difficult. Is it possible for those working nights to take pills at 12 midnight, 4 AM, and 8 AM to avoid missed doses? Also, diarrhea would be a huge interruption in my job. It is so busy and fast-paced. Patients tend to "crump" very frequently related to their illness. I fear I would never be able to leave the bedside to rush to the bathroom. I am also realizing that it would be difficult to "hide" your illness when you work as a health care provider. I would definitely have to change my job to a less stressful/demanding environment.

**Day 5:** Worked 7:00 AM to 3:00 PM. Was able to take meds at scheduled times. I am remembering the Sustiva side effects. The nightmares may prevent me from having a good night's sleep. Working the crazy schedule I do between school and work, sleep time is essential. Also, what if it affects my memory at work? It could lead to a decrease in my response time and assessment skills. This could put my patients at risk.

**Day 6:** Today I had jury duty. This was interesting. I was able to take my AM meds without difficulty. I did not take my afternoon meds because I was afraid I would have diarrhea and not be able to sit on the panel. Also, I really didn't have time to eat a full meal. I don't know what I would do if I were to be picked for an extensive trial.

**Day 7:** Took AM meds after breakfast. Took afternoon meds as scheduled. Went to Umi's to volunteer, then to class. Forgot to bring meds with me! Overall, felt this was a good learning experience. Someone who has a schedule as inconsistent and hectic as mine would definitely have an issue with adherence. I would need an easy-to-take, minimal-side-effect regimen. Preferably twice per day. The afternoon dose was a consistent challenge to me because of my night work schedule.

### Student 2

**Day 1:** 6 AM. Took both drugs on time; lots of water. Not used to the water. Side effects: headache, nausea, diarrhea. Took second Crixavan at 2 PM. Couldn't eat lunch until 3 PM—not happy. Took both again at work, 10 PM. Snacked all night, felt a little queer.

**Day 2:** Got up early—5:45—to take first dose. Can't eat now until 7 AM—O.K. Not used to having so much water intake. Had to interrupt work so I could eat by 12:30, took second dose at 2:30. Last dose at 11 PM. Polyuria all night!!

**Day 3:** Got up early (special) to take first dose. Went back to bed. Ate lunch at 1:30. Screws up 2:30 dose, but I'll just be sick! Couldn't eat until 9 PM, so had to take last dose on full stomach at 10 PM to go to bed on time.

**Day 4:** Taking first dose at 7 AM—water, water, water! Ate breakfast at 5:30 AM. Didn't take first dose until 10:20 with indinavir. Work got crazy. Missed second dose of saquinavir. Took last dose of both at 12 midnight with water.

**Day 5:** Missed day 5 completely.

**Day 6:** On schedule, 6:30 AM, 2:30 PM, 9:30 PM.

**Day 7:** Took 6:30 dose and 9 AM indinavir. Missed lunch dose due to friend in town.

### Student 3

**Day 1:** 7:00 AM breakfast of bagel, tea, water. Took dose of 3 RTV. Moderate nausea. 7:00 PM dinner of fish, sandwich, apple cranberry sauce, orange juice, cookie, small ice cream bar (1/4 C.), tea. Took dose of 3 RTV. Mild nausea.

**Day 2:** 7:30 AM breakfast of bagel, coffee, water. Took dose of 4 RTV. Diarrhea and moderate nausea. 8:30 PM dinner of salad, crackers, cookie, tea. Mild nausea. Took dose of 4 RTV. Mild nausea, diarrhea 3 times! today.

**Day 3:** 7:30 AM breakfast of bagel, tea, water. Took dose of 4 RTV. Diarrhea 5 times throughout the day. 10:30 PM—dinner at 9:30 PM of crackers, cheese, fruit, vegetable, chai. Don't feel well enough to take medication.

**Day 4:** 7:30 AM breakfast of bagel, tea, water. Took dose of 5 RTV. Moderate nausea. Diarrhea throughout day. No evening dose of RTV. 7:30 PM dinner of black bean burrito, water, tea, orange juice. Took dose of combivir only.

**Day 5:** 8:30 AM breakfast of bagel, coffee, water. Took dose of 5 RTV. Diarrhea 8 times; bought Immodium. 7:30 PM dinner of sweet potato, salad, bread, tea, water. Took dose of combivir.

**Day 6:** 10:00 AM breakfast of bagel. Took combivir. No RTV. Used Immodium. Lunch at 1:00 PM. Dinner of toast with small amount of black beans.

**Day 7:** Stopped taking. Need a new regimen where I won't have diarrhea.

### Student 4

**Day 1:** O.K. Well, I missed my first doses, but I have many reasons. First, earlier in the day I had decided to start my new meds that night with my other meds. However, as I was getting ready for bed, I brushed my teeth and then went to take my meds (which is my normal routine). But then I remembered that I had already cleaned my teeth and I didn't want to take the candy. I could have just eaten the candy and then rebrushed my teeth, but I was cold and tired and I just wanted to climb into bed. So I then decided I would start them tomorrow. Interestingly, though, I did consider what Inge would think and say, and I actually considered whether she would be disappointed in me.

**Day 2:** Today I decided to leave the meds/candy on the kitchen table so I would remember to take them after dinner. This would hopefully decrease the chances of cleaning my teeth before taking the meds. Also, I found that it takes me a while to suck on the meds before I can chew them, and therefore I don't want to leave them until I'm ready for bed because then I end up not wanting to take them at all.

**Day 3:** No problems. My boyfriend has even started to remind me to take the meds—he never did that with my real meds!

**Day 4:** No problems.

**Day 5:** No problems.

**Day 6:** No problems P.S. I hate root beer!

### Discussion

Students agreed that after this learning experience, they would work differently with patients regarding the question of medication adherence. They understood the importance of appreciating the patient's daily activities in order to prescribe a regimen that would fit with the particular patient's life. All too often, the expectation is that the patient needs to fit his or her life to a particular medical regimen. That such an approach will not be successful over the long term has not adequately been appreciated.

The one-week experience for these student nurse practitioners enhanced their skill in working with persons living with HIV/AIDS to a degree that would not have been feasible with didactic approaches only.

---

**NOTES**

1. C.M. Hess and N. Gilgannon, Gaming: A Curriculum Technique for Elementary Counselors (Paper presented at the Annual Convention of the American Association of Counselors, New York, 1985), 10. ERIC document 267322.

2. D. Alden, Experience with Scripted Role Play in Environmental Economics, *Journal of Economic Education* 20, no. 2 (1999):127–132.

3. R. Domazzo and P. Hanson, Community Health Problems, Apparent vs. Hidden: A Classroom Exercise To Demonstrate Prioritization of Community Health Problems for Programs, *Journal of Health Education* 28 (1997):383–385.

4. J.B.P. Shaffer and M.D. Galinsky, *Models of Group Therapy and Sensitivity Training* (Englewood Cliffs, NJ: Prentice-Hall, 1974), 108.

5. J.L. Moreno, *Psychodrama*, Vol. 1 (Boston: Beacon Press, 1946).

6. S. Sharon and Y. Sharon, *Small Group Teaching* (Englewood Cliffs, NJ: Educational Technology Publications, 1976), 160–161.

7. R.J. Corsini, *Methods of Group Psychotherapy* (New York: McGraw-Hill, 1957).

8. G.K. Gordon, Human Relations—Sensitivity Training, in *Handbook of Adult Education*, eds. R.M. Smith, G.F. Aker, and J.R. Kidd (New York: Macmillan, 1970), 427.

9. K.M. DeNeve and M.J. Hepner, Role Play Simulations: The Assessment of an Active Learning Technique and Comparisons with Traditional Lectures. *Innovative Higher Education* 21 (1997):231–246.

10. M. van Ments, *The Effective Use of Role Play: A Handbook for Teachers and Trainers* (London: Kogan Page, 1983).

11. W.J. McKeachie, *Teaching Tips: A Guidebook for the Beginning College Teacher*, 7th ed. (Lexington, MA: D.C. Heath & Co., 1978): 137–139.

12. F.E. Rabinowitz, Teaching Counseling through a Semester Long Role Play, *Counselor Education and Supervision* 36 (1997):216–223.

13. van Ments, *The Effective Use of Role Play*, 44–45.

14. Ibid., 45.

15. Ibid., 29.

16. Ibid., 48.

17. McKeachie, *Teaching Tips*, 139.

18. van Ments, *The Effective Use of Role Play*, 98–104.

19. Sharon and Sharon, *Small Group Teaching*, 179.

## SUGGESTED READING

Alden, D. 1999. Experience with scripted role play in environmental economics. *Journal of Economic Education* 20, no. 2:127–132.

Chester, M., and R. Fox. 1996. *Role-playing methods in the classroom*. Chicago: Science Research Associates.

Greenberg, E., and P. Miller. 1991. The player and professor: Theatrical techniques in teaching. *Journal of Management Education* 15, no. 4:428–446.

Kourilsky, M., and L. Quaranti. 1987. *Effective teaching: Principles and practice*. New York: Scott, Foresman.

Newble, D., and E. Cannon. 1995. *A handbook for teachers in universities and colleges: A guide to improving teaching methods*. 3rd ed. London: Kogen Page.

Silberman, M. 1996. *Active learning: 101 strategies to teach any subject*. Boston: Allyn & Bacon.

van Ments, M. 1983. *The Effective Use of Role Play: A Handbook for Teachers and Trainers*. London: Kogan Page.

# CHAPTER 11

# High-Fidelity Patient Simulation

*Alfred E. Lupien and Beverly George-Gay*

## DEFINITION AND PURPOSES

High-fidelity simulation has been used in fields such as aviation, maritime operations, and nuclear power management since the early 1930s, when Edwin Link introduced the first aircraft simulator.[1] Realistic, whole-body patient simulators were first developed in the health care industry for use in anesthesiology in the early 1990s, as a means of improving education and studying human performance. Since the narrowly focused introduction of patient simulators, a wide variety of health care applications has been developed to include procedure training, evaluation of individual response to critical incidents, equipment evaluation, task analysis, and team training.[2,3] Common educational applications of simulation include theme-based workshops on ventilation, pharmacology, airway management, or conscious sedation; ongoing skills development (such as progressively complex anesthesia techniques); and practicing clinical decision making. The first nursing users of high-fidelity simulators were nurse anesthetists; however, applications of simulation have expanded to include acute care, critical care, perioperative, and emergency nursing.

Features of the simulators include a functioning cardiovascular system with palpable pulses, heart sounds, measurable blood pressure (by palpation or oscillometry), electrocardiographic output, and invasive parameters such as arterial, central venous, and pulmonary artery pressures. Respiratory system components include self-regulating spontaneous ventilation, measurable exhaled respiratory gases, and breath sounds. Other simulator features include a pharmacological "system" capable of responding to more than 50 anesthetic, analgesic, and vasoactive agents; a urologic system; reactive pupils; and the ability to accept defibrillation, needle cricothyriodotomy, jet ventilation, needle thoracocentesis, chest tube insertion, and pericardiocentesis.

This chapter describes the use of patient simulators such as the Human Patient Simulator® (Medical Education Technologies, Inc., Sarasota, Florida) and the

PatientSim® Training Simulator (MedSim-Eagle, Inc., Binghamton, New York). The simulator is composed of four components: a lifelike mannequin, a free-standing console containing many of the simulator's components, a computer to integrate the function of simulator components, and an interface that allows the user (either student or faculty depending on the objectives of the exercise) to control the simulation and modify physiological parameters (see Exhibit 11–1). Current simulators have both a portable interface to allow instructors to control simulations from the bedside as well as a stationary console that can be positioned away from the mannequin so that changes in the simulation can be made without the knowledge of trainees. To initiate a simulation, the user selects a patient profile (such as healthy adult male or full-term parturient) and scenario (such as ana-

---

**Exhibit 11–1** Modifiable Parameters of High-Fidelity Patient Simulators

| *Cardiovascular* | *Respiratory* |
|---|---|
| Baroreceptor response | Breath sounds |
| Cardiac rhythm | Bronchial resistance (right and left) |
| Cardiac tamponade | Chest wall capacity |
| Heart rate (fixed or baseline) | Chest wall compliance |
| Heart sounds | Functional residual capacity |
| Hemoglobin | Inspiratory:Expiratory ratio |
| Intravascular volume | Intrapleural volume (right and left) |
| Ischemic sensitivity | Lung compliance (right and left) |
| Pericardial fluid | Oxygen consumption |
| Pulmonary vascular resistance | Partial pressure of venous $CO_2$ |
| Pulses | pH (baseline) |
| Systemic vascular resistance | Respiratory quotient |
| Valve resistance (aortic, mitral, | Shunt fraction |
|    pulmonic, and tricuspid) | |
| Venous return | *Other* |
| Venous capacitance | Chest tube air leak |
| Ventricular contractility (right and left) | Chest tube flow |
| | Eyes (open, closed, blinking) |
| | Intracranial pressure |
| | Pupil size (right and left) |
| | Plasma concentrations of bicarbonate, |
| |    glucose, potassium, and sodium |
| | Urine output |
| | Temperature |
| | Weight |

*Note:* Not all features are available on every simulator.

phylaxis) if desired. Once a simulation has been initiated, the instructor may allow the simulation to run as programmed or may make modifications to emphasize specific teaching points.

Through simulation, a predictable environment can be created to allow health care providers to practice under realistic conditions in "real time" using actual clinical supplies. Practical advantages of simulation include the ability to:

- represent serious or uncommon clinical problems
- allow management errors to develop or multiple treatment options to be explored without injury or discomfort to actual patients
- manipulate time (compression, expansion, and replication).

Educational advantages of simulation include the ability to:

- actively involve the learner
- provide relatively consistent experiences for all students
- collect physiological, video, and audio data for use in reflective sessions following the simulation session.[4,5]

The simulated environment may also be used to create a standardized setting for testing critical-thinking and decision-making skills.

Disadvantages of simulation include the costs of starting and maintaining a simulation program, extensive faculty time commitment, and the tendency for the simulated environment to induce "hypervigilance" or exaggerated caution. Moreover, despite a significant amount of human physiological, pharmacological, and phenomenological data, anatomical and physiological models are incomplete and imperfect.[6] Finally, the transfer of learning from the simulated environment to actual clinical practice is not well documented.

## THEORETICAL RATIONALE

The landmark Flexner Report to the Carnegie Foundation in 1910 established the dominant paradigm for health care education in the 20th century.[7] Two key components of the model were a university-based scientific curriculum and a clinical practicum.

The scientific curriculum historically featured lecture-based instruction where students were passive recipients of factual knowledge. Information was imparted by domain experts according to a predetermined timetable. Although the lecture format ensured that important educational material was disseminated, the passive/uninvolved student may not develop the conceptual links necessary for effective, long-lasting learning.

By contrast, the clinical practicum involved the student more effectively as an active participant in the learning process as experience was gained in discipline-specific care. Unfortunately, because of the random nature of clinical experiences, it was impossible for educators to construct the comprehensive array of experiences that allowed a student to gain knowledge across the broad spectrum of required activities.

Achieving a successful balance between academic and clinical education has been a challenge for educators as health care institutions demand graduates with both broad-based knowledge and improved specialty clinical skills.[8] The result is often competition between classroom learning and clinical experiences, with one educational component occurring at the expense of the other (see Figure 11–1).

Instead of concentrating on the struggle between classroom and clinical teaching, focusing on the educational issue of *passive-controlled* classroom instruction versus *active-random* clinical instruction reveals two distinct pedagogical dimensions: learner involvement and content control. New educational activities become available as these dimensions are maximized. Figure 11–2 illustrates options within each dimension. Traditional lecture and clinical formats are represented as quadrant I and IV activities. In this representation, two additional educational states, passive-random and active-controlled, become manifest. Of particular relevance to this chapter is the active-controlled quadrant, which allows the instructor to control the material to be disseminated yet encourages active participation by the learner. Educational formats that can be classified within this quadrant include both problem-based learning and high-fidelity simulation. Both of these methods emphasize the central tenet of situated cognition, specifically that information is most useful when it is learned in contextual schema.[9]

Critics of situated cognition often focus on the role of the instructor. Tripp noted that the teacher was often used as a coach rather than a master teacher.[10] He argued that the teacher must act as a master of the domain and expose students to the abilities

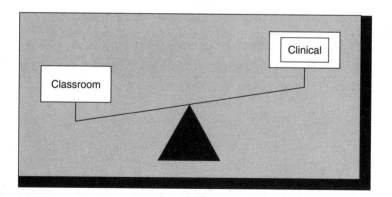

**Figure 11–1** Traditional Concept of Nursing Education. In the traditional educational model, classroom and clinical education are often in competition for limited student time.

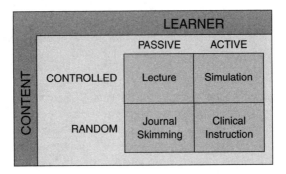

**Figure 11–2** Two-dimensional Concept of Nursing Education. This representation allows educational activities to be classified according to learner involvement as well as the instructor's control over content and illustrates how simulation can be used to control content while using active learning methods.

of master practitioners rather than assume the role of motivator or critic. Additionally, Tripp suggested that some content is taught more effectively in a controlled classroom setting rather than what he characterizes as "on-the-job training."

Instruction through high-fidelity simulation can be designed to address these criticisms. The simulated environment can promote the role of teacher as active participant and role model. Because clinical situations may be repeated as desired, the teacher can act initially as a role model by demonstrating a procedure or decision-making process, then allow the student to practice in an identical or similar situation. By contrast, in the actual clinical area, the faculty member who actively models a procedure, such as insertion of an intravenous catheter, often does so at the expense of the student, who will not be able to repeat the process. In fact, the timing of simulated experiences can be designed so that "clinical" experiences can be introduced to reinforce what has recently been learned in the classroom, with the level of difficulty adjusted to match student capabilities. The ability to create an active learning environment that has been customized for each student is a compelling argument for the addition of high-fidelity simulation to the instructional armamentarium of nurse educators.

## CONDITIONS

Because of the ability to create customized learning scenarios, high-fidelity simulators can be used in a wide variety of situations for all types of students. Simulation can precede, complement, or replace actual clinical experiences.

Prior to clinical experiences, simulation can be used to orient students to an unfamiliar unit. For example, the simulation laboratory can be configured to resemble a surgical intensive care unit. Students are introduced to the types of monitoring equipment, life support devices, dressings, tubes, and drains that might be encountered during an actual clinical rotation. Chatto and Dennis used this method to desensitize physical therapy students prior to a critical care rotation.[11] As students performed physical therapy on the simulator, common events were simulated to include sudden vital sign changes, gradually increasing intracranial pressure, cardiac alarms, and ventilator disconnection. Together with physical therapy and nursing faculty, students implemented safe and effective therapy, identified problems unique to the critical care environment, and practiced collaborative patient care.

In contrast to a one-time orientation session, simulation can also be used to allow students to practice technical skills and decision making before actual clinical experiences. For example, students in an anesthesia nursing program may accrue up to 100 hours of simulation practicing sequences of technical skills and decision making prior to their first clinical experience as a nurse anesthetist.[12,13] In the authors' experience, students who have practiced using simulation prior to real clinical experiences are received more positively by clinical preceptors, and the students receive more efficient and constructive clinical education.

Used concomitantly with clinical practice, simulation provides students and faculty with the opportunity to replicate real clinical experiences and then use the simulator to explore different methods for handling the situation. Students also have the opportunity to create "custom" patients based on their knowledge of physiology and pathophysiology and then compare the responses of their simulated patients to actual patients observed in clinical practice.

Although the fidelity of patient simulators is not developed sufficiently to suggest that training with simulators can replace contact with human patients, simulation can be used to create learning opportunities that are unavailable in the real clinical environment. For example, students can practice high-risk technical procedures, such as defibrillation, in "real time" using actual equipment. Beyond technical skills, students can gain experience in critical clinical situations (e.g., cardiac life support or anaphylactic reaction) that might not occur during scheduled clinical times for all students.

Simulation has also been used to develop "higher order" skills in a fashion that exactly parallels applications of simulation in commercial aviation. Aviation simulation has expanded beyond its use as a teaching/training tool for individual pilots to encompass team training through a program called Crew Resource Management.[14] Similarly, in the field of anesthesiology, programs such as Anesthesia Crisis Resource Management (ACRM) (developed in the United States by Gaba) and Team Oriented Medical Simulation (developed in Switzerland at the University of Basel by Schaefer and Helmreich) focus on the actions of all members of a health care team with the goal of improving team performance. Recently, Fletcher extended the concept of ACRM by developing ERR Watch, which is a program focused specifically on the role of nurse anesthetists in crisis management.[15]

In addition to its uses as an instructional tool, simulation potentially can be used for both formative and summative evaluation. Techniques for formative evaluation of student skills and abilities include using simulation as a mechanism for providing feedback on current skills and decision-making processes or to observe the evolution of a student's abilities. Applications of simulation in summative evaluation are more controversial because the relationship between the performance of nursing students in a simulated environment and actual clinical performance has yet to be demonstrated. Elements of the simulation puzzle are currently being resolved. For example, Monti, Wren, Haas, and Lupien described the use of a rudimentary instrument to evaluate the performance of beginning students in a limited clinical scenario.[16] Both Devitt et al. and Gaba et al. have recently reported excellent indices of inter-rater reliability for instruments to evaluate performance in simulated environments.[17,18] Descriptions of the psychometric properties of the actual instruments are limited. Devitt, Kurrek, Cohen, K. Fish, P. Fish, Noel, and Szalai reported estimates of internal consistency as high as .66 with their instrument for evaluation of anesthesiologist performance.[19] Although these reports describe initial forays into the evaluative use of simulation, there remain considerable limitations to its use. Most notably, because simulators provide an incomplete representation of a patient to the trainee, the implications of inadequate performance during simulation remain unclear.

**TYPES OF LEARNERS**

The Russian psychologist Vygotsky believed that learning was most effective when it occurred within what he termed the "zone of proximal development," where what was to be learned was just beyond the current knowledge level of the student.[20] By altering the underlying physiological parameters, each simulation session can be adjusted to the optimal level of difficulty for a particular student or group: from beginner through expert and technical, undergraduate, and graduate. For example, beginning nursing students can practice taking vital signs or listening to heart and lung sounds. Nurse anesthesia and acute care practitioner students who are learning basic principles of airway management can use the simulator as a part-task trainer to refine fundamental skills such as insertion of pharyngeal airways and bag-valve-mask ventilation. As the student's knowledge level increases, he or she may be expected to maintain ventilation in an apneic patient using oxygen saturation and respiratory gas measurements to guide ventilation. Advanced students may be expected to perform sophisticated airway procedures to include tracheal intubation and needle cricothyroidotomy in simulated patients with abnormal airway anatomy. In a similar fashion, beginning critical care students who are learning to recognize the signs of acute myocardial infarction may be asked to provide care for a patient with a robust cardiovascular system where signs of myocardial ischemia develop gradually without precipitating a cardiac arrest. Advanced students would be expected to recognize subtle physiological clues quickly and to initiate prompt, effective interventions.

## RESOURCES

Perhaps the most critical aspect of a successful simulation program is the designation of dedicated physical space for the simulator and its support equipment. To accommodate the simulator, instructor, and four to six students requires approximately 250 square feet of floor space. A sample floor plan for a simple simulation room is presented in Figure 11–3.

Simulators require both electricity and gas sources. Depending on the type of simulator chosen, there may be requirements for a complete range of respiratory gases, including air, oxygen, carbon dioxide, and nitrogen. Nitrous oxide is optional for the simulation of general anesthesia. Electricity requirements include two to four outlets for the simulator, plus additional sources of power for patient care equipment.

Patient care equipment depends on the types of simulations involved and may include physiological monitors, infusion pumps, ventilators, anesthesia machines, and a defibrillator. Support equipment includes airway devices, needles and syringes, dressings, chest tubes, urinary catheters, scrub wear, gloves, surgical masks, caps, and gowns.

The efficacy of simulation can be enhanced through the video recording of sessions with subsequent debriefing. Recording systems range from a single video camera to complex recording systems that allow multiple camera views, superimposed physiological tracings, and audio recordings from participants and faculty. Dedicated simulation centers include a debriefing room where the videotaped sessions can be reviewed by students and faculty. The debriefing room may also have the ability to receive live video and audio transmissions from the training room.

Some simulation centers also include a control room adjacent to the training room. One-way glass between the rooms allows individuals in the control room to observe simulation sessions as the operator and faculty communicate via headsets with microphones. A technician or faculty member in the control room is responsible for monitoring the simulator, making adjustments as necessary, and selecting video and audio sources for recording.

Because simulation is so resource intensive, personnel support is essential. Depending on the type of simulators and simulation, key faculty with moderate computer skills may be sufficient to support simulation activities on an as-needed basis, although many centers have found it beneficial to designate one faculty member, or an associate, to coordinate simulation activities and maintain the simulator.

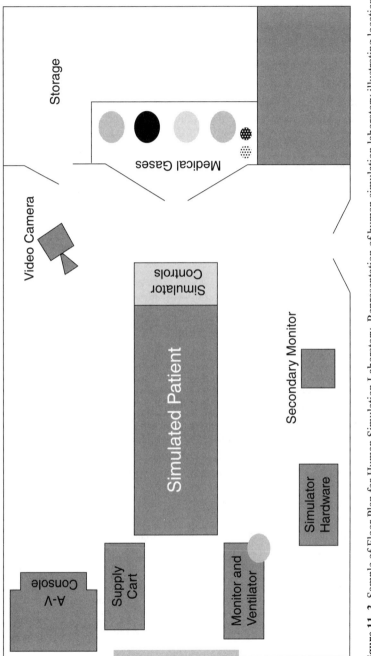

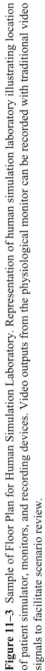

**Figure 11-3** Sample of Floor Plan for Human Simulation Laboratory. Representation of human simulation laboratory illustrating location of patient simulator, monitors, and recording devices. Video outputs from the physiological monitor can be recorded with traditional video signals to facilitate scenario review.

## USING THE METHOD

Successful simulation sessions depend on carefully planned scenarios and clearly defined roles for faculty. The primary instructor is responsible for setting the scenario, guiding students through the simulation, providing important information and clinical cues not available through the simulator, providing transition cues to the simulator operator, modeling behaviors, monitoring or correcting student performance, and correcting simulator errors. In some situations, the instructor may be assisted by another faculty member or technician serving as the simulator operator. The operator's responsibilities include activating the simulation system, starting patient software, overlaying clinical scenarios, monitoring the progress of the scenario, and adjusting the scenario as dictated by the primary instructor. Depending on the expertise of the faculty, complexity of the scenario, and type of simulator being used, one individual may serve as both the faculty member and operator. Complex scenarios may require not only an instructor and operator but also other faculty, students, and/or assistants to role-play as members of the health care team and family.

To develop and implement a new simulation scenario, the seven-step process listed in Exhibit 11–2 is recommended. The following example illustrates how simulation was used to reinforce concepts of respiratory assessment and nursing care.

A critical care nursing elective consisting of 40 didactic hours was designed to compliment a 200-hour critical care clinical practicum for senior students. The elective course focused on pulmonary, cardiovascular, and neurological critical care; advanced hemodynamic monitoring; and critical care pharmacology. The respiratory care section of the course included lectures on respiratory gas exchange, advanced assessment techniques, arterial blood gas analysis, airway management, and ventilatory support. To complement the lectures, the seven-step process described in Exhibit 11–2 was used to develop a simulation session.

---

**Exhibit 11–2**  Seven-Step Process for the Development of Simulation Session

1. Define educational objectives.
2. Construct a clinical scenario.
3. Define the underlying physiological concepts.
4. Modify programmed patients and scenarios, as necessary.
5. Assemble the required equipment.
6. Run the program and collect feedback.
7. Reiterate steps 2–6 until satisfied.

1. **Determine educational objectives.** The simulation session was designed so that the student would be able to achieve the following objectives:
   - Complete and continuously revise the assessment of a patient who is acutely and dynamically ill.
   - Select appropriate oxygen therapy devices for a specified clinical situation.
   - Collect and prepare the appropriate equipment and medications for emergent tracheal intubation.
   - Administer appropriate medications to facilitate emergent tracheal intubation and to assess the drug effects.
   - Perform airway management procedures, as indicated, to include bag-valve-mask ventilation, tracheal intubation, and endotracheal suctioning.
   - Confirm appropriate placement of an endotracheal tube.
   - Prepare an unstable patient for transport from an inpatient unit to a critical care unit.
   - Initiate positive pressure ventilatory support for an acutely ill patient and adjust ventilatory parameters (to include mode, $FiO_2$, tidal volume, respiratory rate, and positive end expiratory pressure) as indicated by patient condition, arterial blood gases, capnography, and spirometry.

2. **Construct a clinical scenario.** A scenario was constructed to facilitate attainment of the educational objectives. Specifically, learners were required to assess a patient with respiratory compromise and to initiate interventions for resuscitative and critical care. Students were told that they were going to evaluate a patient with pneumonia hospitalized on an inpatient medical unit. A brief patient history was provided.

   Students were given the opportunity to assess the patient, including observation of respiratory effort, lung auscultation, estimation of arterial oxygenation by pulse oximetry, and measurement and analysis of arterial blood gases. At the time of initial contact, the patient demonstrated signs of moderate hypoxia, to include rapid shallow breathing, mild oxyhemoglobin desaturation, and rales on chest auscultation. Upon a signal from the instructor to the simulator operator, the patient experienced a significant oxyhemoglobin desaturation.

   The scenario was designed so that the patient initially would require oxygen therapy, then would require more aggressive treatment, including tracheal intubation and positive pressure ventilation using a bag-valve device with both face mask and tracheal tube. Once transferred to the critical care unit, ventilatory support using various modes such as assist-control, intermittent mandatory ventilation, positive end-expiratory pressure, and pressure-support ventilation could be explored.

3. **Define the underlying physiological concepts to be manifest through scenario: patient and events.** The physiological concepts underlying pneumonia include decreased lung compliance and increased shunt. Manifestations

of these alterations include an adaptive respiratory pattern with increased rate and smaller tidal volume, increased peak inspiratory pressure, hypoxemia, mild hypercarbia, rales, tachycardia, and cardiac dysrhythmias. Patient deterioration within the scenario results from progressive reductions in lung compliance and increases in shunt.

4. *Modify programmed patients and scenarios, as necessary.* Program modification generally consists of determining three components: (1) describing the underlying patient, (2) preparing the scenario to include optional modifiable states, and (3) defining transitions between states. Although the simulator includes a series of representative adult patients, for this session, a geriatric model developed by faculty and master's-level nursing anesthesia students was used.* To exhibit signs of pneumonia, rales were introduced, lung compliance was decreased, shunt fraction was increased, and the $CO_2$ set point was increased slightly (to produce mild hypercarbia). Temperature was increased slightly to reflect an underlying infective process. As a result of these changes, tidal volume decreased automatically and respiratory rate increased to compensate for the reduced tidal volume. Physiological alterations were also manifest automatically through changes in vital signs and arterial blood gases.

So that the patient would initially appear to be stable and then deteriorate upon the instructor's command, baseline and decompensation states were created. Although an automatic transition could have initiated the decompensation at a predetermined time, a manual transition was selected to ensure that the destabilization occurred when intended by the instructor.

5. *Assemble the required equipment.* Because the patient is not physically transported from the medical unit to the critical care unit, the simulation lab was originally configured with equipment available to acute care personnel. Items included a resuscitation cart with cardiac monitor and defibrillator, oxygen source, oxygen therapy devices, various airway management devices such as a bag-valve-mask device, pharyngeal airways, endotracheal tubes, laryngoscopes, and suction equipment. Once the scenario shifted to the critical care unit, a positive pressure ventilator was also available for student use.

6. *Run the program and collect feedback.* Prior to use with students, the scenario was run several times to establish an appropriate balance of physiological changes so that the patient would be stable initially yet sufficiently compromised to exhibit symptoms of hypoxemia and to entice the learner to initiate oxygen therapy. Once the deterioration sequence was initiated, the decompensation needed to be sufficient to warrant more aggressive therapy yet sufficiently stable that novice nurses with limited skills and therapeutic options could stabilize the patient.

---

*Development of the geriatric model was supported, in part, by a grant from the Department of Health and Human Services Bureau of Health Professions.

To implement the simulation, the instructor selected the customized geriatric patient from the *Patient Options* menu of the user interface and respiratory exercise from the *Scenario Options* menu. The simulator immediately began emulating the pneumonia patient in the stable baseline state. Progression to the decompensation state required only one additional keystroke or mouse-click.

Once the simulation starts, the instructor has many options in terms of his or her involvement, including whether to serve as (1) role model where critical thinking, decision making, and nursing interventions are modeled; (2) a coach who is available to help students functioning in their nursing roles; or (3) a passive bystander who observes the scenario with minimal involvement. Regardless of the level of participation during the simulation, one of the instructor's key functions is to actively "debrief" the session with students, describing and interpreting the scenario, clarifying learner thoughts and actions, critiquing performance, and generating possible alternative decisions and actions. Depending on the educational goals, the simulation may be repeated to increase the level of student involvement, to explore alternative courses or actions, or to improve student performance.

## POTENTIAL PROBLEMS

Perhaps the most significant potential problem with simulation is its dependence on faculty support. Most commercially available simulation scenarios were developed for medical education. Although many of these scenarios are directly applicable in nursing education, there is also a need for development of nursing-specific scenarios. Scenario writing does not require specialized computer programming skills, but the process of creating and refining scenarios to illustrate specific learning objectives is time intensive. The intimate nature of instruction through simulation also necessitates a small-group format for instruction, which also extends faculty time.

A second limitation of simulation is its incomplete presentation of reality. Although quite lifelike in representing human beings, simulators do not exhibit a complete range of signs and behaviors. Participants in a simulation session are expected to "suspend disbelief" and to respond to the patient based on what they see. For example, the simulated patient experiencing a myocardial infarction will not exhibit diaphoresis. In this situation, the instructor must provide any missing cues that are necessary for appropriate use of the scenario. Although it is surprisingly easy to engage in a simulation, instructors need to be aware of critical cues that are absent or contradictory with the intended signs.

Another potential problem with simulation is controlling the "overgeneralization" of findings to the real world. At least two types of generalization errors can occur. The first type is the generalization of an observed response in one situation to all patients. For example, whenever the baseline healthy 70 kg patient receives an intravenous bolus of 20 µg epinephrine, the heart rate is raised approximately 20 beats per minute. Caution must be exerted to avoid the conclusion that "to increase any patient's heart rate by 20 beats, a dose of 20 µg epinephrine can be administered." To overcome this limitation, faculty can create a series of similar-appearing patients with slightly different physiological parameters such as body weight, oxygen consumption, or baroreceptor responses. By using these similar patients interchangeably, students see variations in drug responses.

The second error of generalization is an incorrect attribution of simulator responses. As an incomplete representation of a human patient, simulators do not present a completely accurate or comprehensive clinical portrait. For example, the simulator, when breathing spontaneously, does not create high negative pressures like a human is capable of generating. Therefore, using the simulator to practice measuring inspiratory effort would lead to inaccurate results. Faculty who understand how the simulator functions will quickly recognize which clinical findings are "real" and which are artifact. Simulation sessions can then be designed to take advantage of areas where the simulator is a reasonable portrayal of a real human and to avoid involving students in activities that are different than would be expected under actual clinical conditions.

Finally, during simulation sessions, participants are often "hypervigilant" because they anticipate the onset of a clinical problem. Although hypervigilance cannot be avoided completely, its effect can be minimized by either mixing routine and critical event simulations or developing a series of potential events that evolve from a common "stem" scenario.

## CONCLUSION

Simulation is a new and exciting application of advanced technology in nursing education. Used correctly, whole-body, high-fidelity patient simulators can effectively bridge the gap between static classroom-based instruction and the dynamic, unpredictable clinical environment. Although most experience with simulators in nursing education has been limited to anesthesia and critical care, on-going refinements in simulators, such as the introduction of pediatric models and open architecture for the development of new simulation applications, will gradually allow the application of high-fidelity simulation across the nursing curriculum.

**NOTES**

1. D.M. Gaba, Simulators in Anesthesiology, in *Advances in Anesthesia*, vol. 14, ed. C.L. Lake et al. (St. Louis: Mosby, 1997), 55–94.

2. D.M. Gaba and A. DeAnda, A Comprehensive Anesthesia Simulation Environment: Re-Creating the Operating Room for Research and Training, *Anesthesiology* 69 (1988):387–394.

3. S.K. Howard, D.M. Gaba, K.J. Fish, G. Yang, and F.H. Sarnquist, Anesthesia Crisis Resource Management: Teaching Anesthesiologists To Handle Critical Incidents, *Aviation, Space, and Environmental Medicine* 63 (1992):763–770.

4. J.L. Fletcher, Anesthesia Simulation: A Tool for Learning and Research, *AANA Journal* 63 (1995):61–67.

5. D.M. Gaba, Simulators in Anesthesiology, 55–94.

6. Ibid.

7. F.J. Papa and P.H. Harasym, Medical Curriculum Reform in North America, 1765 to the Present: A Cognitive Science Perspective, *Academic Medicine* 74 (1999):154–164.

8. P. Manuel and L. Sorensen, Changing Trends in Healthcare: Implications for Baccalaureate Education, Practice, and Employment, *Journal of Nursing Education* 34 (1995):248–253.

9. J.S. Brown, A. Collins, and P. Duguid, Situated Cognition in the Culture of Learning, *Educational Researcher* 18 (1989):32–42.

10. S.D. Tripp, Theories, Traditions, and Situated Learning, in *Situated Learning Perspectives,* ed. H. McLellan (Englewood Cliffs, NJ: Educational Technology Publications, 1996), 155–165.

11. C. Chatto and J.K. Dennis, Intensive Care Unit Training for Physical Therapy Students: Use of an Innovative Patient Simulator, *Acute Care Perspectives* 5, no. 4 (1997):7–12.

12. A.E. Lupien, Simulation in Nursing Anesthesia Education, in *Simulators in Anesthesiology Education,* eds. L.C. Henson and A.C. Lee (New York: Plenum, 1998), 29–37.

13. E.J. Monti, K. Wren, R. Haas, and A.E. Lupien, The Use of an Anesthesia Simulator in Graduate and Undergraduate Education, *CRNA: The Clinical Forum for Nurse Anesthetists* 9 (1998):59–66.

14. R.L. Helmreich and H.C. Foushee, Why Crew Resource Management? Empirical and Theoretical Bases of Human Factors Training in Aviation, in *Cockpit Resource Management,* eds. E.L. Weiner et al. (London: Academic Press, 1993), 3–46.

15. J.L. Fletcher, ERR Watch: Anesthesia Crisis Resource Management from the Nurse Anesthetist's Perspective. *AANA Journal* 66 (1998):595–602.

16. Monti, Wren, Haas, and Lupien, Anesthesia Simulator.

17. J.H. Devitt, M.M. Kurrek, M.M. Cohen, K. Fish, P. Fish, P.M. Murphy, and J. Szalai, Testing the Raters: Inter-Rater Reliability during Observation of Simulator Performance, *Canadian Journal of Anaesthesia* 44 (1997):925–928.

18. D.M. Gaba, S.K. Howard, B. Flanagan, B.E. Smith, K.J. Fish, and R. Botney, Assessment of Clinical Performance during Simulated Crises Using Both Technical and Behavioral Ratings, *Anesthesiology* 89 (1998):8–18.

19. J.H. Devitt, M.M. Kurrek, M.M. Cohen, K. Fish, P. Fish, A.G. Noel, and J. Szalai, Testing Internal Consistency and Construct Validity during Evaluation of Performance in a Patient Simulator, *Anesthesia and Analgesia* 86 (1998):1160–1164.

20. L.S. Vygotsky, *Mind in Society: The Development of Higher Psychological Processes* (Cambridge, MA: Harvard University Press, 1978).

# CHAPTER 12

# Expressive Techniques: Movement As Embodied Knowing

*Carol Picard*

## DEFINITIONS AND PURPOSES

Expressive techniques are activities to assist students in bringing to awareness some aspect of their understanding or experience that is grounded in immediate, personal knowing. The techniques build on other learning activities within the curriculum such as lecture content, reading assignments, or clinical experiences. Through a process of expression and reflection, a deeper understanding of the knowledge of nursing can occur. The practice of nursing is enriched by reflecting on practice as described by Benner, Tanner, and Chesla.[1] Although nursing has a rich tradition in reflective practice, pioneered by Orlando and further advanced by Johns and Freshwater, the educational activities have been primarily text and dialogue-based.[2,3] Nursing education has been enhanced by expressive techniques, such as poetry and art.[4,5]

Movement is an example of another expressive technique. Bateson and Bateson suggested that movement might be a basis for metaphorical thinking by shifting between modes of expression, stating, "Can I, for instance, change my understanding of something by dancing it?"[6] This mode of expression has not been reported as a teaching strategy with nursing students. The author's experience with students and movement and the potential to enhance learning is the focus of this chapter.

The purpose of the expressive technique of movement is to use embodied intelligence in its wholeness to help students understand selected aspects of the process of nursing care and knowledge in practice. These activities create opportunities for students to (1) enhance self-awareness, (2) explore conceptual learning through embodied reflective action, (3) appreciate dimensions of clinical situations, (4) develop an appreciation of the patient/family experience, and (5) come together in community as students/faculty for this learning.

Dance movement therapy literature has described the transformational potential of movement for insight and understanding, as well as its use in fostering an experience of wholeness of mind/body/spirit.[7] Although it is a universal mode of expression, with capacities for heightened self-awareness, modern Western society does not routinely incorporate movement as a mode of expression in learning. In Western culture, embodied movement experiences have been disconnected from reflection and valued knowledge. Yuasa, who explores the modern Western perspective through an Eastern philosophical lens, states: "The mind body issue is not simply theoretical speculation, but a practical, lived experience, involving the mustering of one's whole mind and body. The theoretical is only a reflection on this lived experience."[8] This technique for embodied knowing makes use of what Bryner and Markova call *physical thinking*, or an underused intelligence resource.[9] They use movement activities in teaching corporate executives creative strategies for understanding management issues. Creative movement as a technique changes the learning context and shifts perceptions as students move to know.

The movement component may be guided and structured by the teacher, with specific instructions about the form of the movement. The activity may also take the form of creative movement, where the invitation is to respond to a particular theme, concept, or issue using movement first, instead of words, and then adding words later to enhance the group's understanding of the individual's movement expression. Creative movement is defined as the intentional creative expression of self in dance, gesture, and posture. This form of movement is intended to convey meaning and can be considered a form of embodied reflection.[10] Embodiment refers to meanings, expectations, styles, and habits expressed and experienced by the body-self. Rawlinson described the body as a system of possibility rather than a simple physical entity.[11] Body-subject is lived through in movements, desires, attentions, and gestures. By embodying conceptual knowledge, a richer integration can occur. Current interest in embodiment in the nursing literature highlights the value of student attention to this orientation to themselves, patients, and families.[12,13]

## THEORETICAL RATIONALE

This technique is grounded in Newman's theory of health as expanding consciousness. According to Newman, health is expanding consciousness, and the capacity for self-reflection, expression, and pattern recognition are aspects of expanding consciousness.[14] Consciousness evolves toward increasing complexity in one's relationship to the world. Newman emphasizes the process of becoming, the evolutionary nature of consciousness, and the importance of meaning in appreciating pattern. Newman described movement as the fullest expression of consciousness. Through movement, we come to know our world, others, and ourselves. Exploring a mode of expression that supports wholeness can illuminate and uncover aspects of self-knowledge and meaning.[15]

The use of Newman's theory to ground this pedagogical strategy supports the students' growth as part of their own expanding consciousness. Learning through creative movement gives students an opportunity to address the issues of embodiment, relationship, and reflection both for themselves and issues related to the health care environment and their patient/family's experiences. Very little time is spent in nursing education helping the student reflect on his or her own embodied experiences. Nurses attend to the embodied human health experiences of their patients and families, but it is important to explore the untapped resources in the students' physical being. This rediscovery of the wisdom of the body can support a reflective attitude toward others and an enhanced awareness of one's own body potential, as well as being in a mindful relationship with the environment. The use of expressive techniques also provides an opportunity for students to appreciate directly the potential health-promoting effects of these expressive techniques for patients as well. The impact of these strategies with patients through creative movement and art demonstrates this important dimension of expanding consciousness.[16,17]

The teacher-student relationship can be a mirror of the student-patient relationship in this regard. In both cases, collaboration leads to appreciate the unfolding nature of knowledge of our person/world experience. Using Newman's theory as a ground from which to practice, the goals are awareness of process, appreciation of pattern, relatedness, and transformational change. Each aspect of this exercise can present an opportunity for learning about the whole.

This technique can also be examined in relation to Carper's four patterns of knowing in nursing: personal, empiric, ethical, and aesthetic.[18] Expressive techniques present an embodied mode of knowing of all four patterns.

### Personal Knowing: Self-Awareness

Through expressive techniques, students have an opportunity to engage in understanding nursing science with a sense of immediacy through embodied activities. The exercises give them an opportunity to take the knowledge and make it their own. This is an opportunity to reflect on the questions: Who do I bring to my practice? How does who I am influence the care given? How do I come to understand the ways I embody my attitudes, feelings and beliefs, and new knowledge?

### Empirical Knowing: Integrating Nursing Science

Creative movement techniques provide an opportunity to "play" with concepts and theories, and clinical knowledge, as is described in the exercise. These activities create body metaphors, or body-stories, and move out of analytic, text-based approaches to understanding. The knowledge gained is then reintegrated with prior learning in the reflective dialogue.

### Ethical Knowing: How Should I Act with This Knowledge?

Every component of these exercises provides moments to engage the moral imagination of nursing students. For example, if a student chooses to "pass" on a certain portion of the activity, then the principle of respect for their choice can be discussed, not only in relation to the group but also in relation to patients' choices.

### Aesthetic Knowing: How Do I Express My Understanding of This Knowledge?

Through expressive techniques, the students have an opportunity to create, in movement or gesture, answers to this question. They also have the opportunity to share their creation with the rest of the group. The group component provides a way to come together in a community of creation. The process and the outcome of the activity are equally emphasized.

In summary, creative movement with reflective dialogue is an invitation to students to integrate the four ways of knowing in nursing, grounded in nursing theory, with an emphasis on the student's own expanding consciousness.

## CONDITIONS

The teacher constructs a general framework of exercises for the students that relate to a particular topic or issue. Examples of issues might be professional role, the lived experience of illness such as pain, immobility, or alteration in embodied action as a result of an injury. Other topics that lend themselves to creative movement are the elements of a relationship: trust, security abandonment, loss, and vulnerability. Every learning situation provides some opportunity for embodied reflection.

## TYPES OF LEARNERS

All types of learners may participate, including both graduate and undergraduate students. All exercises may be adapted for students with physical disabilities. It is helpful to suggest that the student is free to pass on any part of the activity because this experience may be new for most students. Creating a safe space will support all learners. Moving in space without any clear expectations may make some students anxious. By framing the exercise with Carper's ways of knowing, students are invited to reflect on their responses to each part of the process. For example, if a student becomes anxious, then the anxiety is processed. The knowledge of how and what would create that response can help the student later in the clinical area. Each student can reflect on his or her own experiences with anxiety. What does it feel and look like? If you couldn't use words, what would its shape be? How does the experience differ from person to person? Have they met any patients whose anxiety was manifested in movement?

With each part of the movement experience, teachable moments and insights are available to students. The leader simply opens with a question, such as: If we are anxious about moving when all is uncertain, what is it like for the patient in strange surroundings, being asked to do things that seem unnatural in some respect?

## RESOURCES

Any space with movable desks or, if possible, a dance studio is a good site for the exercise. In good weather, the use of outdoor space may also be effective; however, if the space is not private, many students may feel uncomfortable with that degree of exposure. For teacher preparation, creative movement workshops are often taught in major cities. Many colleges have dance departments, which offer courses to non-dance majors. Interested faculty members might participate in creative movement workshops because a direct experience of this process with guidance is helpful; however, the faculty member could also walk through the exercises alone, or with a friend or colleague and process the experience directly. In the group with students, the teacher also participates, setting the stage for this process as one of full engagement.

## USING THE METHOD

Consider what the goals are for the experience, keeping in mind to trust the process because insights and developments will arise during the activity and become an important part of shaping the activity. Some exercises may be highly structured, such as trust falls described in a following section, whereas others are a purer form of creative movement generated from within the students. If the exercises are tied to a specific issue or learning objective, then select what calls to you and the students as a beginning. The creative impulse is there in each teacher and student. Talk with students ahead of time and give them a brief explanation of the activity. Let them know that the class will involve a movement activity and to dress in comfortable clothes.

With a movement activity, a generalized structure is used to set the learning. First, identify the time parameters for the session. One to two hours is recommended for a group of eight to ten students. This time frame allows for the process to unfold. As previously mentioned, an important part of the activity is creating a safe place. In order for students to take a risk with a new mode of expression, they must feel safe with the teacher and their peers. Each session begins with warm-up activity to create this safe environment. The following activities are suggestions:

1. ***Warm-up activity.*** Begin with introductions. Invite students to remove their shoes and to stand in a circle. If they do not know each other yet, ask for names all around and then proceed with having each person shake the hands of the others, saying the other's name until everyone can identify his or her classmates. This simple beginning also makes a connection through the handshake. One lesson here is the importance of introductions in any clinical setting. Emphasize the mutual respect and mindfulness necessary for this exercise, even though it has a feeling of play. This concept is important in

the activities that follow because attention to good body mechanics when supporting the weight of another makes it important for attention to be focused. Respect and mindfulness also support a safe place in which to share.

2. A *centering meditative exercise* follows. Widen the circle and ask participants to close their eyes, focusing on their breathing. Suggest that as they breathe, they notice the contact of their feet with the floor. This should take three to five minutes, as you continue to cue them to notice their breathing pattern. Ask that they shift their weight from one foot to the other and notice the subtle changes they must make to accommodate and stay balanced.

3. Have the students *explore their kinesphere*, or their movement potential space. Ask the group to imagine a bubble surrounding each one of them, extending out in all directions as far as they can reach. Invite them to explore this kinesphere in all directions, including behind them, to become aware of the movement potential they possess. Process this activity in dialogue. What can they learn about their own movement patterns? What is it like to explore the range of space? Stretching exercises help the students to notice their bodies and where they are in space. In order to create a safe environment, it is helpful to have students explore not only their own kinesphere, or space potential, but also the studio or room space itself. With each exercise, process the activity with the students. These exercises are done without much contact interaction at first. To create a sense of group cohesion, simple exercises in pairs begin to build the sense of safety with each other. The group can then explore movement activities as a group. As the trust in the group builds, students will feel safer to share their own creative movements with one another.

## POTENTIAL PROBLEMS

### Anxiety

Because of the newness of this teaching technique, students may be anxious. The teacher may be anxious! Giving simple instructions and an overview of the time period will help. Many students think the movement is about traditional forms of dance and may feel uncomfortable, particularly if they have had no dance training. It is important to emphasize that this movement is not like other dance forms with which they may be familiar. Also, emphasize that each student's process will be different and deserving of respect. It helps for students to hear that self-awareness is the key; that the work will not be graded or measured according to some external standard. Rather, the students are invited to engage in a reflective dialogue during the activity. Anxiety may be expressed as laughter or over-talkativeness during the experience. Encourage students to center themselves and to talk only when the activity requires it. Silence when moving allows for a heightened awareness of one's embodied consciousness. Attention to the activity is important for safety reasons.

### Uncovering Painful Material

When an activity is related to a painful topic such as loss, an embodied approach may put the students in touch with their own experiences, which may be difficult or painful. The instructor must be available for processing such content. As with any other triggering that might occur for students either in the clinical area or in the classroom, refer the student for assistance as indicated.

### Avoidance

If a student feels uncomfortable with some part of the exercise, that student can become the observer of the process. In the author's experience working with students in this format, only once did a student find the process so uncomfortable that she could not participate, and only in the creative movement portion of the activity. Students are told that they can pass on any part of the activity.

---

# EXAMPLE
## Students in Maternal Child Nursing Rotation

Baccalaureate students came together to engage in a creative movement reflective dialogue about their new clinical experience as part of a curriculum component called "awareness group." Up until this point, all activities in the group had been discussions. The teacher posed the possibility of a movement activity, and the students agreed.

The students had begun their classroom lectures and reading on topics related to maternal child health, and on this particular week, they were in the newborn nursery and maternity unit. The students identified care of the new family as the learning of the week. The teacher asked what they thought was the most important thing new parents and infants needed. The group agreed that the baby needed a safe holding environment and that first-time parents needed to feel safe and confident in their new roles. Warm-up centering meditative exercises were used to set the stage for the activity. Once the students were able to focus on themselves and their own movement, they were able to begin other exercises that required group activity.

*Walking blind:* This is a trust exercise as well as an invitation to intently notice one's body in space while moving. One student leads the other, whose eyes are closed. Students pair off, switching roles after three to four minutes. Pairs then change partners and repeat the exercise until each person has walked with everyone in the room. The students reflected on each pairing on leading and blindness. The students explored insight into their own comfort level with trust and responsibility for others. The variations in their response with different classmates led to insight regarding patients' comfort level with different staff. Dialogue about comfort ensued, and students planned to read Morse and Bottorff's research on comfort for the following week.[19]

*Trust fall:* The students were invited to take turns standing rigid in the center of a very narrow circle (like a bowling pin) and give their weight to their classmates. The leader demonstrated how to support the center person's weight while maintaining good body mechanics. At first the circle is very small, so the degree of movement is small. As the group and the person in the center become comfortable, the circle can widen. Ask that they do this in silence. After the exercise is completed, the teacher invited the group to reflect. Creating a holding environment, being supportive, letting go of control, and receiving care were themes brought up by the students. With this group, the compelling issue of trust in the group to support their weight gave an immediacy to a discussion of what it must be like to need the kind of care a newborn needs and how trust might be experienced. Participating gave them insight into the uniqueness of a person's response. Several students shared their individual experiences with newborns in their own families, as well as personal family experiences as new mothers, or with relatives or friends who have newborns. They then related their experience to the class lecture that week.

*Rocking in space:* To experience a holding environment, students were invited to give their weight to classmates and be rocked in space. One student at a time would lie on the floor, and the nine other students and teacher would lift the person in silence and rock them slowly. After one to two minutes, they would be gently lowered to the floor. All of this movement was done in silence. Many students described a feeling of peace and safety. One student passed on this exercise, saying that she could take great risks when she felt in control, such as skydiving, but that she could not bring herself to give up control to be lifted four feet off the ground. Students reflected on this lesson of not assuming what another person would want, but rather asking and responding with what was needed.

*Creative movement:* Students were invited to go to a spot in the room by themselves and, after doing a centering exercise, to express in movement or gesture what their feelings about this clinical rotation might be. When they were ready, the group came together in a circle and, one by one, shared the creative movement. They then told the group about the movement's meaning, did the movement again, and then the group would try the movement. As each student in sequence shared her movement, the group would try it and then add it to the movement repertoire of the whole. At the end of 11 movements, including the teacher's, the group had a piece of choreography, which spoke to the collective wishes of this clinical cohort. They had also formed a sense of community, appreciated how much they had in common, and how each of them was unique. Some of the movements related to caring, being able to help, learning not to fear, becoming strong, and being knowledgable. When the creative movement group was over, the students expressed enthusiasm for this model of reflection. Although the group time was over, students stayed in the studio to continue their discussion of what the activities offered.

*Conclusion:* This expressive technique of using creative movement, movement exercises, and reflective dialogue supported student-embodied knowing. Students reported experiencing a heightened sense of themselves in space and an enthusiasm for understanding concepts in action. They reflected on the knowledge acquired as it related to patients and what should happen in a caring environment. They used the time and activities to form a cohesive group, which would work together most effectively over the course of the semester. Subsequent group meetings also used more expressive techniques generated by the students.

---

**NOTES**

1. P. Benner, C. Tanner, and C. Chesla, *Expertise in Nursing Practice* (New York: Springer, 1996).

2. I. Orlando, *The Dynamic Nurse Patient Relationship* (New York: National League for Nursing, 1990).

3. C. Johns and D. Freshwater, *Transforming Nursing through Reflective Practice* (London: Churchill Livingstone, 1997).

4. C. Picard, C. Sickul, and S. Natale, Healing Reflections: The Transformative Mirror, *International Journal of Human Caring* 2, no. 3 (1998):29–37.

5. A.L. Wagner, *A Study of Baccalaureate Nursing Students' Reflection on Their Caring Practice through Creating and Sharing Story, Poetry and Art* (Lowell, MA: University of Massachusetts at Lowell, Doctoral dissertation, UMI #72699, 1999).

6. G. Bateson and M.C. Bateson, *Angels Fear: Toward an Epistemology of the Sacred* (New York: Bantam, 1988), 195.

7. J.L. Hanna, The Power of Dance: Health and Healing, *Journal of Alternative and Complementary Medicine* 1, no. 4 (1995):323–331.

8. Y. Yuasa, *The Body: Toward an Eastern Mind-Body Theory* (Albany: State University of New York Press, 1987), 18.

9. A. Bryner and D. Markova, *An Unused Intelligence* (Berkeley: Conari Press, 1996).

10. C. Picard, Uncovering Patterns of Expanding Consciousness in Mid-Life Women: Creative Movement and the Narrative as Modes of Expression, *Nursing Science Quarterly* 13, no. 2 (2000):150-158.

11. M. Rawlinson, Medicine's Discourse and the Practice of Medicine, In *The Humanity of the Ill*, V. Kestenbaum, ed. (Knoxville: University of Tennessee Press, 1982).

12. J. Watson, *Postmodern Nursing and Beyond* (New York: Churchill Livingstone, 1999).

13. M. Wilde, Why Embodiment Now? *Advances in Nursing Science* 22, no. 2 (1999):25–38.

14. M. Newman, *Health as Expanding Consciousness* (Sudbury, MA: Jones & Bartlett, 1994).

15. Ibid.

16. C. Picard, *Uncovering Patterns of Expanding Consciousness in Mid-life Women: Creative Movement and the Narrative as Modes of Expression* (Chestnut Hill, MA: Boston College, Doctoral dissertation, UMI #9828038, 1998).

17. E. Predeger, Womanspirit: A Journey into Healing through Art in Breast Cancer, *Advances in Nursing Science* 18, no. 3 (1996):48–58.

18. B. Carper, Fundamental Patterns of Knowing in Nursing, *Advances in Nursing Science* 1, no. 1 (1978):13–23.

19. J. Morse, J. Bottorff, and S. Hutchinson, The Paradox of Comfort, *Nursing Research* 41 (1995):14–19.

---

## SUGGESTED READING

Bryner, A., and D. Markova. 1996. *An unused intelligence.* Berkeley, CA: Conari Press.

Cricket, B., and L. Keegan. 2000. Exercise and creative movement. In *Holistic Nursing*, B.M. Dossey, L. Keegan, and C.E. Guzzetta, eds., 453–465, Gaithersburg, MD: Aspen Publishers.

Hanna, J.L. 1995. The power of dance: Health and healing. *Journal of Alternative and Complementary Medicine* 1, no. 4:323–331.

Johns, C., and D. Freshwater. 1997. *Transforming nursing through reflective practice.* London: Churchill Livingstone.

Picard, C., C. Sickul, and S. Natale. 1998. Healing reflections: The transformative mirror. *International Journal of Human Caring* 2, no. 3:29–37.

Picard, C. 2000. Uncovering pattern of expanding consciousness in mid-life women: Creative movement and the narrative as modes of expression. *Nursing Science Quarterly* 13, no. 2, 150–158.

Predeger, E. 1996. Womanspirit: A journey into healing through art in breast cancer. *Advances in Nursing Science* 18, no. 3:48–58.

Samuels, M., and M. Lane. 1998. *Creative healing.* San Francisco, CA: Harper.

# CHAPTER 13

# Debate As a Teaching Strategy

*Martha J. Bradshaw and Arlene J. Lowenstein*

## DEFINITION AND PURPOSES

A traditional view of debate may be that of argument for the purpose of persuading the audience toward a clearly identified position. Political debates have been used as opportunities for candidates to make their perspectives known on key issues. Debate has been defined as "a systematic contest of speakers in which two points of view of a proposition are advanced with proof."[1] Based on this definition, debate becomes a useful teaching strategy.

Debate provides opportunities for students to analyze objectively an issue or problem in depth and to reach an informed, unbiased conclusion or resolution. Debate encourages participants to identify quickly the essential nature of the issue as substantiated by the literature, to establish criteria for judging its successful resolution, and to weigh, compare, and contrast the merits of alternative strategies for resolution. The process of formulating the debate issue and preparing the arguments enhances critical-thinking skills.[2]

> Having to examine and debate an issue brings students to a new level of awareness and helps them to develop the ability to recognize and appreciate the contextual complexities that exist. Although some initial views are adhered to throughout the exercise, others become modified or even changed radically. In either case, students' skills of inquiry are practiced and their world view is broadened by the experience (p. 18).[3]

In addition, presentation of the debate allows students to practice oral communication skills, express professional opinions, and gain experience in speaking to groups.

## THEORETICAL RATIONALE

Two important components of the professional role are the analysis of significant issues and the ability to communicate in efficient and effective ways. Professional communication is seen in many forms: scholarly publication, oral presentations, and electronic networking are a few examples. Similar to other skills, the development of effective communication skills must be fostered by nursing faculty. The ability to communicate one's thoughts clearly and concisely evolves from the formulation of a perspective on a topic, analysis of that perspective as well as other views, and development of sound conclusions. Debate enables students to participate actively in a meaningful communication exercise.

DeYoung differentiates debate from general discussion by pointing out that general discussion is based on open-mindedness and a free flow of ideas. Discussion usually aims toward some sort of conclusion and often is a cooperative compromise. Debate, on the other hand, is argumentative, with each team competing to establish its position as the most correct one or the one that should be upheld.[4]

One of the purposes of debate is for the learner to go beyond merely identifying an issue. Learners must analyze the issue: What are its key elements? What historical precedents have contributed to the issue? Who are the key proponents and opponents of the issue? What is the future of the issue? Analysis on this level leads to powerful learning, calling for the use of reasoning and other forms of higher-order thinking.[5]

## CONDITIONS FOR LEARNING

Debate is most useful as part of a course or seminar in professional and academic settings. Because of the nature of this strategy, it should be employed in a course that centers around issues or topics that raise debatable questions. This strategy can be used to facilitate students' ability to implement thinking skills, to systematically critique an issue and arrive at salient points, and to demonstrate more professional development related to group process.

The learning goals for the debate strategy include improving oral communication and library skills, structuring and presenting an argument, and exercising analytical skills. The process for formulating and presenting the debate should facilitate these goals as much as possible; therefore, the faculty should provide as much freedom as possible for the students to reach these learning goals independently. Students should be given enough structure or direction to help them plan and organize their work, but they also should understand the responsibility they must take for researching debate positions, analyzing key issues, and practicing speaking skills. In the debate strategy described by Lowenstein and Bradshaw, students were encouraged to take the viewpoint opposite the one they (personally) held.

This approach promoted an understanding of existing oppositional perspectives and enhanced the ability to respond to opposing views.[6]

Preparation for the debate should begin early in the course to provide adequate opportunity for library research and exploration of issues. Faculty facilitation is an essential part of the learning process. Conditions central to use of debate as an effective strategy include the following:

- Students need to be introduced to key issues in the course and have been able to identify controversial points suitable for debate.
- Students need to be familiar with one another in order to form working groups.
- Students need knowledge of existing resources to use in formulating debate. This includes increased familiarity with the faculty member(s) as a source of support and information.

## TYPES OF LEARNERS

Debate can be used with all levels or types of learners, including undergraduate students, graduate students, and practitioners, because the learning goals of debate are suitable for all groups. Lowenstein and Bradshaw used debate with registered nurse students who were completing their BSN.[7] Debate is a particularly success-ful strategy with this group because these students combine personal experience with actual patient or practice problems with the need to refine communication and analytical skills. Thus, debate provides a true opportunity for professional growth in this type of student.

By creating the need to objectively analyze an issue, debate is useful for a student who is strongly influenced by personal values or certain work experiences. An undergraduate who has not formed a world view about sensitive ethical dilem-mas, for example, can have the opportunity to examine the issues and how deci-sions are made. A practitioner who has been receiving negative influence in the work environment has the opportunity for objective analysis of the situation.

## RESOURCES

Faculty members serve as an important resource by assuming the role of facili-tator. Formal debate questions and positions can emerge from class discussion about important issues. Faculty members can assist students in formulating the debate question and can direct them to resources related to the issue.

The library offers many resources for debate preparation. By using the profes-sional literature to support the debate position, students are introduced to a wide range of journals, books, and other printed material. Electronic information sys-tems are extremely helpful to students as they identify debate issues and develop related positions. Database searches enable students to consider related topics, which may generate additional support for a position. The electronic media access most current information, which may be particularly helpful for students who have timely political topics. Electronic bulletin boards and other communication networks provide students with the opportunity to interact with individuals outside their own institution who are involved with the issue.

The debate can be presented in any planned classroom setting. The environment should be such that the debate teams can be seen and heard by the audience.

## USING THE METHOD

In the Lowenstein and Bradshaw method, faculty members define broad (topical) areas from the course outline and identify an advisor for each area. Students choose the general area in which they are interested and form groups of four or five members. At least one group is formed for each topical area to guarantee that course objectives or topics are addressed. Depending on student interest and enrollment, a second group may be formed in certain areas. For example, two groups may choose to address the area of professional roles and responsibilities. Specific debate questions are formulated by the group in keeping with the objectives or broad topics of the course and personal interests of group members. Many of the topics are those currently being debated by our colleagues in all levels of nursing. Health care reform, nursing care delivery systems, use of restraints, and euthanasia are a few examples.[8]

Each group should meet with the faculty advisor as needed to organize the debate presentation, gain insight into the points being presented, and receive assistance with resources. For each debate group, two students select the affirmative position, two select the negative, and the fifth serves as moderator. In groups of four, the faculty advisor serves as moderator. Each group develops a reading list of significant articles related to the issue under debate. The list is circulated to the entire class at least one week prior to the debate. Students not involved in the presentation are expected to be prepared to discuss the issues under consideration.

The debate consists of opening remarks by a moderator, two affirmative and two negative presentations, rebuttal, and summary. Following the presentation, the floor is opened to the class for discussion. Questions and comments based on the presentations and readings are generated by the class. The debate moderator facilitates discussion and provides a final summary of the issues and discussion. With some issues, it may be appropriate to develop a resolution plan upon conclusion of the formal debate. This plan can incorporate some ideas from both positions to encourage "win-win" negotiation. This process gives students experience in developing workable solutions to practice-related issues.

Class members not participating in the debate are asked to evaluate each presenter based on a rating scale. Students evaluate the analysis of the issue, the evidence presented, supporting resources, organization of the presentation, the argument presented, interaction with the audience and opponents, and response to questions (Exhibit 13–1). An overall effectiveness score is given, and the evaluators indicate if their stand on the issue changed as a result of the debate. All faculty members participating in the seminar also evaluate the presenters. Debate grades are based on preparation, individual performance, and group efforts that were reflected in the effectiveness of the debate.

To reinforce the learning from the debate, students may be asked to write a formal paper on one of the professional issues discussed in the course. The paper can be evaluated on the presentation of the issue, arguments for both sides of the issue supported by literature, the student's position and rationale for selection of the position, application of ideas to practice, and use of references and format.

---

**Exhibit 13–1**  Grading Tool Debate

Date: _____ Subject/Topic: _____

Evaluate each speaker using the following scale:

**Superior = 5; Excellent = 4; Good = 3; Fair = 2; Below standard = 1**

| *Team A* | | *Team B* |
|---|---|---|
| 1 2 3 4 5 | Bibliography (4 max) | 1 2 3 4 5 |
| | Overview of Problem (1–2) | |
| 1 2 3 4 5 | Representing Side of Debate (1–2) | 1 2 3 4 5 |
| _____ | Opening Remarks | _____ |
| *Debater* | | *Debater* |
| 1 2 3 4 5 | | 1 2 3 4 5 |
| _____ | Resolution Plan | _____ |
| *Debater* | | *Debater* |
| 1 2 3 4 5 | | 1 2 3 4 5 |
| _____ | Response to Opposing Team | _____ |
| *Debater* | | *Debater* |
| 1 2 3 4 5 | | 1 2 3 4 5 |
| _____ | Concluding Statement | _____ |

## POTENTIAL PROBLEMS

The debate strategy calls for significant student responsibility and preparation, for both debaters and the audience. Debaters are required to thoroughly research the issue and the position taken for the argument. From this preparation, they formulate a succinct and effective presentation. Debaters are expected to practice speaking skills and to prepare supporting materials for the oral presentation. The debate group provides an appropriate reading list for the other class members. Those students take the responsibility to read about the issue prior to the presentation in order to understand the issue and participate effectively in discussion. Lack of preparation leads to inadequate presentation of the issue and superficial discussion.

The debate causes students to clearly classify an issue as one that is right or wrong, or answered "yes" or "no." Students may have to defend a position to which they are not clearly committed. Students with strong moral beliefs about an issue may have difficulty defending a specified position or accepting the views of others. At some point during the presentations, it must be made very clear that there are no right or singular answers to most issues.

Nervousness about speaking in public can be a major concern. Some students have had little or no speaking experience, or they may have had negative experiences that generated anxiety. Students need encouragement and need to view the debate as an opportunity to speak to an open, receptive group in order to gain experience. What some students look upon with apprehension often results in being uplifting and beneficial. For example, one student was timid about speaking in groups and was extremely nervous before and during her debate presentation. Her nervousness was manifested in physical symptoms, such as sweating, flushed face, tremulous voice, shaking hands, and rapid blinking. She received appropriate support from faculty and students, which encouraged her to work on this problem during the rest of her academic work. Three years later, she successfully defended her Master's project in a dignified and professional manner. Her public speaking skills have now advanced to the point that she is able to address both groups and individuals effectively in her current employment as a clinical specialist.

The argumentative or confrontational nature of the debate may create anxiety. In addition, debate or public speaking may be a new strategy on which students are graded, thus heightening anxiety. Faculty and students must continually place emphasis on the debate as a learning experience. The excitement of defending a position, stressing key points, and deriving a workable solution should be presented as positive outcomes of the debate. Faculty members should stress that students will not be condemned or inappropriately criticized for taking unpopular viewpoints during the debate. Faculty members are prepared to handle strong emotional viewpoints and to help students understand that there is room for conflicting opinions in our society. Students need to be encouraged to see the benefit of the opportunity to practice speaking skills, research skills, and group work.

## CONCLUSION

Debate is a strategy that promotes student interaction and involvement in course topics. There are many advantages to using this strategy. Debate expands the student's perspective on a given issue, creates doubt about the existence of one clear answer, and requires much thought and further evidence before deriving a solution. Debate also increases awareness of opposing viewpoints. As an interactive strategy, debate develops techniques of persuasion, serves as a means by which students confront a controversial issue, and promotes collaborative efforts and negotiation skills among peers. This strategy promotes independence and participation in the decision-making process, as well as enhancing writing and organizational skills. Debate allows for examination of broad issues that influence professional practice. Critical thinking is enhanced by the scrutiny of more than one position on the issue. Debate allows the student a wider forum than writing a paper and may give a greater sense of accomplishment.[9]

Selection of debate as a teaching strategy requires a strong commitment to preparation and guidance from faculty. Faculty members will have to deal with emotions that can be elicited by the arguments. Faculty members will need to provide support for students who take minority or unpopular positions and for those who have limited public speaking skills. Following the debate, those students whose ideas are not accepted by the majority should be encouraged to recognize those parts of their work that were of value, even if others disagreed with their position. Those students whose ideas reflected the majority view should also recognize that public consensus can change quickly and, as more information becomes available, opinions may be swayed. Finally, faculty members can help students to recognize that the debate is just a start to exploration of professional issues. Students will need to be encouraged to incorporate their newly learned and practiced skills into their professional practice.

---

**NOTES**

1. C.L. Barnhart, *The American College Dictionary* (New York: Random House, 1966).
2. C.S. Green and H.G. Klug, Teaching Critical Thinking and Writing through Debates: An Experimental Evaluation, *Teaching Sociology* 18 (1990):462–471.
3. N.E. White, N.Q. Beardslee, D. Peters, and J.M. Supples, Promoting Critical Thinking Skills, *Nurse Educator* 15, no. 5 (1990):16–19.
4. S. DeYoung, *Teaching Nursing* (Redwood City, CA: Addison-Wesley, 1990).
5. M.L. Colucciello, Creating Powerful Learning Environments, *Nursing Connections* 1, no. 2 (1988):23–33.
6. A.J. Lowenstein and M.J. Bradshaw, Seminar Methods for RN to BSN Students, *Nurse Educator* 14, no. 5 (1989):27–31.
7. Lowenstein and Bradshaw, Seminar Methods.
8. Lowenstein and Bradshaw, Seminar Methods.
9. DeYoung, *Teaching Nursing*.

# CHAPTER 14

# The Tree of Impact

*Richard L. Sowell*

## DEFINITION AND PURPOSES

The *tree of impact* is a shorthand analysis of the possible consequences of a policy decision or event. This technique does not provide an in-depth analysis; it only looks at the relationship among options. The tree of impact provides an overview of possible relationships as the consequences of alternative futures are developed. It is important to realize that this technique provides a view of possible alternative futures but does not tell the future. The technique is a method of helping the futurist to determine where, when, and how significant elements of change can occur. It also helps the futurist to understand the logic of specific systems of change.[1] The tree of impact is also referred to as a *futures wheel*,[2] or a *relevance tree.*[3]

The purpose of this strategy is to provide an overall framework that organizes ideas or actions and subsequent consequences over time. The technique provides a method by which the impact that an idea might have on the future can be simulated. Additionally, this technique provides a method that readily organizes the large number of diverse ideas that can arise from group discussions or brainstorming sessions. The construction of a tree may be desirable to accomplish any of the following:

- structure the problem
- identify the system alternatives
- identify the possible impact of the focus problem
- help evaluate the impact of various approaches to the focus problem
- identify decision makers
- identify possible action options for decision makers
- present results[4]

This technique, when used with students, gives the student the opportunity to interact with a large volume of knowledge through preclass preparation and in-class participation. It furthers the logical application of knowledge to anticipate the long-term consequences and interactions of ideas.[5] Once initiated through classroom participation, it can serve as a guide for more in-depth study by the student. Each branch of the tree can serve as the focus of further investigation and analysis as the student works toward the alternative future that is determined to be most appropriate or desirable.

## THEORETICAL RATIONALE

The theoretical foundation for the tree of impact is brainstorming. Brainstorming is based on the free-flowing generation of ideas within an innovative and non-restrictive atmosphere. This technique employs not only the application of knowledge in problem identification and problem solving but creativity and intuitive insight as well.[6] Such an approach is designed to overcome the tendency for absolute patterning of thought identified by Edward de Bono in 1971. De Bono stated that the mind develops patterns from early acquired knowledge and then filters out all new information that does not fit that pattern.[7] The innovation and free association of brainstorming help overcome obsolete patterning, allowing the acquisition of new modes of thought.

This teaching strategy, as derived from brainstorming, acts to organize the ideas that are generated. It provides a visual frame of reference for the session that can further stimulate the participants' imagination and provide insight into crucial elements as possible points of impact or consequence. The tree, as an organized overview of alternative futures, is supported by Clark and Cole as a model of value in that it provides simplification and structuring of potential realities.[8]

## CONDITIONS

The use of this method is based on the need for a group or individual to

- anticipate the long-term consequences and interactions of current events or trends,
- foresee the long-term results of present policies and actions,
- compare the possible long-term consequences of other options or alternative futures, and
- identify the elements of alternative courses of action and potential opportunities for intervention before undesirable consequences are realized.[9]

This teaching-learning technique is used when innovation, creativity, and flexibility are desired in an approach. This method is particularly well suited for use in viewing complex trends and alternative futures that are subject to contradictory pressures, change, and duplication. The construction of the tree is a versatile technique that can be adapted to a variety of situations. It is especially valuable for nursing staffs planning for future technology, or studying issues that have an impact on nursing.

In the brainstorming, any consequence may be proposed by any group member as the branching of the tree is developed; once a consequence is proposed, it is included as part of the developing tree. This process is a quick and free-wheeling approach to problem solving that encourages innovation.

Because the tree of impact can be used in conjunction with the beginning or final stages of the Delphi survey, guidelines for choosing topics of interest, as well as expert panel members, are often the same.[10] Because an in-depth presentation of such guidelines is provided under the Delphi technique, these guidelines will not be repeated in this section.

A modification of the technique can be used as the final stage of the Delphi technique, serving to further narrow the focus elements obtained from the Delphi survey to something more specific. In contrast to the application of the tree within brainstorming, the rules for developing the tree in this procedure are essentially reversed.

In developing the tree, any group member may propose a consequence related to the determined focus concept, but every other group member maintains potential veto power over inclusion of that consequence. To be included in the tree as a consequence or event, the item must receive the group's unanimous approval.[11] In this manner, the results of a Delphi survey can be narrowed and critical elements examined in depth. The results of this approach do not allow for the richness of unrestricted individual input found in brainstorming, but they make the probabilities of the resulting outcome consequences more accurate.

The tree of impact technique can also be used to provide schematic representation of the critical points of interest for future scenario development. Although it is not as comprehensive as the scenario technique, it does have the advantage of providing a precise visual representation of the critical information found within a futures scenario.[12]

It is important to remember that the lines used to form the branching of a tree of impact do not necessarily represent a cause-and-effect relationship. Rather, they signify a relationship that may or may not represent a time sequence, depending on the guidelines provided for the specific tree being developed. This ability to develop individualized trees makes this technique applicable in a wide variety of situations and settings.

The objective of the tree of impact technique is to free the learner from the restrictions of old knowledge patterns and develop an innovative method of viewing potential futures. The technique incorporates elements of creative problem solving, including fact finding, problem finding, idea finding, and acceptance finding.[13]

The learner goes from an examination of what is or has been to an exploration of what might be. From this perspective, the learner is able to develop modes of critical-thinking and decision-making skills that permit attainment of the goal of determining what will be.[14]

This method of learning facilitates the flow of ideas from both individuals and groups that can be logically ordered into a meaningful system of understanding; however, the learner must be aware of the principle of "counter intuitive"—that is, events that seem to defy common sense and logic.[15] The learner must guard against constructing faulty alternative futures by not considering the possibility of the occurrence of such counter-intuitive events. Such a situation challenges learners to look beyond themselves and to use their mental abilities to their fullest.

## TYPES OF LEARNERS

This technique can be used with any individual or group who has knowledge of the focus topic or who has access to such knowledge. This technique is particularly suited for adult learners who are able to apply knowledge gained from life experiences to the exercise. The construction of a tree stimulates the informed learner or expert by providing a fast-moving exercise that provides opportunity for short-term feedback in viewing potentially long-term consequences or trends.

## RESOURCES

The tree of impact technique can be used within various types of futuristic programs, including the following:

- *The academic futuristics program*—within this setting the tree of impact is employed in an educational context to teach individuals about futurism and techniques that are used to predict alternative futures. Construction of the tree is designed to develop the learners' skill in creative thinking. The learner usually cannot implement the results of the exercise.[16] The exercise teaches the student how to identify critical factors and analyze their impact.
- *Strategic planning program*—such strategic planning usually takes place within the work setting. Strategic planning allows organizations to develop strategies to meet organizational goals. The tree of impact is an important tool in developing alternative futures as strategic planners explore the consequences of various ideas and actions. In this situation, results are often put into action, so predicting the future significance of trends is a major part of the organizational planning process.[17] Strategic planning would be aided by this process, for example, when studying environmental trends that would impact on a proposed ambulatory care unit.
- *Personal futuristic program*—here an individual or group uses the predictive technique in developing alternative futures from which the desirable can be chosen. The chosen future may be implemented in whole or in part by

devising relevant action plans.[18] The participant, for example, can test consequences of pursuing a master's degree in nursing as opposed to a degree in education or business.

The most important resource required in the development of a tree of impact is the participants' time; however, the time investment can be limited by the number of participants in the sessions and the time allotted for each accomplishment. The development of a tree should be a fast-moving process that involves a limited number of sessions of no more than approximately one hour each. This time limit keeps the process fresh and spontaneous.[19]

The actual equipment needed to implement the technique consists of a flip chart or chalkboard and a marker with which to draw. In the educational setting, however, adequate library resources must be available so that student participants can investigate topic areas as part of their preclass preparation.

## USING THE METHOD

The initial step in implementing the tree of impact technique is preparation. The individual or group wishing to use this approach must first determine the topic of interest.

Second, they must establish specific objectives to be achieved by use of this technique. For teaching, topics of interest should be chosen that are familiar to both the instructor and students; once the steps of the technique are mastered, the strategy may then be applied to more complex or unfamiliar problems.

Once the topic of interest and exercise objectives have been established, the third step is information gathering and synthesis. When the tree of impact technique is used with a group of experts, this step may include activities such as review of present knowledge, analysis of recent events and trends, or investigation of new technology. When the technique is employed in teaching, however, the scope and time commitment of preclass preparation will most likely be more extensive. The students must familiarize themselves with the topic area before participating in the class exercise. Student preclass preparation should include the following:

- review of historical developments in the topic area[20]
- past examples of logical and counter-intuitive trends or events in the topic area[21]
- identification of critical factors or elements related to the topic[22]
- present knowledge in the topic area[23]
- opinions of experts in the area[24]
- other topic areas that will potentially have an impact on the topic area of focus

The implementation of the technique can begin once the participants have acquired the necessary knowledge base. The rules related to specific trees should be clearly stated and enforced. The group leader or instructor is responsible for ensuring that participants understand the technique and the specific guidelines for this particular exercise. The guidelines may be adjusted regarding use or nonuse of a time relationship in developing branching; an individual or unanimous group approach to inclusion of proposed consequences; or the time allowed each participant in the construction process. By clearly stating and adhering to the exercise guidelines, the exercise procedure will be kept on target and arguments and misunderstandings will be prevented.[25]

After the guidelines for the exercise are established, the actual tree of impact is constructed. The tree is built from the central topic statement by initially adding a single row of consequences related to the topic statement. Each of these first-row consequences serves as a focus as other related consequences are added to the tree. In this manner, each level of the tree becomes more complex while serving as a focus.

The tree development occurs as each group member provides a consequence or impact event in turn. Each proposed consequence may or may not be included in the tree's development, depending on the guidelines established for the exercise. In either case, the next participant proposes an item. A group member who is unable to contribute an item for the specific branch under consideration passes, and the process continues with the next participant. This process is continued for the time allotted for the exercise or until the desired level of investigation is reached.

The construction of a tree can be simple or quite complex. When broad topics such as racial issues are explored, duplication and contradiction often occur among various branches of the tree.[26] This result is to be expected and may be desirable. It is often necessary to indicate relationships both vertically and horizontally between the elements of various branches of the tree, as the complexity of the topic issue is explored.

When completed, the tree of impact provides immediate feedback to group participants; however, it also provides the basis for further analysis of specific elements identified during the exercise. The developed tree can serve as the foundation for further refinement of trends or events and be the inspiration for construction of still other trees of impact.

---

# EXAMPLE
# Plotting the Future of AIDS

The development of the tree of impact described in this example was undertaken as part of the coursework for a graduate-level course in sociopolitical issues. The goal of the course was to examine forces that have an impact on the nursing profession as well as the larger health care system.

The overall learning objective emphasized the use of futurcasting techniques as a method of examining alternative futures that may evolve from present events or trends. The objectives were specifically that, upon completion of this exercise, the student would be able to

1. define the tree of impact technique
2. evaluate the purpose of the technique as a tool for planning
3. identify incidents in which the technique would be appropriately used
4. analyze the advantages of the tree of impact technique over other futurcasting techniques
5. discuss the steps necessary to fully initiate and develop a tree of impact
6. apply the technique to a selected topic of interest to develop a method of viewing alternative futures
7. defend the role of the tree of impact as a method of generating further research and analysis within a study area
8. defend the importance of exercise guidelines as a means of individualizing the technique to meet specific situational objectives

The initial step in the exercise was selection of a focus topic, acquired immunodeficiency syndrome. AIDS was especially suited for the exercise because the issues surrounding this health care problem are complex, yet familiar to the group.

The topic provides adequate challenge for students at the graduate level as they implemented the tree of impact technique within a learning setting. To assist the student in obtaining needed knowledge during the preparatory phase of the exercise, a reading list was provided. The student was required to read a minimum of seven articles from the list before participating in the exercise. The following terminology was necessary:

| | |
|---|---|
| 1. Tree of impact | 11. Futurist |
| 2. Futures wheel | 12. Creative problem solving |
| 3. Relevance tree | 13. Trend |
| 4. Consequence | 14. Academic futuristics |
| 5. Branching | 15. Strategic planning |
| 6. Relationship linkage | 16. Personal futuristics |
| 7. Futurcasting | 17. Impact |
| 8. Counter-intuitive | 18. Panel of experts |
| 9. Topic of focus | 19. Delphi survey |
| 10. Alternative futures | 20. New knowledge |

The exercise in which the actual tree was constructed took place near the end of the academic term. The student consequently had adequate time to obtain an understanding of the futurcasting techniques, as well as knowledge in the topic area to be explored. The exercise was conducted in a classroom setting with all members of the sociopolitical class. Rules for the exercise were established by the group prior to beginning the exercise. It was determined that the overall goal of the exercise would be to construct a tree of impact that would organize the many diverse issues related to AIDS. This approach was designed to provide a logical framework for viewing the topic issues and to help predict the potential impact of specific events in the future. It was determined that the branching links developed among concepts and events in this exercise would not signify actual cause-and-effect or true relationships. Rather, these links would indicate only that the items were related within the framework.[27]

During the initial phase of the exercise, four subtopics related to AIDS were determined by the group: (1) public action, (2) HIV infection, (3) education, and (4) research. These subtopics were to help focus the exercise despite the broad scope of the AIDS topic.

Once the four subtopics were identified, it was clear that each of these concepts formed the center of a new individualized tree of impact under the broad topic of AIDS. The initial level of the framework was constructed to reflect this situation (Figure 14–1) and the exercise proceeded.

At the second level of the exercise, group members were able to propose a consequence for any of the four trees of impact being developed from the subtopics. All proposed consequences were included in the branching process as the exercise progressed through the various levels of the technique, and the overall outcome is shown in Figures 14–2 through 14–5.

The tree developed during this exercise features examples of both duplication and contradiction.[28] The concept of "life style change" was identified as a potential consequence within both the HIV infection and education subsystems. Likewise, both an increase and decrease in the number of AIDS cases were predicted by different branches of the research subsystem. The inter-relationship among the elements of the developed over-

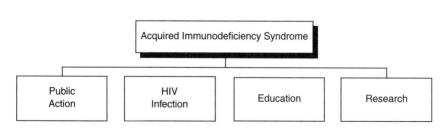

**Figure 14–1** Initial Framework for the Tree of Impact for AIDS Developed during the First Phase of the Exercise

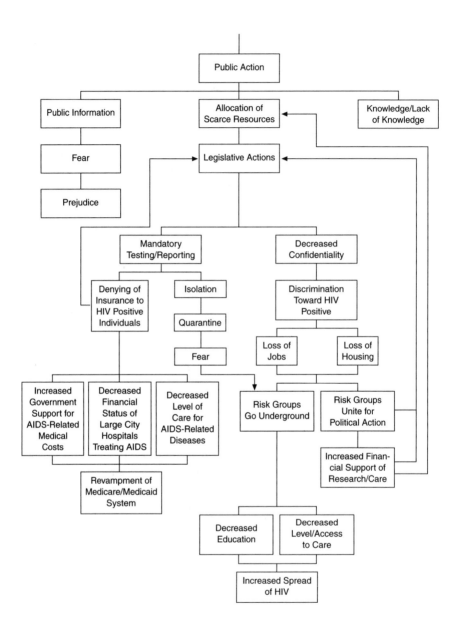

**Figure 14–2** Public Action

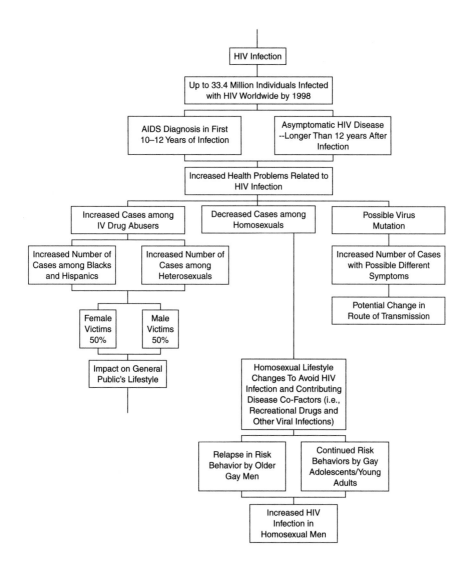

**Figure 14–3** HIV Infection

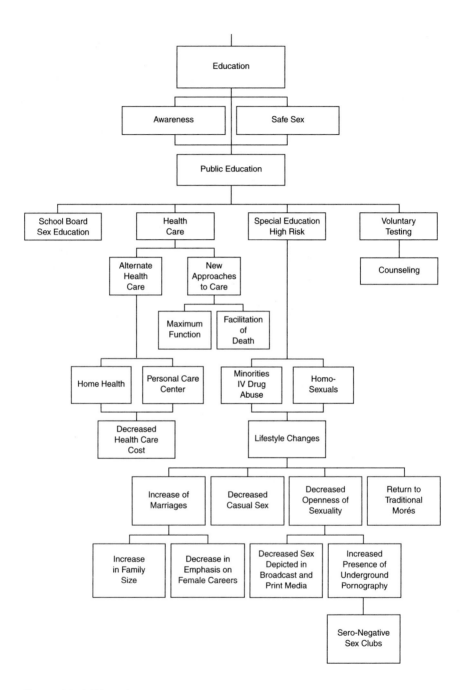

**Figure 14–4** Education

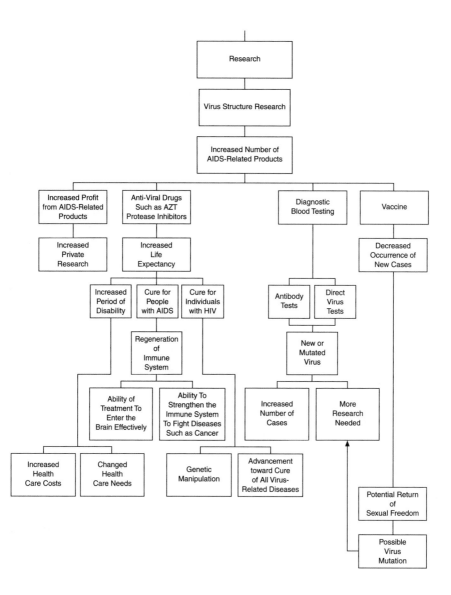

**Figure 14–5** Research

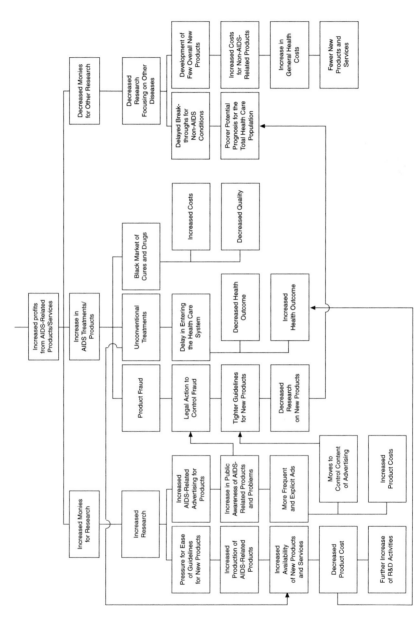

**Figure 14–6** Tree of Impact for Further Analysis of a Specific Consequence Generated during the Initial Learning Exercise

all system gives insight into the topic issues and adds to the tree's ability to provide an adequate framework with which to view the future. The beginning student may be encouraged to know that when this exercise was conducted, several of the proposed consequences were not seen as likely by most participants. Such a consequence was the development of zero-negative dating clubs, included within the education subsystem; however, since this tree of impact was constructed, such organizations have become reality. In this instance, the technique was successful in predicting the future.

This particular exercise was concluded with the construction of the tree depicted in Figure 14–6; however, this end product has the potential for generating further analysis of this topic as items or systems identified in this exercise are further explored using futurcasting techniques. Figure 14–6 shows how the consequence of "increased profit from AIDS-related products" can become the topic of focus of a new tree of impact.

---

**NOTES**

1. J.J. Kurtzman, *Futurcasting: Charting a Way to Your Future* (Palm Springs, CA: ETC Publishing, 1984), 29.

2. P.H. Wagschall, Judgmental Forecasting Techniques and Institutional Planning: An Example, in *Applying Methods and Techniques of Futures Research,* eds. J.L. Morrison et al. (San Francisco: Jossey-Bass, 1983), 44.

3. J.F. Coates, Technology Assessment, in *Handbook of Futures Research,* ed. J. Fowles (Westport, CT: Greenwood Press, 1978), 408.

4. Ibid., 415.

5. J.M. Richardson, Jr., *Making It Happen: A Positive Guide to the Future* (Washington, DC: U.S. Association for the Club of Rome, 1982), 19.

6. Coates, Technology Assessment, 417.

7. J.S. Mendell,The Practice of Intuition, in *Handbook of Futures Research,* ed. J. Fowles (Westport, CT: Greenwood Press, 1978), 150–154.

8. M. McLean, Getting the Problem Right—A Role for Structural Modeling, in *Futures Research: New Directions,* eds. H. Limestone and W.H.C. Simmond (Reading, MA: Addison-Wesley, 1977), 149.

9. Richardson, *Making It Happen.*

10. Wagschall, Judgmental Forecasting.

11. Ibid.

12. I.H. Wilson, Scenarios, in *Handbook of Futures Research,* ed. J. Fowles (Westport, CT: Greenwood Press, 1978), 234.

13. S.J. Parnes, Learning Creative Behavior: Making the Future Happen, *The Futurist* 18, no. 4 (1984):30.

14. Ibid., 32.

15. Kurtzman, *Futurcasting,* 33.

16. Parnes, Learning Creative Behavior.

17. Ibid.
18. Ibid.
19. Wagschall, Judgmental Forecasting.
20. Kurtzman, *Futurcasting*.
21. Ibid., 33.
22. Coates, Technology Assessment, 415.
23. Kurtzman, *Futurcasting*.
24. Ibid.
25. Wagschall, Judgmental Forecasting.
26. Ibid.
27. Kurtzman, *Futurcasting*.
28. Wagsehall, Judgmental Forecasting.

## SUGGESTED READING

Fowles, J. 1978. *Handbook of futures research.* Westport, CT: Greenwood Press.

Glenn, J.C., ed. 1999. *Futures research methodology.* CD-ROM. The American Council for the United Nations University/The Millennium Project.

May, G.H. 1996. *The future is ours: Foreseeing, managing and creating the future.* Westport, CT: Praeger.

Hicks, D., and R. Slaughter, eds. 1998. *Futures education.* In World Year Book of Education. London: Kogan Page.

Kauffman, D.L., Jr. 1976. *Teaching the future.* Palm Springs, CA: ETC Publishing.

Kurtzman, J. 1984. *Futurcasting: Charting a way to your future.* Palm Springs, CA: ETC Publishing.

Limestone, H., and W.H.C. Simmond. 1977. *Futures research: New directions.* Reading, MA: Addison-Wesley Publishing.

Morrison, J.L. et al. 1983. *Applying methods and techniques of futures research.* San Francisco, CA: Jossey-Bass Publishers.

Naisbitt, J., N. Naisbitt, and D. Phillips. 1999. *High tech—High touch: Technology and our search for meaning.* New York: Broadway Books.

Nirenberg, J. 1997. Power tools: *A leader's guide to the latest management thinking.* Old Tappan, NJ: Prentice Hall.

Sullivan, T.J. 1997. *Introduction to social problems.* Needham Heights, MA: Allyn & Bacon.

# PART IV

# Technology Assisted Strategies

Educational technology continues to grow by leaps and bounds and has changed the complexion of the world of education. The technology can be as simple as communicating by e-mail, or as complex as presenting a full degree-granting program by distance learning. The Internet has opened a new and extensive world of information that was not available five or ten years ago. Teaching in a technological world requires faculty collaboration with information specialists to learn how to use the ever-changing systems, but also to keep abreast of new resources as they become available.

The discussion in these chapters provides a look at different ways of utilizing available technologies and discusses strengths of the system and problems that can occur. Technology may be used to assist learning, but does not replace the instructor. Learning objectives must be the main focus for the decision to use technology. Teaching methods require adaptation to be effective in this new environment and should be evaluated for that effectiveness. The amount of Internet information may be overwhelming, and it is critical that faculty and students learn to cull the material to a reasonable amount and to validate accuracy. The use of educational technologies may require extra time and effort from faculty, but can be very effective in enhancing learning, and rewarding for students and faculty alike.

# CHAPTER 15

# Teaching by Distance Education

*Martha S. Tingen and Linda A. Ellis*

## DEFINITIONS AND PURPOSES

Distance education is a process of providing instruction within a synchronous system. Synchronous implies interaction between faculty and students occurring in "real time" or simultaneously.[1] This is a different teaching strategy than asynchronous processes, such as Internet delivery or traditional correspondence/home study in which interaction between faculty and students does not take place at the same time. The traditional class, which is also a synchronous learning environment, typically involves one classroom setting. With the traditional classroom, students are at one location with the faculty teaching the course.

The use of "distance education" in its original format of correspondence/home study is nearly 300 years old.[2] Currently more than 100 million Americans have completed course work by the original distance education method.[3] With the technology explosion, however, a new reference to distance education emerged that incorporates both human and technological capabilities. Over the last 10 years, schools of nursing have begun to use this new strategy of distance education.

Distance education offers many possibilities for interactivity. Through the use of telephone lines, different locations are connected for the educational process. As faculty and students at separate locations communicate, they can see and hear each other on a monitor similar to a television screen. Typically, the number of locations (sites) that can be connected is determined by the state within which the university resides or the university offering the course work and is due to technology limitations. There are numerous configurations for distance education. For example, faculty may be at one location with students at one or more different locations. Or, faculty may be with students at the same location, called the home site, and connected with additional students at other locations. A distinguishing feature of distance education is that faculty and students at multiple sites can see, hear, and participate in the same class at the same time; however, the "requirement" of traveling to the location of the faculty teaching the course is removed with this strategy. Many students, traditional and nontraditional, view this as a significant asset when pursuing educational goals. Additionally, distance education provides many students in rural areas with the opportunity to engage in an interactive classroom, which was not available prior to the computer age and the recent advances in technology.[4]

Technology has been identified as facilitating learning through different lenses. According to Goldsworthy,[5] the five lenses through which learning can occur are (1) from technology, (2) with technology, (3) around technology, (4) supported by technology, and (5) through technology. While learning from technology, students can be taught directly by a software package, similar to a computer-assisted instruction (CAI). Learning with technology occurs as students use a wide range of supportive products and programs to complete course requirements, whether it be word-processing systems, statistical packages for research projects, or computer testing programs. With learning through the lenses of around technology, students learn not only with the technology of using a computer, for example, but they also learn from the interactions that occur in the environment around the computer they are using such as the peer interactions occurring. With learning being supported by technology, Goldsworthy refers to electronic grade books and resources that foster the management aspect of learning. With the lenses of through technology, learning occurs through the interaction of the students at a distant site as mediated through technology. The faculty instruction is facilitated through technology, as are online chat lines, electronic bulletin boards, and electronic mail (e-mail). The computer serves as a "conduit" for interactions that contribute to the learning process.[6] This interaction is the focus of the strategy of distance education, a process of delivering courses that results in learning, through the use of numerous technology mediums.

## THEORETICAL RATIONALE

As early as 1956, there was some agreement among learning theorists as to the manner in which people learn.[7,8] This agreement stemmed from aspects of stimulus-response theory and Gestalt-field theory. Stimulus response theory is frequently associated with Pavlov and the classic conditioning of the salivating dog. Although this idea has made significant strides since Pavlov, behavioral learning theorists support the premise that providing a meaningful reward to the learner for a specific action results in an increased probability of the action occurring again. Students in distance learning classes who receive verbal and nonverbal positive reinforcement for an action often will continue to repeat the action. For example, in discussing a specific topic within the distance classroom, a student who contributes a comment that is highly praised (rewarded) by the faculty is more likely to continue to speak up and to participate verbally than the student who is criticized for his or her comment. While this aspect of distance learning may seem no different than for the traditional classroom, the real difference is that distance students do not always feel connected, which makes praise more important.

In Gestalt theory, behavior is considered to be intelligent or purposive. People have the ability to pursue short-term and long-term goals in order to fulfill their needs. Self-cognition is important in Gestalt theory, and goals are accomplished by one's own efforts through interactions with other people. With distance education, many students are able to accomplish their short-term and long-term educational goals as well as interact with others. Distance education fosters personal autonomy, motivation, contextual learning, and collaboration, all of which are important components supportive of either stimulus-response theory or Gestalt theory.[9]

Recently, Fishbein and Ajzen's Theory of Reasoned Action was tested for predicting behavioral intentions of completing a baccalaureate degree through distance education.[10] This theory proposes that behavior is a result of intention. Intention consists of three antecedents: attitude toward the behavior, subjective norm (personal and social), and perceived behavioral control. According to the theory, attitude is personal in nature and, in the referenced study, reflected what the person believed and felt about completing a baccalaureate degree through distance education. Subjective norm is a concept with a personal and social aspect. From the social perspective, what the person's significant others (parents, siblings, marital partner, friends) believe about them completing a degree by distance education impacts the person's decision. The personal aspect of the subjective norm is reflected by the individual person's motivation to comply (agree) or not comply (disagree) with what their significant others believe about them pursuing a baccalaureate degree offered through distance education. Perceived behavioral control is the amount of control the person perceives to have over the behavior at hand—pursuing a baccalaureate degree by distance education. Results of the study were that attitude and subjective social norm are significant predictor variables for completing a baccalaureate degree by distance education.[11] Although a relatively new teaching modality for nursing, distance education has strong theoretical underpinnings.

## CONDITIONS

Distance education has been taught effectively at all levels of higher education.[12] Whether a student is pursuing a baccalaureate, master's, or doctoral degree, teaching strategies that can be used in distance education facilitate many types of learning objectives and outcomes. Because distance education allows students and faculty to interact simultaneously, teaching from the concrete to the abstract is possible and can be implemented well.[13] Students can be divided into groups and given case studies for collaboration and solving. Problem-based learning, which has been hailed as an effective strategy for building critical-reasoning skills, can occur within a distance education class. Activity-based learning, which encourages concept building, can also be incorporated into the distance learning environment. Demonstration of psychomotor skills and evaluation of return demonstrations can occur in the distance learning classroom, as well as student-led presentations.[14] Distance learning provides several options similar to the traditional classroom. Students can be given immediate instructional feedback in the distance learning classroom. Also, with faculty addressing course objectives, requirements, and evaluation methods at one time to all students enrolled in the course, there is a decrease in student complaints of discrepancies or inequities among classes.

Distance education is a highly desired option for numerous types of potential students. Although some faculty members perceive the obstacles to teaching using distance education exceed any opportunities it affords the students, many faculty members who engage in this strategy express that the required extensive preparation necessary for distance education improves their teaching skills and results in empathy toward their students.[15] Faculty have also identified that teaching materials (handouts, computer applications, etc.) developed for distance classes are superior to those used in their traditional classes.[16] Other opportunities that distance education offer include (1) reaching a broader student population that is often underserved, (2) meeting the needs of students who are prohibited from traveling to the "main" campus location, and (3) connecting diverse students with different sociocultural, economic, and experiential backgrounds.[17]

Additionally, exposure of students to doctorally prepared faculty is often not available in small towns or rural areas. Residents of rural areas often seek to further their education through a degree or continuing education units, which are often required for initial certification and for maintaining certification. Rural students with a distance education option are able to avoid travel to the originating location of their course work. This possibility may foster the rural student's growth by preventing an undesired relocation or employment change. Professionals, who are often employed full-time and juggling multiple roles, can access course work through distance education for continuing education requirements. The paradigm that academic institutions will always have students arriving at their location has changed with rapid technological advances. The new paradigm is educational opportunities on demand.[18] Institutions of higher education need to participate in this new paradigm shift by taking opportunities to potential students.

Students and faculty at multiple locations who are connected in a distance education classroom have many opportunities and assets to facilitate learning. First, all students can see, hear, and interact with the expert faculty, even though some or all students may be at physically different locations. Second, the interaction of students from multiple sites brings the richness of collaboration and discussion based on the unique environment and background of each student learner. Third, distance learning always has an accompanying component of communication during "off-class" time. For example, students may communicate with faculty or their peers using other electronic media such as the telephone, facsimile, e-mail, electronic bulletin boards, or chat rooms. These communications should occur frequently during the week between class sessions and should foster learning.[19]

## TYPES OF LEARNERS

Distance learning is appropriate for many types of learners, to include the auditory, visual, and kinesthetic. Although distance learning occurs in an electronic classroom, all students at multiple locations view the faculty in person or over a monitor that is similar to a television screen, and see students at each of the locations over a monitor. All students hear the same information from faculty and student peers, who participate verbally in the class regardless of the location. With a demonstration, all students see the same procedure as it is presented and are able to see it clearly because the equipment in a distance learning classroom enables students to see in more detail because of the magnification that can be done with technology. Many faculty seasoned in teaching by distance education use study guides or note-taking guides that are distributed or purchased prior to class sessions.[20] These guides serve several purposes: (1) the guides serve as a roadmap for the specific class as to where the instructional content is headed and where it will end; (2) for students who are kinesthetic, this guide is an instrument that facilitates their learning style as notes are taken from the presentation, and (3) the guides are adjunct visual aids that are completed as the content is delivered verbally by the faculty.

Willis[21] and Ostmoe et al.[22] suggest that faculty should consider the learning styles of students when using different teaching strategies. This reinforces the importance of using multiple strategies in the distance learning classroom. Willis and Ostmoe et al. also recommend that the student should actively participate in the learning process and that communication between student and faculty is important. This idea is reiterated by Hannafin and Hannafin[23] in their distance education teaching checklist. They stress that teaching methods for distance education should "engage" students, requiring active participation from them. Research reveals that effective learning with distance education occurs with (1) frequent collaboration among students and faculty, (2) students who have positive attitudes toward computers and the distance learning method, and (3) students who are highly motivated and self-disciplined.[24-26]

## RESOURCES

Equipment and personnel that are required to teach using distance education may vary among institutions, but some basics are essential.[27-29]

- *Transmission (usually through telephone lines or satellite) that connects multiple sites.* The primary communication path is typically referred to as the "backbone."

- *Technology*
  — Hardware
    - Computers (for presentations, Internet access)
    - Document camera (shows printed text, pages in a book, actual items, models, demonstration of procedure)
    - Slide projector
    - Video pointer
    - Video monitor(s)
    - Video players
    - Facsimile
    - Cameras
    - Codec necessary for transmission of signals from multiple sites
  — Software
    - Computer programs, CD-ROMS (for teaching and learning)
- *Infrastructure* (located at all sites—originating and receiving—represents networks and telecommunications, servers, electronic mail, etc.)
- *Personnel*
  — Faculty responsible for teaching
  — Technician/facilitator at distance locations

One of the greatest assets to new distance education programs are resource personnel. Resource personnel within the originating institution and at distance locations are invaluable to faculty and students who are using this strategy for the first time. Resource people include faculty experienced in delivering courses by distance education, technicians who are experts with the technology, and facilitators who may be faculty, technicians, or staff at the distance locations. All of these personnel are extremely helpful in problem solving with system errors, decreasing anxiety for faculty and students, and ensuring that the entire process goes well for faculty and student novices of distance education.[30]

## USING THE METHOD

Teaching a distance learning course requires good communication, detailed planning, and organizational skills. Prior to the first class, faculty members should gain an understanding of the delivery system (technology) and the roles and responsibilities of technicians or facilitators at the originating and distance locations. Hands-on practice by the faculty with the technology prior to the first course day is critical for successful implementation. During this practice, faculty members can experiment with different presentation mediums, become familiar with looking at the camera to attempt eye contact with the distance students, and see how the distance students will be visualized in the originating classroom. This is also a time to share with the technician or facilitator any unique aspects of one's own teaching style and the general flow of the classes. Time spent for this intensive practice is extremely important and cannot be overemphasized. This time also provides an opportunity to become better acquainted with the technician and/or facilitator and communicate to him or her a genuine interest on the part of the faculty in the course being delivered well. With upfront preparation by the faculty, the stage is set for a smooth implementation.

Teaching using distance education can be implemented successfully using the following seven principles for Good Practice in Undergraduate Education, by Chickering and Gamson.[31] Although specified for undergraduate education, we believe these principles are also applicable in teaching master's and doctoral courses over distance education.

### 1. Good Practice Encourages Student-Faculty Contact.

Beginning with the first class session, faculty members need to convey an interest in all students at all locations. If class size does not exceed 40 students per location, then have each student introduce himself or herself and share briefly anything he or she chooses. This is an excellent time for faculty to get to know the students better and for students at the multiple locations to have an opportunity to hear from each other. The faculty member begins this process and sets the tone by sharing briefly about himself or herself. If each class size is greater than 40 students, have a printed form that is distributed at each location asking students' names and for them to share briefly about themselves in writing. With all size classes, communicate to each student that faculty want to get to know them, are interested in them, want them to succeed, and are available to them. Announce during the first class faculty office hours, e-mail address, office telephone, and facsimile numbers. Provide this information in print in the syllabus to all students. Encourage students to call, e-mail, or come by the office for clarification as questions arise. This is also the time to share faculty expectations regarding the form and flow of classroom interaction.

Learn students' names at all locations and call on individual students for input during class sessions. If possible, visit the distant sites several times during the school term and conduct the class from a distant site. This communicates faculty interest in the distant students, makes them feel more a part of the whole, and provides the experience to the originating site of how distant students are receiving the class each week. According to Chickering and Gamson, "Frequent student-faculty contact in and out of classes is the most important factor in student motivation and involvement."[32(p.1)]

### 2. Good Practice Encourages Cooperation among Students.

In a distant education environment, increased learning often results with collaboration among students. Planned interaction for students will help facilitate this collaboration. Group activities during class time may include case studies, student presentations, discussion of a research article, debates, or problem-based learning. For classes that are too large to allow for this group interaction, have students from the different sites identify the most important aspect of the day's presentation.[33] Course requirements may include a group presentation to all sites by three to five students followed by feedback from all locations. All students are required to participate in this type of process and will experience interaction and learn more about responsibility in planning a group presentation. "Sharing one's own ideas and responding to others' reactions improves thinking and deepens understanding."[34(p.1)]

### 3. Good Practice Encourages Active Learning.

Faculty members need to engage students in distance learning classes and use strategies that require their participation. Involving students in class discussions, asking questions about the reading assignments, and having students identify any confusing or unclear idea that was presented are all ways to promote students' involvement in the class. Students need to move out of the spectator role and into the participant role in the distance education classroom. Involvement in the learning process promotes understanding and improves outcomes.[35(p.1)]

### 4. Good Practice Gives Prompt Feedback.

Students need to receive verbal and written feedback in a timely and meaningful way. When encouraging students to participate in class, acknowledge and reinforce their enlightening comments, and use extreme tact for addressing inappropriate comments. Evaluation methods, whether by testing, written assignments, or oral presentations, should be reviewed and returned within a rapid time frame (preferably one week or less). Provide oral and written feedback to each individual student. Have a scheduled conference time available to discuss the evaluation with each student either by telephone, e-mail, or in person. This conference needs to occur in close proximity to the written evaluation that the student receives. This feedback helps foster understanding of the course content.[36(p.2)]

### 5. Good Practice Emphasizes Time on Task.

Student expectations need to be well-defined and percentages allocated with consideration of the time involvement. In distance learning classrooms, students are from varied backgrounds and locations. To facilitate a group project, faculty may wish to use a Web-based chat room where all group members can log in and plan the project. If this is not feasible, perhaps 10 to 15 minutes of class time can be released for work on the group project. Faculty creativity and support for the magnitude of the task and its time requirements for completion may engender student enthusiasm and participation in the process.[37(p.2)]

### 6. Good Practice Communicates High Expectations.

Beginning with the first class, be enthusiastic and communicate clearly high expectations. People usually try to "live up" to what is expected of them. This responsibility is mutual for faculty and each student. Faculty members need to role-model exceptional preparedness and teaching, with verbal expectations of the high quality of work anticipated from each student. Expecting exceptional performance can become a self-fulfilling prophecy for students when we, as faculty, demonstrate high standards.[38(p.2)]

### 7. Good Practice Respects Diverse Talents and Ways of Learning.

Within each class, regardless of the location, are students with diverse strengths and ways of learning. Some students may long for an opportunity to present to the class without any hesitation. The thought of this task for other students may be extremely anxiety inducing. Some students may rejoice if it is announced at the first class that all testing will be completed on the computer, whereas others who are uncomfortable with computer technology experience fear. An opportunity exists for faculty with each student: to focus on their strengths and to foster improvement of their weaknesses. For example, if computer testing is being used for all students, identify students who are technologically skilled and ask if they would have time to share their expertise with a student who is "afraid" of the process.[39(p.2)]

Also, when using a new strategy like computer testing, always offer practice sessions that emulate the testing process. This practice decreases student anxiety for the new method. If skilled students agree to assist their peers in practicing on the computer, then the faculty has initiated beginning collaboration within the class. Perhaps later in the course, the students who were helped will return the favor using a strength they possess. This exchange is similar to the old idea of the "barter system." Students should be encouraged to engage in this type of process because it fosters a "win-win" environment. Encourage students to acknowledge their strengths and weaknesses and to take responsibility for seeking help and guidance from faculty and peers when needed.

Recent research supports teaching effectiveness and student satisfaction with distance education.[40–43] Souder[44] evaluated students enrolled in a master's program taking the same course in the traditional classroom versus by distance education. Results of the study support that students at the distant site performed better on examinations and written homework assignments with no significant differences in the quality of term papers. In another study, Naber and LeBlanc[45] measured how distant students performed on course objectives and the resulting grades in a human biology lab course. Eighty-three percent of the students received either an A or a B in the course, and distance delivery was received positively by the students. Other research has included measuring the physical learning environment, course structure, perceptions of student-teacher interaction, and overall enjoyment of the course among traditional, distant-site, and host-site students.[46] Distant and host-site students responded less positively to items that addressed the physical learning environment than traditional students, yet there were no differences in measurements from any of the three student groups in rating student-teacher interactions and course structure. Spooner and colleagues[47] used a standard course evaluation to measure faculty instruction provided in a distance learning graduate course as compared to the same course being taught on campus. Results were similar across settings for rating the course, instructor, teaching, and communication. Although research supports that students can have optimal learning experiences and meet course objectives with distance learning, there are always, as with any strategy, potential problems.

## POTENTIAL PROBLEMS

Three main potential problems are associated with delivering courses by distance education. First, the communication between locations may be interrupted unexpectedly. This situation needs to be planned for well in advance by the faculty. Distant site technicians/facilitators need to know what to do if this interruption occurs and have a backup plan in place. Clear communication between the faculty and technicians/facilitators must have occurred prior to the course beginning concerning this possibility. If this happens, the system is often returned to full communication within a few minutes. This is not much different than a slide or overhead projector not working in a class and taking time to problem solve the situation.

A second problem that can occur is animosity between the different sites. Often, this may occur when faculty are located at only one site and the "distant students" perceive that they are on their own without faculty support and contact. An attitude of the main site (where the faculty is for the entire term) may become one of superiority and of having all the resources available to them, implying that they will achieve a better education than the distant students. This animosity can be prevented if faculty are willing to travel to the distant sites even one to two times during the school term.[48] Additionally, seasoned faculty know that the positive attitude that is engendered with the distant students by traveling to their location typically prevents or diffuses this type of situation. Faculty members who are experienced with teaching by distance education will make all locations feel included as part of one class from the beginning.

A third problem may occur when faculty members who are resistant to the technology are assigned to teach a distance education course. Often, resistance stems from faculty's lack of understanding of the technology and its potential.[49] These faculty members need to resolve their issues prior to using this strategy, which may be partially resolved through education. Also, a "core group" of faculty members who are trained and experienced in the technology and art of delivering classes effectively with the distance learning strategy need to serve as a resource for new faculty assigned to teach with this method. This "core group" should be recognized and rewarded for their efforts. Currently, some universities provide extensive training for faculty members to adapt their teaching styles for distance instruction.[50] A reward system is also in place on some campuses, where faculty members are paid stipends for developing courses to teach by distance education and are given salary supplements for delivering courses by this method.[51] These incentives may lure some faculty members who otherwise would not have been willing to even try it to become experts in this method. Also, this idea rewards those faculty members who take the initiative to develop new options for students, which often increases program enrollments. Any other problems that may occur with using distance learning are similar to those of the traditional classroom.

## CONCLUSION

Teaching by distance education is an exciting new strategy that has occurred as a result of recent advances in technology. Coupled with a new paradigm of higher education that encourages institutions to make courses and degrees more available to potential consumers rather than requiring the consumer to come to the institution, distance education can reach a wide market and accomplish this goal. With excellent communication, planning, and organization by faculty, distance learning courses can be implemented successfully with achievement of optimal student learning within a high-tech environment.

---

### NOTES

1. L.A. Ellis, *A User Friendly Guide to GSAMS* (Medical College of Georgia, School of Nursing, 1996).

2. L.A. Hesser, R.P. Hogan, and R.P. Mozell, The Sum of the Parts Is Greater Than the Whole in On-line Graduate Education, *Lecture Notes in Computer Science* 602 (1992):283–293.

3. *Distance Education and Training Council* (1998), http://www.detc.org.

4. Hesser, Hogan, and Mozell, The Sum of the Parts.

5. R. Goldsworthy, Lenses on Learning and Technology: Roles and Opportunities for Design and Development, *Educational Technology,* July/August (1999):59–62.

6. Goldworthy, Lenses on Learning.

7. R.M. Gagne, *The Conditions of Learning* (New York: Holt, Rinehart and Winston, 1965), 58–89.

8. E.R. Hilgard, *Theories of Learning*, ed. 2 (New York: Appleton-Century-Crofts, 1956).

9. R. Oliver and T.C. Reeves, Dimensions of Effective Interactive Learning with Telematics for Distance Education, *Educational Technology Research and Development* 44, no. 4 (1996):45–56.

10. E.A. Becker and C.C. Gibson, Fishbein and Ajzen's Theory of Reasoned Action: Accurate Prediction of Behavioral Intentions for Enrolling in Distance Education, *Adult Education Quarterly* 49, no. 1 (1998):43–55.

11. Becker and Gibson, Fishbein and Ajzen's Theory.

12. B. Willis, *Distance Education: A Practical Guide* (Englewood Cliffs, NJ: Educational Technology Publications, 1993).

13. R. Martens and M. Valcke, Validation of a Theory about Functions and Effects of Embedded Support Devices in Distance Education Learning Materials, *European Journal of Psychology of Education* 10, no. 2 (1995):181–196.

14. Ellis, *A User Friendly Guide to GSAMS*.

15. Willis, *Distance Education: A Practical Guide*.

16. University of Florida's Institute of Food and Agricultural Sciences Distance Education Task Force Report (1999), http://www.agen.ufl.edu/-fzazueta/de-rep.htm.

17. University of Florida's Task Force Report.

18. University of Florida's Task Force Report.

19. K.M. Hannafin and M.J. Hannafin, The Ecology of Distance Learning Environments: Implications for Design and Evaluation, *Training Research Journal* 1 (1995):49–69.

20. Willis, *Distance Education: A Practical Guide*.

21. Willis, *Distance Education: A Practical Guide*.

22. P.M. Ostmoe, H.L. Van Hoozer, A.L. Scheffer, and C.M. Crowell, Learning Style Preferences and Selection of Learning Strategies: Considerations and Implications for Nurse Educators, *Journal of Nursing Education* 23, no. 9 (1984):27–30.

23. Hannafin and Hannafin, Ecology of Distance Learning Environments.

24. Hesser, Hogan, and Mozell, The Sum of the Parts.

25. Oliver and Reeves, Dimensions of Effective Interactive Learning.

26. Willis, *Distance Education: A Practical Guide*.

27. Ellis, *A User Friendly Guide to GSAMS*.

28. Willis, *Distance Education: A Practical Guide*.

29. P. Theriault, How To Use Distance Education Tools (1999), http://www.mcg.edu/eresources/ode/tips.html.

30. Theriault, How To Use Distance Education Tools.

31. A.W. Chickering and Z.F. Gamson, Principles for Good Practice in Undergraduate Education, *The Wingfield Journal* (1987), Special Insert.

32. Chickering and Gamson, Principles for Good Practice.

33. Ellis, *A User Friendly Guide to GSAMS*.

34. Chickering and Gamson, Principles for Good Practice, p. 1.

35. Chickering and Gamson, Principles for Good Practice, p. 1.

36. Chickering and Gamson, Principles for Good Practice, p. 2.

37. Chickering and Gamson, Principles for Good Practice, p. 2.

38. Chickering and Gamson, Principles for Good Practice, p. 2.

39. Chickering and Gamson, Principles for Good Practice, p. 2.

40. W.E. Souder, The Effectiveness of Traditional Versus Satellite Delivery in the Management of Technology Master's Degree Programs, *The American Journal of Distance Education* 7, no. 1 (1993):37–53.

41. D. Naber and G. LeBlanc, Providing a Human Biology Laboratory for Distance Learners, *The American Journal of Distance Education* 8, no. 2 (1994):58–70.

42. J.D. Thomerson and C.L. Smith, Student Perceptions of the Affective Experiences Encountered in Distance Learning Courses, *The American Journal of Distance Education* 10, no. 3 (1996):37–48.

43. F. Spooner, L. Jordan, B. Algozzine, and M. Spooner, Student Ratings of Instruction in Distance Learning and On-campus Classes, *The Journal of Educational Research* 92, no. 3 (1999):132–140.

44. Souder, The Effectiveness of Traditional Versus Satellite Delivery.

45. Naber and LeBlanc, Providing a Human Biology Laboratory.
46. Thomerson and Smith, Student Perceptions of the Affective Experiences.
47. Spooner, Jordan, Algozzine, and Spooner, Student Ratings of Instruction.
48. Oliver and Reeves, Dimensions of Effective Interactive Learning.
49. University of Florida's Task Force Report.
50. Distance Education, University of Nevada (1999), http://www.unr.edu/unr/edtech/disted.htm.
51. Distance Education, University of Nevada.

## SUGGESTED READING

Palloff, R.M., and K. Pratt. 1999. *Building learning communities in cyberspace: Effective strategies for the online classroom.* San Francisco: Jossey-Bass Publishers.

Willis, B. 1993. *Distance education: A practical guide.* Englewood Cliffs, NJ: Educational Technology Publications.

# CHAPTER 16

# Electronic Communication Strategies

*Arlene J. Lowenstein*

## DEFINITION AND PURPOSES

Educational institutions are increasingly moving toward a "computer-enriched" environment.[1] The use of computers for electronic communication takes many forms, including, but not limited to, bulletin boards, chat rooms, e-mail, forums and threaded discussions around specific topics, electronic libraries, use of the Internet, which is worldwide, and intranets, which are established within one school.[2] E-mail use has been growing significantly in educational settings and has brought about dramatic changes in communication between students, faculty, and staff.[3]

Enrichment is the key phrase. Computer technology is a valuable teaching tool, but it must never replace the teacher. Faculty members can use computers as one strategy to enhance the teaching-learning process, but the need for human contact should also be considered. Effective use of this technology depends on the learning objectives.[4] E-mail journaling may be appropriate for learning objectives that are geared toward the individual, whereas threaded discussions or group e-mail discussion may be more appropriate for objectives that include learning to work with group process.

Computers can be used to stimulate students to become actively involved in the teaching-learning process by giving them tools they can manipulate to control their learning environment.[5] Computer use can be asynchronous, which does not require that both parties communicate at the same time. Students and faculty can read and answer messages at their convenience. E-mail messages can be longer and more detailed than traditional voice-mail messages. The instructor is responsible for introducing students to the resources available, providing guidelines for use, and troubleshooting with the student when technical problems occur.

196

## THEORETICAL RATIONALE

Mitra and Steffensmeier carried out a longitudinal study of students following a university decision to provide a computer network, create an intranet for student use, and provide students with laptop computers.[6] The computer-enriched environment was positively correlated with students' ability to facilitate communication and positive student attitudes toward computers in general. Ease of access was a major influence in fostering those positive attitudes in the teaching and learning process.

Levin studied the use of electronic communication in teacher training.[7] Four types of communication were explored: (1) student-to-peer e-mail journal entries, (2) student-to-keypal e-mail exchanges with teachers in another state, (3) e-mail exchanges between students and instructor, and (4) a threaded discussion using student-to-group messages. Although there were many personal and supportive messages, the most frequent purpose of the student-to-peer e-mail exchanges were messages that provided an opportunity to reflect on their growth as teachers and to discuss teaching resources and planning instruction. Reflective comments were also found in student-to-keypal exchanges, but not as often as in student-to-peer messages. Student-to-keypal messages tended to use more descriptions and comparisons of programs, although supportive feedback as well as reflection were also found.

Student-to-instructor exchanges were often found in addition to journal assignments. The exchanges provided a mechanism for students to have a running discussion with the instructor that lasted for several weeks. These messages tended to revolve around the topic of student development as teachers and included planning lessons and curriculum discussions. Personal issues and technical problems were also discussed. The main purpose of the student-to-group discussions was reflection, which was the content of many of the messages. The discussions also provided a forum for feedback and moral support. Reflective, self-analytical thinking was fostered the most by the student-to-group discussions. Student-to-peer discussions included more than personal and supportive messages; they also shared issues and problems.[8]

Most faculty members are routinely faced with two issues in class. The first issue is that of encouraging students to become more active in preparation for class, including reading assigned material and reflecting on it prior to class. A second issue is to encourage students who are silent during class discussions and who do not offer ideas or opinions. By using technology to serve pedagogy and facilitate learning, Parkyn addressed those issues by developing a discourse community of students who were assigned to use a collaborative electronic journal.[9] Students were assigned to small groups, with no more than 10 to 12 students per group. Each group was responsible for writing a collective, weekly journal. The journal provided an opportunity for students to discuss ideas about the reading assignment, respond to comments of other students, and become aware of how other students responded to the entry. Students were found to be better prepared for class discussions, and peer-mediated learning was higher than that found in the traditional classroom. Some students found the journal to be a safer environment in which to discuss ideas than the open classroom. This safe environment was fostered through the use of a pseudonym or "journal name" by each student, known only by the individual student and instructor.[10] Over all, students were able to share with one another in a way that transformed individual learning into collaborative and effective learning.

## CONDITIONS

Access to the technology and technology support services, along with faculty comfort with computers, are the most important conditions for utilizing this teaching strategy. Students who are not familiar with the equipment or computers can be given a period of time to learn and practice if support is available. Faculty members also need time and support to develop expertise in using e-mail or other computer-assisted strategies. Students should be able to access computers at home or at school. If passwords are necessary, then a process needs to be defined to ensure student access to the needed material.

## TYPES OF LEARNERS

Electronic communication can be used by all levels of students. Electronic communication strategies work well in both graduate and undergraduate educational settings. Computers are rapidly becoming part of the educational landscape. Students are increasingly being exposed to computers well before entering postsecondary education; however, many nursing students seek to enter the profession or graduate school at a later age than the traditional post-secondary student. Although some of these students will be computer savvy, many have not been exposed to computer usage. It is important to determine the students' level of computer comfort when making assignments, and to be supportive as the students work their way through the computer learning curve.

## RESOURCES

Although many faculty members have been exposed to and use computers, others have not and do not, and the same is true for students. Training with technical support follow-up must be made available. Knowledgeable and friendly technical support is very important. Working with computers can be extremely frustrating and stressful for novices unless an adequate support system to troubleshoot problems and encourage the user is in place. Learning to work with computers takes practice and persistence, but the process can be well worth the time and energy. Technical support personnel can alert faculty members to new programs that are available. For example, Oosterhof described a process that can be used by faculty with large classes to individualize e-mail through the use of macros and worksheets.[11]

Universities and colleges are becoming increasingly wired for computer usage, with fiber optic or other cabling systems. They are developing intranet systems as well as Internet links that faculty members are able to access and use for instructional purposes. Coordination between the information systems department and faculty is needed to avoid problems caused by underestimating the use and need for assistance.

## USING THE METHOD

The choice of which technology to be used depends on the learning objectives, the need for asynchronous processes, and the resources available. A bulletin board, chat room, or threaded discussion can be developed for use by a specific class. Choice of communication method also depends on the need for group interaction, peer-to-peer-interaction, or student-to-instructor interaction. Passwords may be necessary to gain access for some venues.

Instructions for use must be clear. It is important to assess students' comfort level with computers and to provide resources to assist them. The process for finding help for technological problems should be developed and communicated to students. E-mail messages can be more informal than student papers or written journals. Typos, spelling, and grammar may not need correction in e-mail messages, as long as students understand that good grammar, spelling, and proofreading are required for paper assignments. Many schools have ethical policies for computer usage and e-mail. Students should be informed of those policies and be expected to adhere to them.

## POTENTIAL PROBLEMS

Faculty and student comfort with the systems is the first major problem that needs to be considered. Many individuals are technologically challenged and avoid using computers, especially if they have had bad experiences in beginning attempts. Technological problems often occur, from full computer crashes to loss of messages that have not been saved or were overwritten. Knowing where to go for help becomes very important in these instances. Remembering passwords when they have not been used frequently can be difficult, and a system needs to be available to retrieve a password without compromising security. Misspelled addresses can be frustrating and time consuming when a minor error, such as an extra dot, causes the message to go astray. Finding the error in an address or message can be difficult because of the tendency to read the word as the reader thinks it should be, thereby reading over the error. Computers are famous for carrying out commands literally. What the user wrote in the command may not have been what the user intended, but computers do not recognize intentions. Small errors can cause major problems and are often difficult to discover. At the same time, however, with the proper support, computers can enhance learning and be fun and enjoyable to use.

Privacy and avoiding embarrassment can be important issues. E-mail messages are not private, even though they feel as if they are. Both students and faculty need to be made aware of that fact. In chat rooms, bulletin boards, and other group venues, it is possible for students to use an alias or pseudonym, as Parkyn had students do in the discourse communities he developed.[12] He found that students expressed more opinions when they were free of personal harassment or disparaging remarks directed at their true self.

Time for e-mail is an important issue for the instructor, especially if the selected method involves one-to-one student-instructor conversations. Class size is an important parameter in deciding if the instructor has the time to respond effectively to students. There are other methods to work with larger classes. Oosterhof's method of individualizing e-mail allowed for consolidating messages and providing some automatic answering options.[13] His method was used successfully with large classes. Replies to students can be brief but need to be meaningful. Both large and small classes can benefit from the use of electronic communication when the technology is geared to meet specific teaching-learning objectives.

---

# EXAMPLE
## Electronic Journaling

The History of Nursing Ideas course was developed to enable graduate students to view nursing theory in the context of nursing history and growth of the profession. The course description and objectives are shown in Exhibit 16–1. A major mission of the nursing program and the school is to prepare students for leadership within the profession. Understanding dynamics of change and recognizing decision makers is important to the development of leadership skills necessary to carry out that mission. The critical-thinking objective is used to prepare students to recognize decision makers and those dynamics of change within the nursing profession and in the provision of health care.

**Exhibit 16–1** History of Nursing Ideas Course Syllabus

---

**Course Description:** This course focuses on the contributions of nursing history, nursing theory, and contemporary issues in the social evolution of nursing as a profession. The nature of nursing theory and the relationship between philosophy, theory, and science are explored. The evolution of nursing knowledge within the social context of history is emphasized.

**Objectives:** *Upon completion of the course, the student should be able to:*

1. Identify major issues associated with the development of nursing as a profession.
2. Examine the influences of hospitals and the rise of medicine in the development of nursing.
3. Utilize critical thinking to analyze the components of theories and the history of development in nursing.
4. Examine the relationship between historical development in nursing, nursing theory, and nursing science.
5. Apply theory in domains of practice. Analyze contemporary nursing within the framework of its historical development.

---

The nursing program offers a generic masters for students who have no nursing background but hold a baccalaureate in another field. This course is taught to those students in the first semester of their first year in the program. This course is also required for all registered nurses (RNs) who enter the graduate program, although they have the option to take the course at any point in their program plan of study. For entry-level students, the course attempts to establish an understanding of the profession in which the students will be entering, and specifically the importance of theory-based practice. This course also emphasizes the use of theory-based practice for the RN student. For both groups, the course sets the groundwork for the development of leadership skills and understanding the expectations of scholarly work in graduate study. Other courses in the curriculum build on the leadership and theory framework of this course, and a scholarly project that requires self-directed scholarly work is the culmination of the program.

These students bring a variety of backgrounds to the course. Entry-level students have included students with a previous master's degree in public health or another field, a heavy science background, or a doctorate in another field; professional musicians; emergency medical technicians; peace corps volunteers; or, at the other extreme, students fresh out of college with a liberal arts or science degree. Some have had experiences with the health care system or cared for an ill friend or relative, and that experience influenced the decision to enter nursing, whereas others have different reasons for their decision. The RNs also have varied backgrounds and enter the program with clinical expertise that they can share with the entry-level students. All of these students have something special to offer their fellow students and the instructor. They range in age from 21 to well over 50, all bringing life experiences with them. It is a wonderful group to work with, but it is challenging because of the students' expertise and status as adult learners. Principles of adult learning must be considered in the design of teaching strategies for this course.

The course is presented along a timeline, looking at past to present to future. Influences on the development of the profession are explored over that timeline. Students look at such issues as the impact over time of sociocultural influences and changes, war, religion, economics, immigration, new diseases, new technologies, the development of medicine and health care, nursing practice, and nursing education. The era of the late 1960s and 1970s brings in the impact of the civil rights, women's rights, and consumer rights movements and the reaction of nurse leaders in recognizing the need for a stronger professional view of nursing and the development of nursing science. The development of a nursing body of knowledge becomes a major focus of the course for many weeks. Students conduct group presentations for their colleagues, explaining a specific nursing theory, including appropriate research, critiques, and applicability to practice.

No single reference book can be used for the content of this course. In order to effectively contribute to class discussions, students must read various articles and book chapters and become familiar with other sources, which may include the Internet. Students must be actively involved in the learning process to benefit from this course. Students must carry out a certain amount of discovery on their own, with instructor assistance in finding appropriate resources.

In designing the course for my first time teaching, I followed the format that other instructors had used—the development of weekly topics with reading assignments for each. A book of readings, developed for purchase and adhering to copyright laws, was made available to provide students with easy access to the articles. Special attention was given to the reading selections to be sure they would provide different perspectives for discussion and new information applicable to course objectives. In addition, students formed groups in which they were responsible for a nursing theory presentation. They were expected to conduct a literature review for the particular theory and present a bibliography to the class. A term paper was also required, which presented another aspect of the students' theories or discussed the historical issues that were presented in class.

The group presentation and paper assignments required students to seek out literature and be able to discuss it orally or in their term paper. Preparing for class discussions was problematic, however. Some students took advantage of the reading collection and contributed well to the class discussion, whereas others were quiet or contributed general knowledge that did not relate to readings. These students were missing out on the richness that the readings provided. Another problem was finding ways for the instructor to assist students in preparing their presentations and papers. Although regular office hours were available, many students used the time just before or after class to talk with me. The time was rushed, and, although I was aware of some resources that could help, I did not have time to explore additional resources that would have been helpful to them.

All students in the school had access to an e-mail account that could be used within the learning resources center, but it was a new experience for many of them. I had become quite comfortable in using e-mail and found it to be a valuable form of communication. The next time the course was offered, I decided to require an electronic journal that would allow students to discuss readings with me prior to class and to turn in their term paper outlines and/or project for feedback and assistance (see Exhibit 16–2). My objectives

---

**Exhibit 16–2** E-mail Journal Examples

**Student #1**

In Carper's article, "Fundamental Patterns of Knowing in Nursing," the author states the importance of wholeness and incorporating all of the Patterns of Knowing in Nursing. The American Nurses Association Policy Statement states that, "Nursing is a scientific discipline as well as a profession" (ANA Policy Statement, 7). I concur that all of the components stated above explain the profession of nursing well; however, I do not believe the theorists have put enough emphasis on the synergistic effect of the different components that constitute the profession of nursing. Although placing the branches of nursing together is great, one needs to look beyond that and see what happens when they work together and create this new dimension of nursing. The sum of these components truly makes the nursing profession unique. I believe it is important for nurses to be aware of the synergistic effect of the wholeness of nursing.

**Student #2**

Hello Dr. Lowenstein, This is —— from your Nursing History class. I'm e-mailing this from my house, but if you need to reply to anything, I use my —— —— e-mail more.

*continues*

**Exhibit 16–2** continued

Well, I'm not sure if anyone had picked this one either, but I read "The Seeing Self: Photography and Storytelling as a Health Promotion Methodology" by Mary Koithan. I enjoyed how this article addressed the issue of our world being too fast-paced and impersonal these days because I believe this is very true. It also cited that more and more diseases today are related to stress, which is obviously detrimental to our well-being. The author stresses the importance of finding other ways to block out the confusion and busyness of everyday life and to center ourselves and concentrate on our wellness. She referred to these methods as aesthetic modalities that would promote health, empower the person, and make them aware of the connection between mind, body, and spirit. Such aesthetic modalities must work wonders for some people who are skeptical about modern medicine. It is good that we have these additional ways of healing because it is very individual and self-promoting. I found this article very interesting and hope to read more on similar subjects. I will see you in class on the 18th!

**Student #3**

The article I found dealt with the use of drawing to gain information about children and their experiences and feelings. The article "Children's Drawings: A Different Window" by Judy Malkiewicz and Marilyn L. Stember discussed that children will offer more of their feelings and experiences through drawings than through conversation with a health care provider. It is thus very useful for nurses to use this artistic technique to help them understand their younger patients and know how to address their needs, especially since younger children cannot express themselves well through verbal communication. The only obstacles that the authors presented were those involved with the interpretations of such artwork. Many times health care providers overanalyze these pieces, as well as underestimate their significance.

The article also discussed several different types of drawing exercises that can be used. Draw-a-Person, Kinetic Family Drawing, House-Person-Tree, Draw-a-Situation, and others provide the means to enter the child's world in various situations and roles that the child encounters. Each specific type of drawing serves a unique and specific purpose.

On a personal note, I worked at —— for three years as a Child Life Assistant. In this position, I worked with the kids to keep them occupied with arts and crafts, tutor them on schoolwork, help them understand procedures using medical play, and educate them and their families on the things that were happening during their hospital stays. Most of the children on the unit were experiencing chronic illnesses such as cystic fibrosis, cancer, AIDS, spina bifida, and others. Thus, we saw the children repeatedly and for long durations of time. Among our many activities and tools was the use of drawing. It provided a great release for the kids, and it told us a lot about how

*continues*

**Exhibit 16–2** continued

> they were feeling about their care. It tuned us in to their fears, how we could reduce them, and how we could prevent them. I thought it was a wonderful thing. Also, the drawings were a source of pride for the kids. We displayed them all over the units and entered them into national competitions within the hospitals of the Children's Miracle Network. That was why my interest was struck by this particular article, but I can attest to the fact that these drawing exercises are valuable for both caregiver and patient. The article was from the book *Art & Aesthetics in Nursing*.

were to encourage students to read before class, to encourage students who found it difficult to speak in class to discuss what they had read, and to be available for questions about assignments. In addition, papers from the previous class had shown that students were not comfortable with the format for citing references and needed feedback prior to turning in the final paper. I added an annotated bibliography to the assignment to help them understand citation formats and to gain skill in abstracting information from a journal article.

This was only one of four courses that the entry-level students took as part of their program. They were beginning basic nursing, with clinical experience that took time and was their primary interest. It was important to keep the assignments at a manageable level and to keep their interest in the topic. The basic nursing course was designed so students would begin to recognize and use a theory base in their practice. For that class, they were able to use the information they worked with in History of Nursing Ideas, which helped them to see the relevance of what we were doing.

The use of theory-based practice was not as clear for the RN group, which was a factor that I needed to acknowledge in my responses to their e-mails. The RNs were encouraged to read articles relating theory to practice, and to comment on how they viewed using the theory in their own nursing practice.

Instruction to students included the following:

A journal and annotated bibliography are responsible for 20 percent of the course grade. A **weekly journal** discussing your reactions to the readings and class discussion should be submitted by e-mail. For the weekly journal, pick out the major points within the reading and comment on them. This can be somewhat informal, I do not need the whole citation for that reading, and try to keep your comments to two or three paragraphs in length. Of course, if you feel that a reading deserves more depth, I will gladly look forward to reading your comments. I will respond to each message, to acknowledge receipt or to discuss some of your points. I may also ask you to bring up the point you are making in the class discussion, so the rest of the class can benefit from your thoughts. I understand that you may not be able to read every article every week in advance of class, but that should be the exception, not the rule. If that happens, please read the article after class and comment on your reactions to the article in light of the class discussion.

An **annotated bibliography**, consisting of a minimum of four articles over the course of the semester, should also be submitted by e-mail, in addition to the weekly journals. The annotated bibliography should follow the following guidelines:

> The content of the article should be relevant to the course objectives; include one article from the journal *Advances in Nursing Science*; and include the article citation in APA format, an abstract of the article including major issues and findings, and a brief critique and reaction to the article. The selection of articles is in addition to the assigned readings but may include articles to be used in the presentation or final paper.

> You are also encouraged to use e-mail to correspond with me regarding any questions you may have about your presentation, paper, or any other issue you feel the need to discuss. I will be pleased to give you feedback in these areas. Of course you may schedule an appointment if you wish further assistance with these projects.

I have been very pleased with the response from the journals and annotated bibliography. Students who were not familiar with e-mail found it to be very helpful by the end of the semester and were often proud of their new skill. They usually became comfortable after a few tries, although it may have been stressful at first. Although technical problems did arise periodically, most students were successful in using the system. Technical problems included difficulty getting an e-mail address and being unable to open attachments, especially when different operating systems were being used. To address that problem, I suggested that students not use the attachment feature, but rather paste the text directly into the e-mail message, which was usually successful. Computer crashes and lost messages occurred sporadically, but most students were able to cope. To avoid complaints about needing to be on campus to use e-mail, I accepted e-mails from school or home addresses.

The responses added much to the class discussions. Students did contribute experiences or ideas that they had expressed in the e-mails and that I felt would benefit the class discussion. Students demonstrated a deeper understanding of issues and content. I did not penalize students for missing a week or two, but instead worked with them to be sure they had met the course objectives.

An added advantage to using e-mail was the ability to discuss e-mail and other computer applications during the technology topic discussion. Class discussion included looking at the present and future, identifying the technology issues and how they have and potentially will influence both nursing practice and nursing education.

The amount of e-mails can be difficult to manage for the instructor. With a class of 35, I needed to set aside time to read and respond to e-mails in a timely fashion. In some cases, no long response was necessary; I was able to acknowledge the e-mail with few words. For others, a longer conversation was in order. I have learned to pay attention to the e-mail as soon as I receive it, and to respond immediately, and not allow it to pile up. I was able to move the e-mails into a permanent file, sorted by student, with a separate permanent file for my responses. This allowed me to return to the messages if questions arose, and to be sure students had met course objectives.

Although some students do read early, most of them wait until it is close to class. There were times when I was unable to read all of the messages before the class discussion, but these instances were usually spread out enough to allow me to at least acknowledge and possibly bring something up in the class discussion that I was not able to comment back in the message. Overall course and professor evaluations have improved with use of the e-mail journals (see Exhibit 16–3). Students have felt a closer rela-

---

**Exhibit 16–3** Evaluation Comments

"I liked the structure of the course in regards to the group project on theorists rather than doing a lot of heavy reading. I also liked the seminar/discussion style of the course. The reading was intensive, though, but the e-mail system was <u>great</u>!"

"I really enjoyed the readings and found the journal keeping and e-mailing very rewarding. I felt I definitely learned a lot about nursing that I didn't know about. Acceptance of my comments and experiences made the work very unthreatening."

"Enjoyed use of e-mail, very effective, allows for better student/teacher interaction. Thank you."

tionship with me, and I have been able to assist students with problems or issues that would not have surfaced in other formats. Students have demonstrated improved skills and benefits from the course content. I will continue to use journals to achieve those learning objectives.

---

### NOTES

1. A. Mitra and T. Steffensmeier, Changes in Student Attitudes and Student Computer Use in a Computer-Enriched Environment, *Journal of Research on Computing in Education* 32, no. 3 (Spring 2000):417–435.

2. M. Kimeldorf, Teaching Online—Techniques and Methods, *Learning and Leading with Technology* 25, no. 2 (September 1995):26–31.

3. L.B. Gatz and J.B. Hirt, Academic and Social Integration in Cyberspace: Students and E-Mail, *The Review of Higher Education* 23, no. 3 (Spring 2000):299–318.

4. D.L. Little, W.H. Hannum, and G.B. Stack, *Computers and Effective Instruction: Using Computers and Software in the Classroom* (New York: Longman, 1996).

5. T. Morgan, Using Technology To Enhance Learning: Changing the Chunks, *Learning and Leading with Technology* 25, no. 2 (September 1995):50–55.

6. Mitra and Steffensmeier, Changes in Student Attitudes.

7. B.B. Levin, Analysis of the Content and Purpose of Four Different Kinds of Electronic Communications among Preservice Teachers, *Journal of Research on Computing in Education* 32, no.1 (Fall 1999):139–155.

8. Ibid.

9. D.L. Parkyn, Learning in the Company of Others: Fostering a Discourse Community with a Collaborative Electronic Journal, *College Teaching* 47, no. 3 (Summer 1999):88–90.

10. Ibid., p. 90.

11. A. Oosterhof, Efficiently Creating Individualized E-Mail to Students, *Journal of Computing in Higher Education* 11, no. 2 (Spring 2000):75–90.

12. D.L. Parkyn, Learning in the Company of Others.

13. A. Oosterhof, Efficiently Creating Individualized E-Mail.

---

### SUGGESTED READING

Bachman, J. A., and S. Panzarine. 1998. Enabling student nurses to use the information superhighway. *Journal of Nursing Education* 37, no. 4:155–161.

Barber, K., K. Wyatt, and F. Gerbasi. 1999. On-line interactive evaluation in course and clinical instruction. *Nurse Educator* 24, no. 2:37–40.

Deets, C. 1999. Electronic theses and dissertations—The wave of the future. *Journal of Professional Nursing* 15, no. 6:330.

Korn, K. 1999. Nutrition information on the Internet. *Journal of the American Academy of Nurse Practitioners* 11, no. 8:355–356.

Little, D.L., W.H. Hannum, and G.B. Stack. 1996. *Computers and effective instruction: Using computers and software in the classroom.* New York: Longman.

Morersund, D. 1997. *The future of information technology in education: Learning and leading with technology.* Eugene, OR: International Society for Technology in Education.

Oosterhof, A. 2000. Efficiently creating individualized e-mail to students. *Journal of Computing in Higher Education* 11, no. 2:75–90.

Parkyn, D.L. 1999. Learning in the company of others: Fostering a discourse community with a collaborative electronic journal. *College Teaching* 47, no. 3:88–90.

Zwim, E.E. 1998. Media, multimedia, and computer-mediated learning. In *Teaching in nursing: A guide for faculty*, eds. D.M. Billings and J.A. Halstead, 315–329. Philadelphia: W.B. Saunders.

# CHAPTER 17

# Web-Based Instruction

*Judith Schurr Salzer*

## DEFINITION AND PURPOSES

The information explosion has precipitated the rapid incorporation of technology into educational institutions, influencing how teaching and learning are being accomplished. Integrating the Internet into distance education changes our information delivery system, impacts instructor and student communication, and creates challenges for instructors and students. With the percent of higher education institutions offering distance education courses increasing from 33 percent in 1995 to 44 percent in 1998, every indication is that continued technological advancement will have a direct impact on education in the future.[1]

The Internet may be used in a course that is totally Web-based asynchronous (no face-to-face or real-time interaction), totally Web-based synchronous (no face-to-face interaction but class meets online in real time), partially Web-based with some face-to-face class meetings (plus asynchronous or synchronous class interaction), or a traditional class with supplemental Web-based components (e-mail, forums, chat rooms, class content). The most controversial application of the Internet in higher education is the emergence of "virtual" colleges (Open University, Western Governors University) and consortiums of colleges or groups (University of Phoenix, Southern Regional Electronic Campus) offering online courses and degrees.[2] Some people believe that "virtual" colleges, which exist only in cyberspace, are the means by which all higher education will be delivered in the future. Others believe that a combination of traditional and Internet delivery systems will best meet future educational needs. Pragmatically, Web-based educational programs may provide the means for achieving the long-standing goal of increasing access to higher education. With the number of institutions offering asynchronous Internet-based courses increasing from 22 percent in 1995 to 60 percent in 1998, the Internet clearly offers a teaching strategy that cannot be ignored.[3]

Rather than the Internet being used as an "all or none" strategy, it is more likely to be integrated into courses as one of many teaching strategies. Educators are currently struggling to learn what subject matter is appropriate for the virtual classroom. Although some courses may effectively be delivered as asynchronous and Web-based, the learning gained from student interaction is lost. For courses not appropriate for the virtual classroom, the ratio of distance to face-to-face contact and the mode of distance contact must be determined. Although educators recognize the opportunities and challenges inherent in the rapid technological innovations of the Internet, implementation of the technology is in the era of early research and trial-and-error.

## THEORETICAL RATIONALE

Web-based instruction is a distance education tool. Emerging with the development of correspondence courses, distance education eventually added videotapes and computer-assisted instruction (CAI) to its repertoire of available tools. Applying the Internet as an educational delivery system is the newest and most controversial innovation in distance education. Only in the past few years has technology advanced to the point where personal computer memory, modem speed, and bandwidth support Web-based education to most individuals with computer and Internet access.

As with any innovation, use of the Internet to provide or enhance courses has proponents and detractors. As technology continues to develop at an accelerated pace, many educators are venturing into the unfamiliar, untested territory of Web-based teaching and learning. Anecdotal studies and publications abound, but there is a dearth of research supporting Web-based instruction. Therefore, there is little consensus on whether Web-based instruction is a tool to be embraced or shunned, and instructors who incorporate online components into their courses do so without a reliable body of research on which to base their decisions. Regardless, most educators agree that Internet resources can enrich curricula and enhance learning when integrated into courses as one of a variety of teaching strategies.

Much discussion about Web-based instruction in the literature and on campuses centers around the controversy over implementation. Administration's push for technology in the classroom raises the concern that "technology is driving pedagogy," whereas educators contend that "pedagogy should drive technology."[4,5] Some faculty members are being required to implement Web-based instruction against their better judgment, although others believe that "online learning is superior to anything going on in traditional education."[6(p.A43)]

Fundamental questions are yet to be answered about Web-based instruction. What are the defining differences between Internet-mediated instruction and learning and that in the traditional classroom? Some educators question what pedagogical model is guiding online course development and postulate that a whole new pedagogy is required for online instruction. Others contend that teaching is teaching regardless of the delivery system. Experiential evidence suggests that effective instruction through the Internet is less about technology and distance and more about defining effective education, regardless of the delivery system.[7] If quality education involves helping students to make meaningful connections with content, then the power of the Internet enables students to make rapid connections through readily available information. Simultaneously, educators are faced with the new challenge of directing students to appropriate-quality Web sources within the vast collection of easily accessed material of varying quality.

Although some educators are intimidated by the rapid development of Web-based educational applications, the impact of the Internet on all courses cannot be ignored. It is reassuring that experience seems to be demonstrating that a new way of teaching is not required to incorporate innovative technology into the classroom. As many have postulated, it seems likely that the teacher, not the technology employed, makes a good course.

## CONDITIONS

An evolving instructional method with innumerable variations in its use, Web-based instruction may be integrated into any course. The fundamental principles of good teaching and learning are merely applied in a new and different setting.[8] Defining how online instruction is to be used in a course prior to its implementation helps to avoid the mistake of applying the technology simply because it is new. Web-based instruction offers a wide range of uses depending on how it is integrated into a course.

Specific elements of Web-based teaching may be appropriately incorporated into different levels of education. At the undergraduate level, students require extensive discussion with peers and faculty to develop critical thinking skills. As a result, virtual courses lacking student-to-student and faculty-to-student interaction could be counterproductive; however, supplementing traditional courses with communication tools such as asynchronous forums or synchronous chat rooms can provide students with ongoing dialog between scheduled classes. In addition, posting class outlines prior to classes may increase students' level of preparation for more meaningful discussions. Web-based teaching at the graduate level may eliminate the need for some or all same-place classes, depending on the type of course content.

At the other end of the spectrum, entire programs and schools are now available through the Internet. In fact, some schools have no brick and mortar existence but are found only on the Web. Web-based programs span the range from offering little interaction with faculty, a "do-it-yourself" type of program, to frequent faculty communication and specific, concentrated on-campus requirements.

Although it is impossible to say with certainty where the trend toward Web-based instruction will lead, using the Internet to teach and learn is clearly here to stay. What subjects are most amenable to Web-based instruction or what parameters cause use of the technology to be counterproductive are yet to be definted.[9] Employing creative ways of integrating Web-based instruction into courses helps to determine the limits of this developing technology.

## TYPES OF LEARNERS

Although courses with integrated features of Web-based teaching are appropriate for all types of students, courses taught wholly online should be aimed at the adult, nontraditional student. Adult and traditional adolescent learners differ in motivation, purpose, learning styles and preferences, and intellectual skills.[10] Participation in any form of distance learning requires students to be self-directed and able to function in an environment with limited faculty feedback and lacking face-to-face interaction. For online courses, students must also have basic computer skills and feel comfortable in a computer-based environment.[11]

Whereas few students are prepared to be self-directed and conscientious about completing assignments when they leave high school, not all adult learners possess the required characteristics for distance learning success either.[12] Several institutions have developed online self-assessment questionnaires to assist students in determining whether online courses are a reasonable alternative for them. Exhibit 17–1 is one confidential questionnaire that is completed online and submitted for "grading." The student receives feedback on the questionnaire with an assessment of his or her probability of success in a distance-delivered course.

## RESOURCES

Any instructor with a computer and Internet access is able to add several helpful online components to courses. Instructor Web pages with links to course-related material may be created by novice computer users with specialized software. Free software is available for download to provide chat rooms for synchronous student discussions, and new applications are under continuous development. To take advantage of online course features, students must have computer and Internet access.

Courses that are developed and managed online require institutional support in the form of equipment, services, and faculty time and recognition. The necessary infrastructure is expensive to set up and maintain. Faculty members require computers, supporting software, and Internet access. A server and an online commercial teaching and learning environment must be purchased. An expert staff specializing in using and maintaining the environment must be trained and available at all times. Faculty training on how to develop courses to take advantage of vari-

**Exhibit 17–1** Example of On-Line Self-Assessment Questionnaire

**Thinking about enrolling in a course or program at WGU?**

Answer the following questions by selecting one answer to each question. This quiz can help you decide whether a distance-delivered course is right for you. It is for your own use only, so try to be as honest and as accurate as possible. When you have answered all 10 questions, click the "Submit" button that appears at the bottom of the page.

1. **Having face-to-face interaction with my instructors and fellow students is:**
   (a) not particularly important to me.
   (b) somewhat important to me.
   (c) very important to me.

2. **I would classify myself as someone who:**
   (a) is good at prioritizing tasks and often gets things done ahead of time without being reminded by my instructor.
   (b) is sometimes poor at prioritizing, needs to be reminded of assignments once in a while, and often does assignments at the last minute.
   (c) is poor at prioritizing and sometimes forgets to complete assignments if I'm not reminded about them frequently.

3. **Classroom discussion is:**
   (a) rarely helpful to me.
   (b) sometimes helpful to me.
   (c) almost always helpful to me.

4. **When an instructor hands out instructions for an assignment, I prefer:**
   (a) figuring out the instructions myself.
   (b) trying to follow the directions on my own, then asking for help as needed.
   (c) having the instructions explained to me.

5. **When it comes to assessing my own progress, I:**
   (a) feel as if I can keep tabs on my progress, even without immediate or frequent feedback from my instructor.
   (b) prefer to receive regular feedback from my instructor, but don't mind if I can't get that feedback immediately after turning in a test or assignment.
   (c) need feedback from my instructor immediately and often.

6. **My need to take a distance delivered course is:**
   (a) High—I need it immediately for a degree, job advancement, or other important reason.
   (b) Moderate—I could take it on campus or substitute another course.
   (c) Low—It's a personal interest that could be postponed.

7. **Considering my professional and personal schedule, the amount of time I have to work on an online course is:**
   (a) 7–9 hours per week.
   (b) 4–6 hours per week.
   (c) 1–3 hours per week.

*continues*

**Exhibit 17–1** continued

8. **When I am asked to use software or technologies that I haven't used before (such as e-mail, voice mail, a VCR):**
   (a) I look forward to learning new skills.
   (b) I feel apprehensive, but try anyway.
   (c) I put it off or try to avoid it.

9. **If I had to describe my predominant learning style/preference, I would say it is:**
   (a) Auditory—I learn best when I can listen to an explanation of a concept.
   (b) Visual—I learn best when I can read the course materials or view graphics and other visuals.
   (c) Tactile—I learn best by "doing" (for instance conducting an experiment in a lab).

10. **My personal and professional schedule is:**
   (a) Predictable. I can generally plan, well in advance, blocks of time to devote to my coursework.
   (b) Generally predictable, but sometimes last minute meetings or events come up that I cannot reschedule.
   (c) Kind of crazy. I rarely know when I'm going to have free time that I can set aside for my coursework.

Courtesy of Western Governors University.

ous teaching strategies in the online environment is essential. In addition, innovations in the environment must be communicated to faculty through periodic training updates.

Because not all faculty members adapt to the technical environment at the same pace, support and mentoring groups help those who may be overwhelmed or intimidated by the technology. Support groups also provide a forum for sharing experiences on what worked well on the Internet and which content proved inappropriate for online presentation.

Institutional administrative support is required for faculty release time to develop online courses. Administrators must understand that an online course with any faculty-student communication component requires a lower student-to-faculty ratio than a traditional course. Monitoring and guiding online communication among class members in addition to direct faculty-to-student communication requires a significant faculty time commitment. Institutions that commit the resources to support online course delivery will likely require faculty to effectively use the resources provided. Administrative policies for merit and tenure need to be adjusted to recognize the knowledge, skills, and time required to develop and teach courses in an online environment.

## USING THE METHOD

This discussion will focus on the practical integration of Web-based instruction into traditional courses. Other resources are available to guide educators in creating and maintaining virtual courses. Regardless of the format, any course must be carefully planned, including identifying which online components will enhance the teaching and learning environment. During course development, instructors must keep in mind that online tools do not improve teaching and learning. A tool's effectiveness is determined by the manner in which it is integrated into a course to support the objectives and to create a community of learners.[13] Web-based tools generally impact communication through the transmission of information or by enabling two-way communication. Information may be transmitted to students by posting the syllabus, class outlines, or other resource information to be electronically accessed by the student at a convenient time. Chat rooms, e-mail, electronic bulletin boards, forums, and quizzes provide means for two-way electronic "talking" between instructor and students and/or among classmates. Faculty members should become comfortable with using new tools prior to their implementation and should provide students with an orientation to the technology, new tools, and expectations for their use.

Although basic information transmission may be accomplished through instructors' personal Web pages created on the World Wide Web, tools available in commercial structured learning environments provide a standardized system for transmission of specific types of information. Information paths and pages enable instructors to offer the full syllabus online, to provide class content outlines, and to establish direct links to appropriate Web sites. Students may print out all or parts of the information provided. Pages created for faculty and student profiles help class members get to know each other and course faculty. Management tools enable instructors to track students' hits and identify students who may be falling behind. Students may track their grades and view statistics on each test or assignment, such as grade range, median, and mode. A calendar tool may be used by both instructors and students. Information about class schedules or content may be posted by instructors. Students may post clinical activities for instructor review or personal schedules that can be made visible only to the posting student. Although posting and viewing videos and slideshows is possible, current technology does not provide readily available quality and speed to support their general use. These and other as-yet-undeveloped means of information transmission will be commonplace and expected by students within a few years. New user-friendly tools that are continuously under development are incorporated into frequent updates of commercial structured learning environments.

Two-way synchronous or asynchronous communication is facilitated by e-mail, bulletin boards, forums, chat rooms, and quizzes. Because student access to the tools is available 24 hours a day, 7 days a week, faculty members must inform students what limits have been established for faculty input. Some faculty members prefer to use the tools only during the traditional work week, whereas others also "check in" during evenings and weekends. The more often faculty communicate with students, the more often students will take advantage of the communication tool. This additional two-way communication results in a greater than usual faculty time commitment.

E-mail is familiar to most faculty and students. Either personal e-mail accounts or e-mail embedded in commercial structured learning environments may be used for asynchronous communication. E-mail embedded in commercial structured learning environments may be used to communicate only with course faculty and those students who are registered in the course. Faculty members may send the same message to all class members or communicate with individual students. Students may provide information, clarify content, or ask questions directly to the instructor. Successful use of e-mail requires an agreement among users on the frequency of checking for messages.

Electronic bulletin boards are used by instructors and students to post messages to the entire class. Similar to a bulletin board, a forum provides for asynchronous communication among members of a designated group. In large classes, forums provide for more productive conversation among students in smaller groups. Forums may be used by students to work through an assigned discussion question between scheduled classes. Forum discussions may be monitored by instructors for both content and student participation. Instructor comments provide positive feedback to the group, redirect the discussion, or suggest resources. Students have the opportunity to think about their answers or to do some reading prior to posting comments. Exhibits 17–2 and 17–3 demonstrate a student-initiated, faculty-monitored forum discussion. Again, expectations and rules must be communicated to students to avoid rambling pages that lack substance. The expected minimum number of postings per student needs to be clearly stated and understood by students. Postings may be graded, counted as class participation, or used as a critical-thinking exercise.

Real-time or synchronous conversations may be conducted in chat rooms that are commercially available for free download, with some Internet service provider (ISP) services, or within a commercial structured learning environment. Use of a chat room requires setting a date and time to "meet" in a designated room. Student groups may use chat rooms to discuss projects or class content. Instructors may meet with small groups of students for topical discussions, to discuss problems, or to clarify content between scheduled class meetings. Some chat rooms permit the instructor or all participants to print conversations out at the completion of the chat session. A printed record of the discussion and action agreed upon is helpful to both instructors and students.

Online testing is widely available, often with immediate grading and student feedback. Although essay questions generally require hand-grading at this time, programs for computer grading are under development. Quiz-type tools in commercial structured learning environments have several uses. Student self-administered quizzes with immediate feedback aid students' study of online content. Graded tests assess students' knowledge throughout the course. In addition, a quiz tool may be used as another form of asynchronous communication. Open-ended

**Exhibit 17–2**  Forum Listing on Bulletin Board

Interesting case [Forum: Group 1]
- ☐  144. Kathy Benton (Thu, Mar. 2, 2000, 16:40)
- ☐  145. Instructor (Thu, Mar. 2, 2000, 20:40)
- ☐  146. Annie Freund (Sat, Mar. 4, 2000, 15:24)
  - ☐  147. Instructor (Sun, Mar. 5, 2000, 12:32)
    - ☐  148. Donna Rider (Sun, Mar. 5, 2000, 13:38)
      - ☐  149. Annie Freund (Sun, Mar. 5, 2000, 14:03)
- ☐  150. Kathy Benton (Sun, Mar. 5, 2000, 16:18)
  - ☐  151. Instructor (Mon, Mar. 6, 2000, 08:45)

**Exhibit 17–3**  Forum Dialog under Exhibit 17–2 Forum Listing

Subject: Interesting case
[Prev Thread] [Next Thread]

[Prev Thread] [Next Thread]
Article No. 144: posted by Kathy Benton on Thu, Mar. 2, 2000, 16:40

I saw something this week that I haven't seen before and wanted to ask you guys about it. I saw a 3-year-old who we diagnosed with a right otitis media. She presented with serosanguineous drainage from the ear, but she did not have myringotomy tubes. She did have a perforated ear drum. We treated her with Floxin 6 drops twice a day and Amoxicillin by mouth. I have not looked at the literature yet, but I wanted to know if you guys have seen this presentation of otitis media and how you treated it. Kathy

[Prev Thread] [Next Thread]
Article No. 145: [Branch from no. 144] posted by Instructor on Thu, Mar. 2, 2000, 20:40

What was the history on this child? Did she have an upper respiratory infection symptoms, ear pain, fever? What dose of Amoxicillin did you use? Prof. Sanders

[Prev Thread] [Next Thread]
Article No. 146: [Branch from no. 144] posted by Annie Freund on Sat, Mar. 4, 2000, 15:24

I saw a similar case this week. The child presented with bloody ear drainage and was diagnosed with acute otitis media with perforation. We treated the child with Amoxil and Floxin. I haven't had a chance to look at the literature yet, but will let you know if I find anything. Annie

*continues*

**Exhibit 17–3** continued

---

[Prev Thread] [Next Thread]

Article No. 147: [Branch from no. 146] posted by Instructor on Sun, Mar. 5, 2000, 12:32

It's interesting that each of you have seen this since it is not that common. Makes me wonder if there is an unusual underlying cause like a virus. What was the age of your patient, Annie? What other symptoms did she have? Prof. Sanders

---

[Prev Thread] [Next Thread]

Article No. 148: [Branch from no. 147] posted by Donna Rider on Sun, Mar. 5, 2000, 13:38

Dr. Patton saw a child this week whose mother reported seeing bloody drainage on the sheet when they got up in the morning. The mom described the drainage as a quarter-sized amount or slightly more, and she said she thought it came from his ear. On exam there was no evidence of ruptured ear drum. One tympanic membrane was slightly hazy, but the other was normal appearing. We did not find any evidence of bleeding from the nose, mouth, etc. We did not diagnose as a ruptured tympanic membrane. Kathy, what did the tympanic membranes look like on exam? Donna

---

[Prev Thread] [Next Thread]

Article No. 149: [Branch from no. 147] posted by Annie Freund on Sun, Mar. 5, 2000, 14.03

The child was 20 months and has had 2 previous episodes of otitis media this winter. She also attends daycare. She is the first case like this I have seen and I thought it was unusual. Annie

---

[Prev Thread] [Next Thread]

Article No. 150: [Branch from no. 144] posted by Kathy Benton on Sun, Mar. 5, 2000, 16:18

I found a good article online in Contemporary Pediatrics, May 1999. You can access it from www.contpeds.com and go to past issues. Kathy

---

[Prev Thread] [Next Thread]

Article No. 151: [Branch from no. 150] posted by Instructor on Mon, Mar. 6, 2000, 08:45

Good. Sounds like we need to discuss this further this week. Please see what else you can find in the current literature and bring the references to seminar. Also, make sure you have the relevant history and physical findings of children you have seen with ear drainage. See you Wednesday. Prof. Sanders

---

questions provide a framework for students' clinical journal entries or notes and provide for timely instructor-to-student feedback. At the same time, students' clinical progress may be closely monitored to identify student problems and provide for early intervention (Exhibits 17–4 and 17–5).

**Exhibit 17–4** Sample SOAP Note Using Quiz Tool Construction

---

**Question 1: Enter complete, concise subjective information.**

*Student Response:*

A 21-month-old female comes to clinic today for a sick visit accompanied by her mother. Child has had a fever, runny nose, and cough. The fever has been for 2 days up to 102 axillary. She has had a cough that sounds "hacky" for about 3 days, and she has had a runny nose for about 1 week. Her appetite has been decreased, but she is drinking okay. She has had 6 oz. of juice and 6 oz. of milk today. Her elimination pattern is normal. She has had 3 wet diapers already today. Her activity level has been decreased, and mom thinks that she is sleeping more than usual. Her cough is waking her up some at night, but then she goes right back to sleep. She has not had any vomiting or diarrhea. She is in a small daycare with 4 other kids, and mom does not think that she has had any illness exposures. She has not been to daycare in 2 days. The only medicine she has had is Tylenol for the fever, and it has brought the temperature down, but after it wears off it goes back up. The last dose of Tylenol was 3 hours ago. Dad smokes in the house.

*Comments:*

Allergies? Tylenol dose? The progression of this illness would be easier to follow if you begin at the beginning: well until 1 week ago when she began having a runny nose. Hacky cough began 3 days ago and fever up to 102 axillary began 2 days ago. Add in when her decreased eating, decreased activity level, and increased sleeping began. Work on being more concise.

**Question 2: Enter pertinent objective information.**

*Student Response:*

Weight - 29 lbs. Temperature - 100.8 tympanic
General - ill appearing but in no acute distress; quiet and cooperative for exam
HEENT - normocephalic; sclera clear, conjunctiva pink, right tympanic membrane slightly injected with good light reflex, clear landmarks, good mobility; left tympanic membrane slightly injected with good light reflex, sharp landmarks, good mobility; nares patent, turbinates erythematous wtih purulent white drainage; pharynx clear, tonsils +2 with no erythema or edema; mucoid post nasal discharge
Mouth - mucous membranes pink and moist, lips dry
Cardiovascular - clear S1, S2, without murmur; capillary refill brisk, peripheral pulses strong and equal
Lungs - coarse breath sounds bilateral; crackles in lower lobes bilateral, posterior > anterior; no wheezing or retracting; respirations even, unlabored, rate 28; no grunting
Abdomen - soft, nontender, no masses or hepatosplenomegaly
Genital - normal external female genitalia without discharge or rash
Skin - warm, dry, without rash, good turgor
Lymphs - shotty, nontender, posterior cervical nodes bilateral

*continues*

**Exhibit 17–4** continued

*Comments:*

Was the white nasal discharge really purulent? Was it thick or thin?

**Question 3: Enter your assessment with rationale.**

*Student Response:*

Pneumonia - bilateral, likely viral
Rationale: According to the articles by Schidlow & Callahan and Churgay, crackles and wheezes are sounds that indicate compromise of the lower respiratory tract. Churgay's article pointed out that most pediatric pneumonias are viral in origin, but a bacterial source should be considered because antibiotics would then be crucial to the treatment plan. The articles I reviewed all indicated that children with a bacterial pneumonia are usually sicker, in more respiratory distress, and with higher fevers than those with viral pneumonia. After my reading, I have a much better understanding of how to diagnose and differentiate pneumonia.
*Comments:*

Good job.

**Question 4: Enter your plan with rationale.**

*Student Response:*

My preceptor obtained a chest X-ray that showed patches of consolidation and admitted the child for treatment of pneumonia. After my reading, I would not have done this. Because the child was in no distress and appeared mildly ill, I'm not sure I would have obtained an X-ray. The articles indicated that pneumonia in young child is a clinical diagnosis because X-rays may be unreliable. In addition, obtaining an X-ray would not have changed my treatment for this child. My plan would have been:
1. Amoxicillin 400mg / 5ml, 1 teaspoon by mouth twice a day (60mg / kg / day)
2. Push oral fluids - juices, Gatorade
3. Cool air humidifier at night for the coughing - instruct mom on use and cleaning
4. Instruct mom on what signs to look for that would indicate the child was working hard to breathe - mom to call or go to Emergency Department if they occur
5. Discuss dangers of passive smoke exposure
6. Return in 48 hours if child is still running a fever >101
7. Return in 3 days for follow-up

Rationale: Although 90 percent of childhood community-acquired pneumonias are viral, it is very difficult to distinguish them from the bacterial causes. Because of this, antibiotic therapy is usually given (James, 1999). Aside from viruses, streptococcus pneumoniae, staphylococcus aureus, H-flu, and group A strep are the main pathogens causing pneumonia. Streptococcus pneumoniae is by far the most com-

*continues*

**Exhibit 17–4** continued

mon cause and can be treated with penicillin or erythromycin in those allergic to penicillin (James, 1999). I used Amoxicillin because it can be given twice daily at 60-80 mg/kg/day, and it is generally well tolerated by children and is inexpensive.
*Comments:*

Good. Be specific when you ask parents to "push fluids." How much, how often? I would also have arranged to call the family the next day to see how the child has been doing since the visit. To implement your plan, you need to feel comfortable that the parents are capable of assessing the child accurately at home. In this case, it certainly sounds reasonable. I am not familiar with Amoxicillin that comes 400mg/5ml. Please let me know what your reference is for this.

**Question 5: What references did you use?**

*Student Response:*

Churgay, C. (1996). The diagnosis and management of bacterial pneumonias in infants and children. *Primary Care: Clinics in Office Practices*, 23: 821–835.
Lassieur, S.M. & Jacobs, R.F. (1999). Pediatric pneumonia: Recognizing usual and unusual causes. *The Journal of Respiratory Diseases for Pediatricians*, 1: 42–50.
Latham-Sadler, B. & Morell, V. (1996). Pneumonia. *Pediatrics in Review*, 17: 300–310.
*Comments:*

You refer to an article by James (1999), but it is not listed in references. Please provide this reference. Nice job. I see much progress in your critical thinking on these cases.

**Exhibit 17–5** Sample Student Weekly Self-Assessment Using Quiz Tool Construction

**Question 1: What are your strengths, weaknesses, and areas you need more experience in during your remaining clinical time?**

*Student Response:*

I feel comfortable talking with parents and younger children. Parents seem to be responding to me by asking questions about their children and listening to what I have to say. I'm finally feeling like I know how to answer some of the questions. I'm not as comfortable with adolescents and have had limited experience dealing with them. Because we see few adolescents in this practice, is there somewhere I could get more experience with them?

*continues*

**Exhibit 17–5** continued

*Comments:*

It is good when you start to feel like you know what you're doing! There is a teen clinic not far from you that we have used for students in the past. Let me see if they would be able to have you work with them for some of your clinical. You can also ask around to see if there are other appropriate sites. Let me know if you find anything and I'll look into it.

**Question 2: What problems have you encountered in the clinical setting that are obstacles to your learning? What can you do about them?**

*Student Response:*

The only problem is that Dr. Towner is so busy at times that I don't get to ask him his rationale for a diagnosis or treatment. I don't feel that I can try to slow him down because there are so many patients to be seen. I'm not sure what to do.

*Comments:*

Have you thought about arranging for a routine, 15-minute meeting with Dr. Towner to ask your questions? Take a look at your day and see when 15 minutes might be convenient for him. Write your questions down and be very concise. Make sure you do not take more than the prearranged time. Keep me posted on what you decide to do.

## POTENTIAL PROBLEMS

Although innovative and state-of-the-art, Web-based instruction is not without problems and disadvantages for administrators, faculty, and students. The electronic environment poses several threats to courses dependent on Web-based instruction. Electrical outages eliminate the ability of individuals in affected areas to participate in Web-based courses, sometimes for extended periods. Each user depends on an ISP for a connection to the Internet. ISPs vary in efficiency, reliability, and quality. As Internet users increase, access problems can be anticipated as ISPs become overloaded. Users also depend on the efficient functioning of an institution's server for the commercial structured learning environment. When the server goes down or is undergoing maintenance, all course work ceases. The newest potential problem is the threat of electronic vandalism, although it is difficult to anticipate how extensive the problem may become. Invasion of courses by hackers could compromise student confidentiality or result in the modification or theft of course materials.

Administrators are faced with the expense of continuous maintenance and upgrading of servers, hardware, and software. Far from being a lucrative means of providing education, most institutions are finding that online courses are more expensive than traditional courses to develop and implement. Administrators initially anticipated that online instruction would enable faculty to teach larger classes and to positively impact the bottom line. The increased demand on faculty time arising from the ease of student-faculty communication over the Internet is beginning to be realized. Although Web-based instruction is often an improvement in teaching and learning, most administrators no longer consider Web-based courses an extremely profitable venture.

Faculty members need to learn how to work with a new technology and how to apply appropriate teaching strategies. High motivation and a willingness to invest time in the learning curve are required, but without the expectation of recognition or early reward. Developing online courses is teaching innovation that should be expected, respected, and rewarded, but in most institutions it is ignored as an important scholarly activity. Similarly, current intellectual property policies for Web-based materials are inconsistent and often do not allow for faculty ownership of online courseware.[14]

Students enrolled in Web-based classes with limited or no face-to-face meetings may feel isolated and fail to develop the identity, cohesion, and rapport usually found in face-to-face classes.[15,16] Student isolation may also interfere with learning. Computer access is becoming less of a problem because many institutions began requiring students to have personal computers; however, reliable ISPs with local telephone access numbers may be limited for students in remote areas. Resulting service interruptions may limit students' course participation, and excessive long-distance telephone bills may create an additional financial burden. Even large, well-established ISPs vary in connection speed and quality, with some services consistently disconnecting students after short periods of online time. These problems cause students to lose unfinished online work or prevent them from participating in group synchronous chat sessions.

## CONCLUSION

Adventurous educators are venturing into the realm of Web-based instruction. Although clearly a trend that will continue into the future, the parameters and limits of Web-based instruction are currently untested and unknown. Innovative educators must continue to document and share their experiences as they employ creative uses of the Internet in teaching and learning.

---

**NOTES**

1. G.W. Phillips, The Release of Distance Education at Postsecondary Education Institutions 1997–98, *National Center for Education Statistics* (December 17, 1999), <http://nces.ed.gov/commissioner/remarks99/12_17_99.asp> (26 January 2000).

2. E. Neal, Distance Education, *National Forum* 79, no. 1 (1999):40.

3. Phillips, *National Center*, online.

4. University of Illinois, *Teaching at an Internet Distance: The Pedagogy of Online Teaching and Learning*, The Report of a 1998–1999 University of Illinois Faculty Seminar (December 7, 1999), <http://www.vpaa.uillinois.edu:80/tid/report/tid-final-12-5.doc> (28 January 2000).

5. A. Feenberg, Distance Learning: Promise or Threat, *Crosstalk* (Winter), <http://www-rohan.sdsu.edu/faculty/feenberg/TELE3.HTM> (25 January 2000).

6. S. Jaschik, Historians Differ on Impact of Distance Education in Their Discipline, *The Chronicle of Higher Education* 46, no. 20 (2000):A43.

7. University of Illinois, *Teaching at an Internet Distance*, online.

8. M.D. Milliron and C.L. Miles, Aha! Making the Connection between the Internet and Learning, *League for Innovation in the Community College* 3, no. 1 (2000), <http://www.league.org/publications/abstracts/learning/lelabs0001.htm> (14 February 2000).

9. S.R. Barley, Computer-Based Distance Education: Why and Why Not, *The Education Digest* 65, no. 2 (1999):55–59.

10. Neal, Distance Education, 41.

11. V. Murphree, Using the Virtual Classroom, *Occupational Health & Safety* 68, no. 9 (1999):28–29.

12. Neal, Distance Education, 43.

13. G.M. Funaro, Pedagogical Roles and Implementation Guidelines for Online Communication Tools, *ALN Magazine* 3 (December 1999), <http://www.aln.org/alnweb/magazine/Vol3_issue2/funaro.htm> (26 January 2000).

14. University of Illinois, *Teaching at an Internet Distance*, online.

15. M. Rangecroft, Interpersonal Communication in Distance Education, *Journal of Education for Teaching* 24, no. 1 (1998):75–76.

16. Neal, Distance Education, 43.

# Remote Faculty

The strategies in Part V have a primary aspect in common with the strategies in the previous section on Technology. This commonality is that the faculty and student are not together in the same environment every time a learning experience takes place. However, the teaching-learning relationship is maintained, and faculty give input into student learning whether the faculty are or are not physically present with the student. The participants do meet together as the experience evolves and events warrant face-to-face interaction.

Learning experiences that involve the remote faculty are usually for more advanced learners, and are in unique settings that call for more independence on the part of the learner. Even in remote settings, students engaged in clinical practice will need supervision, often from an active practitioner who serves as a preceptor. For faculty, the nature of the remote setting calls for planning and organization, in order to maximize time on site. When technology is involved, it is imperative that the equipment is functioning properly, in order to maintain needed links.

Learning experiences in which the student is apart from the faculty enable the student to be engaged in real-life events, thus increasing opportunities for independent problem-solving. Learners begin to detach from the instructor, thus preparing themselves for actual practice.

# CHAPTER 18

# Co-Consultant

*Barbara Fuszard and Astrid Hellier Wilson*

## DEFINITION AND PURPOSES

*Co-consultant* is a teaching-learning technique that uses the consultant process and role for student synthesis and application of knowledge in the practice setting. The *consultation process* can be defined in many ways. It can be applied in most professional activity.[1] "In the pure sense, according to Haveloch, the consultant is a facilitator, helper, objective observer, and specialist in how to diagnose needs, how to identify resources, and how to retrieve from expert sources . . . . The underlying rationale for consultant is that only the client himself (the user) can determine what is useful for him."[2] The dependent-interdependent relationship between student and faculty member varies with the knowledge level and experience of the student.

The purpose to be achieved by the co-consultant teaching-learning strategy is to help the student become a true professional. The students are to acquire the approach of facilitator, helper, and objective observer—the ideal client-professional relationship. As the students gain knowledge and experience, they will also be able to offer the expert skills of a professional—data-gathering techniques, diagnosis skills, knowledge of resources, and access to expert sources. The co-consultant approach permits the students to learn with a real problem, and with as much support as they need at a particular level of professional development. The range of faculty support is from role-modeling in the clinical setting to remote support through availability in tutorials. The experienced professional, for example, a doctoral nursing student, would be ready to gain practical experience in the entire consultation process.

## THEORETICAL RATIONALE

This strategy has roots similar to role-playing, with mental health consultation and role theory forming the structure upon which the strategy is built. Caplan's concept of the consultant-consultee-client relationship is most appropriate for the faculty member-student-client relationship of the co-consultant strategy. The concept of process consultation is especially appropriate for facilitator. It is a collaborative approach in which the consultant facilitates the client's use of his or her own strengths to resolve problems. The role of facilitator implies an egalitarian relationship between consultant and client, rather than that of decision maker to troubled client.

Carl Rogers' humanist approach offers client-centered therapy, where consulting approaches are concerned with client desires and feelings rather than finding an ideal problem solution. The skills that Rogers emphasizes for the first stage (entry) of the consultant-client relationship are the approaches the co-consultant process wishes to teach the young professional—"communication of respect, genuineness, and accurate empathy."

Lewin's force-field-analysis model offers the consultant relationship an analytical approach to description of the environment in which the problem is occurring. This knowledge permits indirect intervention by suggesting change in one part of the environment. McGregor's Theory Y offers a basis for measuring group characteristics such as trust, conflict, communication, and team goals. He suggests the consultant use this information to provide clues to the group on how group effectiveness can be improved. Schein, the father of "process consultation," suggests the consultant's role is to provide "insight" into the interpersonal dynamics involved in the problem, so that they can be structured into a workable frame.[3]

Role theory enters the co-consultant teaching-learning strategy in the relationship of the faculty member to the student. With the young professional the relationship is one of role-modeling for the student, with gradual distancing permitting the student to take over more of the responsibilities as knowledge and skills grow.[4]

Nurses are exploring new approaches to create community partnerships in health care delivery both in the United States and throughout the world. Within the framework of consultation, nurses are becoming increasingly autonomous and many are self-employed. Nurse-centered consultation models have been effective in assisting families to care for selected populations such as low-weight infants, the elderly, the handicapped, the chronically ill and mentally ill.[5]

An extensive review (1985–1995) of consultation outcome research was conducted to determine, in part, whether or not consultation is effective. One of the findings was that, in general, consultation services yield favorable results. However, recommendations for future consultation outcome research include increasing the rigor of the research and the need to ascertain the long-term effects of consultation services on clients, consultees, and systems.[6]

## CONDITIONS

Co-consultant strategies are valuable for the very young professional student, to inculcate early the professional relationships expected of the graduate. The master's and doctoral students will benefit by developing skill in the complete consultation role.

A special situation can make the co-consultant strategy a method of choice. When there are no professional role models in the setting, it is incumbent upon the faculty member to meet this need. Sister Dorothy Sheehan contends that in hospitals, where most nursing today is practiced, professional nursing services do not exist.[7] If nursing students are learning in these settings, they must have faculty role models to demonstrate the practice of professional nursing.

This method is also ideal for individualizing instruction based upon the student's level of understanding. The faculty member can maintain direct contact with the student, or any level of distancing, depending upon the learning needs of the student.

The co-consultant teaching strategy is an ideal adult learning tool. The student is permitted to work within the existing level of competence and to grow during the experience. The problems are real life, in a real health care setting, offering experiential problem solving. The relationships among facilitator, student, and client evidence mutual respect. This strategy's greatest contribution to adult learning is probably its adaptability to the needs of the individual student. The exercise also permits evaluation of self, work, personal relationships, and social structure in the process of assisting a real client.

A first requirement of the consultation, of course, is a client with a problem. There must be the ability to travel and relatively unstructured time periods for the consultation interaction, both with the client and between co-consultants. Unless group consultation is possible, such as in the example below, there must be more time allotted to the exercise than normal classroom hours. A consultation relationship that can be evaluated, and that can be completed in the time available, must be planned. A co-consultant activity calls for a great deal of planning, and a certain amount of flexibility on the part of all, to meet both client and educational needs. Within the planning, the relationships and responsibilities must be clearly outlined for all parties.

The co-consultant strategy is applicable to almost any content. As the student advances in knowledge and skill and the faculty member begins to withdraw, it becomes increasingly more important that the problem area be in the expertise of the student. The novice nurse will need to learn professional relationships, whereas the advanced student will be involved with the whole consultation process, including expertise in the content area.

## TYPES OF LEARNERS

This method is appropriate for the senior undergraduate student, especially the RN, master's, and doctoral students. Nurses who are experts in their clinical fields are often called upon to offer consultation (formal or informal) to other nurses in nearby institutions. Staff development through co-consultation would prepare them well for the professional aspects of consultation and the entire consultation process, which would enable their expertise in the content area to be put to best use.

## RESOURCES

Resources needed emphasize time, especially with beginning professional students, as the relationship is usually a 1:1 faculty-student relationship, and at best calls for an individualized approach to each student. Material resources are not indicated, not even classroom space, as consultations take place within the client agency, and meetings between faculty and student are tutorials.

## USING THE METHOD

Frances Lange discusses the five stages of consultation, a logical progression of planned change activities that are followed in the co-consultant method.

1. entry
2. goal setting
3. problem solving
4. decision making
5. termination

*Entry* is accomplished by the faculty member for the novice professional, as described in the example. With faculty guidance, the more advanced student will be able to negotiate this difficult step. In this stage both consultant and client explore the nature of the problem and negotiate the responsibilities and outcomes of the relationship. In this stage a contract is developed.

*Goal setting* provides a blueprint for the consultation relationship. It is the beginning of the planning stage, and includes "approaches, objectives, tactics, and possible activities that will achieve the worthwhile goal."[8] Again with the novice professional, the faculty member will role-model the goal-setting activities, with the students contributing to the degree they are able.

*Problem solving,* and the identification of alternative actions, is the third stage of consultation. *Decision making* involves analyzing the alternative actions and permitting an informed decision to the problem for the next step. The final step, *termination,* should have been part of the initial plan between client and consultant, and should leave both with feelings of satisfaction and accomplishment.

The example shows a slight change from the five stages outlined by Lange. As outside consultants, faculty and students are contracted to assess, evaluate, and recommend. Other than gathering data from the client, the work of the consultants is to compare findings to a national standard, to report these findings, and to make recommendations of how to meet these standards where deficiencies exist.

The co-consultant teaching-learning method has additional steps added to the consultant role, in which the faculty member and student interact to meet the learning objectives. They include study of the consultant role, objectives of the educational experience, and plans for the first interface between student and client. During the consultant stages, the faculty member maintains contact with the student in the setting or through tutorials. This permits the student to raise concerns and problems, and the faculty member to assess the learning level and learning needs of the student during the process. It also permits immediate planning for each subsequent stage of consultation. Final meetings at the end of the consultation permit faculty-student evaluation of the consultation as a learning experience.

The faculty member's role has been identified in the stages of consultation and elsewhere above, and was identified as changing depending upon the knowledge-skill level and growth of the student. The student role moves quickly from passive to active, and from dependent to interdependent in the process of co-consultation. The student may move at an independent rate through the mentioned roles, and this calls for self-direction and self-motivation to take a more active, interdependent role in the consultation.

## POTENTIAL PROBLEMS

There will be confusion of the use of the consultant role as a teaching-learning strategy if the teacher lacks understanding of the consultation process itself. Additional problems will arise if the teacher does not individually assess student readiness for a specific level of dependence-interdependence.

Inappropriate selection of client and/or of student can cause problems in the consultation setting. The faculty member will avoid problems with client selection by spending time and resources to get to know the client well, and to establish a firm contract. The entry stage of the consultation process, therefore, is the critical point for prevention of such problems. Not all students possess the poise and maturity desired for a clinical experience so visible to the public and so dependent on human interaction skills. And not all faculty members have the privilege of choosing the students who will be assigned to this experience. The potential problem student will have to be assigned carefully, after great thought and exploration of client situations available.

A faculty member's expectations for the students and for the agency may be mutually incompatible, causing an ineffectual consultation process and learning process. Again, time and careful study during the entry stage will reduce the chance for such occurrences later in the process. A final limitation of this approach would be in situations offering few consultant opportunities. The faculty member will need to view the catchment area creatively!

The example was modified to offer a group experience to novice consultants, students in master's programs. The group approach with the facilitator co-consultant with the students at all times permits economies of this learning strategy, which otherwise could be prohibitive with novice students.

---

# EXAMPLE
## Consultation for Nursing Service Standards

*Barbara Fuszard*

The co-consultant method offers the novice student an opportunity to develop professional behaviors. It also serves to replace preceptorships when prepared preceptors are unavailable. Such was the case when the nursing faculty sought practicum experiences for nursing administration students in a rural state where there was only one master's-prepared nurse administrator in the entire state. To the benefit of the hospitals of the state, the rural hospitals obtained free, quality consultation services for their nursing departments through this teaching activity.

In a monthly meeting of the Nursing Service Administrators Group, to which this faculty member was a regular invited guest, the faculty member explored with the nurse administrators their interest in having her and her students offer consultation on nursing service standards. The co-consultant group offered to assess nursing departments on criteria from the Joint Commission on Accreditation of Healthcare Organizations[9] (Joint Commission) and the *Standards for Organized Nursing Services and Responsibilities of Nurse Administrators across All Settings*[10] by the American Nurses' Association (ANA). This topic was chosen because the rural hospitals had avoided applying for Joint Commission accreditation because of expense, but the nurse administrators wanted to be assured that they were meeting the same standards as Joint Commission hospitals. They also expressed interest in meeting ANA standards.

Before the faculty member had completed her presentation, one of the nurse administrators had already interrupted, saying "First, first!" All of the nurse administrators expressed interest in having the consultant group work with their departments, even those larger hospitals that had Joint Commission accreditation. One nurse administrator said, "The Joint Commission is coming this fall. Help us see if we are ready." And the nursing home nurse administrators said, "Hurry and finish with the hospitals, so that you can help us."

With this reception, the issue of entry for the consultation group was academic. The faculty member took a strong leadership role, because the students were beginning graduate students. Objectives of the student experience were as follows:

- to offer experience of leadership as facilitator, helper, objective observer, and specialist in nursing service standards
- to develop data-gathering skills through skillful interview and observation
- to synthesize the concurrent roles of the consultant.

While students studied from a reading list on the role of the consultant, the faculty member visited the hospital to meet with the nurse administrator and hospital administrator. In lieu of a consultation contract, the faculty member elected to use the introductory forms of a scientific report. The manual utilized was W. Paul Jones, *Writing Scientific Papers and Reports,* 4th ed. (Dubuque, Iowa: Wm. C. Brown Company, 1960) to give the students a format that they could use in the future for varied reports. The acceptance letter written by the faculty member included the following:

> Thank you again for inviting my students and me to serve as volunteer consultants to your hospital for the purpose of developing guidelines for the Joint Commission and ANA standards in your nursing department. We are tentatively planning to come to your hospital for the entire day, Wednesday, 10 November, and to have a written comprehensive report to you by Christmas. Please let me know if 10 November is open for you and your staff.
>
> Our plans at this time will be to ask you to send us certain documents that you have already prepared, so that we may study them before coming. We then plan to spend as much time as you can give us with you, with the nursing personnel, and any patients who "just want to talk" to us. After our visit we will be in touch with you through the mail or by phone for any additional information or will schedule another visit with you as needed.
>
> Our students right now are studying philosophy, purpose and objectives, budgeting, staffing, labor relations, and orientation of the new graduate. They are very excited about the topics. They will cover all the areas outlined by the Joint Commission before coming to you.
>
> Be assured that we will change nothing at your hospital. We will make recommendations and offer standards only in written form, and you are free to do with these materials as you see fit. Our hope is that they will be of real value to you. I will be available after Christmas to personally work with you if you want help in implementing any of the materials.

A large initial task faced by the first group of students was to review the Joint Commission and ANA standards, and to find a way to mesh these criteria for purposes of the consultation visit. The following is an example of ANA and Joint Commission criteria being grouped for purposes of analysis.

## ANA Standard II

Organized Nursing Services are Administered by Qualified and Competent Nurse Administrators (p. 3).

## ANA Criteria

The nurse executive is a registered nurse who holds a baccalaureate degree in nursing and a graduate degree in nursing or a related field from a program that includes organizational science and management concepts. Certification in nursing administration by a nationally recognized nursing organization is recommended (p. 4).

## Joint Commission Standard

Nursing services are directed by a nurse executive who is a registered nurse qualified by advanced education and management experience (p. 145).

## Joint Commission Criteria

If the hospital utilizes a decentralized organizational structure there is an identified nurse leader at the executive level to provide authority and accountability for, and coordination of, the nurse executive functions (p. 145).

The criteria were organized under the ANA standards because the Joint Commission standards were in various parts of the manual, and under different services, and would have made organization under the Joint Commission standards more difficult. By the time this lengthy process was completed, the students knew well the Joint Commission and ANA standards for nursing services. Future classes of students had the benefit that the coordinated standards were on the word processor. Their task was to update the standards as they were changed by their sponsoring agencies.

The faculty member had some information to share about the hospital after her visit with the administrators. However, most of the material was yet to be gathered, and this data gathering called upon the observational and interviewing skills of the co-consultants. Three approaches were taken to obtain information for analysis.

First, each co-consultant accepted a section of the standards and determined which interview question to ask of the director of nursing. Second, each co-consultant asked to be attached to a member of the nursing staff for the day of visit, and planned to cover all the questions with this person.

Third, each was assigned associated documents and equipment to survey, for final confirmation and information. For example, the student studying the emergency room was responsible for evaluating the classified level of ER service, and the appropriate nurse coverage and equipment appropriate for that level. The sources of information tapped in these ways permitted the co-consultants to verify observations and reporting, and to fill in gaps of information that would not be available from one common source.

Students were also responsible for a level of expertise in the area they would be investigating, such as staffing, budget, philosophy, and organizational charts. Time before the visit permitted these and similar topics to be covered in depth. Students individually searched and organized the literature, providing classmates with a comprehensive bibliography and actual materials that they felt were important for a top position in nursing administration. In addition to reviewing the two sources of criteria that Westwick states are the main criteria for institutional evaluation,[11] they analyzed the standards, using materials such as Cantor's book on the topic.[12] Thus armed with beginning knowledge of the institution, the standards and specific interviewing questions and/or planned observations for gathering data on specific topics, and beginning knowledge of the role of the consultant, the co-consultant experience began.

At the time of the consultation visit, each co-consultant was paired with a member of the nursing staff, and spent the greater share of the consultation visit with that person. Each co-consultant also had interview time with the director of nursing. Questions from the interview schedule, when addressed to the director of nursing, took longer than anticipated, as the director tended to provide richer amounts of data than had been anticipated. Otherwise the day went very much as planned.

The consultants also examined charts and records, and made observations in the specialty areas, such as the emergency room. The director of nursing, the hospital administrator, and the president of the board of trustees met with the entire group of consultants to answer final questions. At the close of the consultation visit, the director of nursing was asked to send copies of all policies and procedures of the department for consultant use.

Content of the interviews, observations, and perceptions of the consultants were shared with one another, and then each consultant assumed responsibility for writing one part of the consultation report. Materials copied and forwarded to the group were used to supplement and/or confirm data gathered from the interviews and observations. Findings and recommendations were then developed for each standard and criterion of the two sets of standards.

An example of an ANA standard, and criteria related to that standard from ANA and the Joint Commission, with the student consultant findings and recommendations follows.

## ANA Standard I

Organized Nursing Services Have a Philosophy and Structure that Ensure the Delivery of Effective Nursing Care (p. 3).

## ANA Criteria

The philosophy of organized nursing services provides to individual nurses the authority and accountability for the clinical management of nursing practice (p. 3).

## Joint Commission Criteria

Registered nurses evaluate current nursing practice and patient care delivery models to improve the quality and efficiency of patient care (p. 146).

## Findings

The philosophy of nursing or the "authority and accountability for clinical management of nursing practice" (p. 3) statement does not clearly define nursing's role in the participation of the management of the division. At the time of the consultants' visit no committees were functioning. The director of nursing did attend the board of directors' meetings, but did not sit at the table with the administrator and board members.

## Recommendations

Committees (such as infection control, pharmacy, medical records, hospital safety, quality assurance) should be established and meetings held on a regular basis. A qualified nurse should be included in the membership of all committees with impact on patient care.

\*   \*   \*   \*

Preparing for the consultation visit, and in the classroom analytical period, students discussed how they could, or did, convey respect, genuineness, egalitarianism, and caring—the interpersonal behaviors that are part of the consultation process. This aspect of the co-consultant experience was the chief teaching-learning objective for this group of students. They evaluated their success by the responses and openness of administrators and nursing employees alike, attested to by the volumes of data gathered.

They also considered these consultant qualities when writing and rewriting the "findings" and "recommendations" sections of the report, endeavoring to offer pertinent, objective data in a nonthreatening, caring, and appropriate way. A sign of the student success both during the visit and in the written report was evidenced by the director of nursing proudly holding aloft at the next Nursing Service Administrators' Group meeting her inch-thick report, and stating, "You know, we're pretty good!"

The letter of transmittal to the hospital and nursing administrators conveyed qualifiers of the work of this young co-consultant group, and offered further expert help. It read, in part:

> We are indebted to you and your employees for your help in gathering data, both printed and verbal. The candidness of both administration and nursing personnel helped to make the data significant and therefore valuable to you.
>
> Problems can be anticipated in working through some of the long-range suggestions of the report. I will be happy to continue to work with you on these items.
>
> Some of the recommendations will not be of value to you because the suggestions have already been implemented, and the consultants were unaware of the existence of materials or misinterpreted them. Other recommendations may be inappropriate to your institution. You are, of course, under no obligation to implement any of the recommendations of the consultants.
>
> Please feel free to call upon us, through me, if we can be of further assistance....

Several classes of graduate nursing students were treated to a similar approach to the co-consultant teaching strategy. The expected benefits of the interpersonal-relationship part of the consultant process were experienced with each group. As members of future classes also differed in clinical backgrounds, individual applications of the teaching strategy were made with each class. Rural hospitals and nursing homes were found to welcome graduate nursing students in the co-consultant role.

---

**NOTES**

1. F. Lange, *The Nurse as an Individual, Group, or Community Consultant* (Norwalk, CT: Appleton & Lange, 1987).
2. M. Kohnke, *The Case for Consultation in Nursing: Designs for Professional Practice* (New York: John Wiley & Sons, Inc., 1978).
3. Lange, *The Nurse as an Individual,* 34–39.

4. M.E. Hardy and M.E. Conway, *Role Theory: Perspectives for Health Professionals* (New York: Appleton-Century-Crofts, 1978).

5. M.M. Styles, Nursing in the Years to Come. *World Health* 48, no. 5 (1995):34–35.

6. S.M. Sheridan and M. Welch, Is Consultation Effective? *Remedial & Special Education* 1, no. 6 (1996):341–354.

7. Lange, *The Nurse as an Individual,* 53.

8. Ibid.

9. 1994 *Accreditation Manual for Hospitals* (Oakbrook Terrace, IL: Joint Commission on Accreditation of Healthcare Organizations, 1993).

10. American Nurses' Association, *Standards for Organized Nursing Services and Responsibilities of Nurse Administrators across All Settings* (Kansas City, MO: 1990).

11. C.R. Westwick, Evaluation of Nursing Organization and Structure, in *The Nurse Evaluator in Education and Service,* eds. A.G. Rezler and B.J. Stevens (New York: McGraw-Hill, 1978), 249–263.

12. M.M. Cantor, *Achieving Nursing Care Standards: Internal and External* (Wakefield, MA: Nursing Resources, 1978).

---

**SUGGESTED READING**

(*Note:* Co-consultant as a teaching-learning method does not appear in the literature. Readings here are limited to materials on consultation, especially consultation in nursing.)

Alphabetical list of consultants and consulting firms 1993. *Journal of Nursing Administration* 23, no. 7-8:70–132.

Brendon, S. and M. Reet. 2000. Establishing a mental health liaison nurse service: Lessons for the future. *Nursing Standard* 14, no. 17:43–47.

Cerda, G.M., D. Hilty, R.E. Hales, and T.S. Nesbitt. 1999. Use of telemedicine with ethnic groups. *Psychiatric Services* 50, no. 10:1364.

Chamberlain, G. 1994. Women consultants (letter). *British Medical Journal* 308:720.

Clark, M.J. Summer 1986. Factors enhancing the success of a consultation. *Nursing Administration Quarterly* 10, no. 4:1–8.

Clark, M.J. 1986. Planning a successful consultation. *The Facilitator* 12, no. 2:1–2.

Coben, S.E., and C.C. Thomas. 1997. Meeting the challenge of consultation and collaboration: Developing interactive teams. *Journal of Learning Disabilities* 30, no. 4:427–432.

Fuszard, B. 1979. Management concepts that work—Consultant in residence. *The Facilitator* 5, no. 6:2.

Grahame-Smith, D.G. 1993. An encounter with Beethoven's cleaning lady. *Lancet* 342:1315.

Kirkbride, M. 1992. A place for infants with HIV. *American Journal of Maternal Child Nursing* 17, no. 5:264.

McKenzie, J. 1983. Basic science department in a government-funded medical school. *Physiologist* 26, no. 5:278–280.

Palsha, S.A., and P.W. Wesley. 1998. Improving quality in early childhood environments through on-site consultation. *Topics in Early Childhood Special Education* 18, no. 4:243–253.

Preston-Whyte, M.E., et al. 1998. Teaching and assessment in the consultation: A hospital clinician's preparatory workshop for integrated teaching of clinical method to undergraduate medical students. *Medical Teacher* 20, no. 3:266–268.

Rosenberg, H., and B. Polonsky. 1990. The role of nonphysician consultants as health-care educators in postgraduate programs of anesthesiology. *Academic Medicine* 65, no. 2:119–122.

Sakauye, K.M., and C.J. Camp. 1992. Introducing psychiatric care into nursing homes. *Gerontologist* 32, no. 6:849–852.

Sheridan, S.M., and M. Welch. 1996. Is consultation effective? *Remedial & Special Education* 1, no. 6:341–354.

Styles, M.M. 1995. Nursing in the years to come. *World Health* 48, no. 5:34–35.

Twardon, C., and M. Gartner. 1992. A strategy for growth in home care: The clinical nurse specialist. *Journal of Nursing Administration* 22, no. 10:49–53.

# CHAPTER 19

# Preceptorial Experience

*Vickie A. Lambert and Clinton E. Lambert, Jr.*

The teaching strategy preceptorial experience allows an opportunity for students to work with clinical experts in a specific health care setting while still under the guidance of a faculty member. This teaching strategy provides socialization into the role of the professional nurse and an opportunity for independent problem solving.

## DEFINITION AND PURPOSES

As a method of clinical teaching for nursing students, the preceptorial experience has grown in popularity over the past 30 years. Both nurse educators and nurse administrators see such an experience as a means of assisting students in the transition from the idealistic academic setting into the reality-based service arena. The experience tends to enhance clinical performance and to facilitate role socialization.[1] A preceptorial experience can be defined as *a clinical learning activity that utilizes unit-based nurses who are engaged in a one-to-one teaching experience with nursing students in addition to carrying out their regularly assigned responsibilities.* The preceptor serves as a role model and resource person and is immediately available to the student within the clinical setting.

## THEORETICAL RATIONALE

Role socialization provides the theoretical basis for the preceptorial experience. Socialization from a role perspective "involves learning to meet, for a variety of situations, the behavior requirements that are delineated by other members of society" (p. 175).[2] Role socialization is successful if the process prepares the individual to respond to a variety of situational demands with the appropriate role characteristics.

242

To obtain appropriate role characteristics, one must acquire knowledge of the role demands, the ability to fulfill the role demands, and the motivation to meet the role demands. A preceptorial experience provides the student with an intense, personalized opportunity to work with a role model on assimilating and acquiring such behaviors. Working alongside a preceptor allows the student to (1) observe and acquire knowledge about the role, (2) work in an environment where the demands of the role can be carried out, and (3) be in a climate that fosters motivation to meet the demands of the role.

Socialization for a given role, during the preceptorship, is a continuous and cumulative process that occurs throughout the entire experience. As a result, any role that a student assumes during the preceptorship will continually evolve with each new clinical experience related to the specific role. For some students, even after completing the preceptorial experience, they chose to utilize a specific preceptor as a role model/mentor for an extended period to assist in further enhancing their professional role socialization.

## CONDITIONS

The preceptorial experience is helpful in assisting students to take knowledge gained in the academic setting and transfer it to the reality-based service world. The experience provides a learning environment in which students can become more self-directed and less faculty dependent.[3] Independent problem solving, synthesis of knowledge, and the use of accumulated clinical skills are the primary outcomes of a successful preceptorial experience.

Although preceptorial experiences often occur during the final phases of students' educational programs, it is not uncommon to utilize preceptors in other aspects of the program (i.e., clinical elective courses). In a clinical elective course, students have the opportunity to be matched with a clinical expert in a specific nursing specialty. This type of clinical experience allows students to accumulate an additional repertoire of role behaviors that are related to a specialty practice.

## TYPES OF LEARNERS

Whereas the preceptorial experience can be used with any student, it appears to be most successful with students who are in the latter part of their educational program. The students who appear most comfortable with the experience are self-motivated, self-directed, and challenged by independence.[4] To enhance the success of the experience, students must be able to identify and deal with their own strengths and limitations, to develop appropriate objectives and strategies for addressing specific learning needs, and to maintain open and appropriate communications with the preceptor and the faculty.

## RESOURCES

The preceptorial experience can take place in any health care agency. It can be of any length, as long as sufficient time is provided to meet the student's specific learning objectives. One limitation to the success of a preceptorial experience is the availability and accessibility of qualified individuals to serve in the role of preceptor.[5] Working with a student is not desirable or manageable for all individuals. In addition, many health care agencies, because of budgetary constraints and patient acuity, are limiting the number of preceptorial experiences that they can provide to schools of nursing.

## USING THE METHOD

The keys to a successful preceptorial experience are an orientation about the experience for students and preceptors, and the selection of appropriate preceptors. The orientation needs to focus on the goals and expectations of the experience; the responsibilities of the preceptors, the students, and the faculty; communication procedures; methods of evaluation; possible problems that can occur during the experience and their related solutions; and student and preceptor perceptions about expectations related to the preceptorial experience.

So the preceptor can successfully fulfill the responsibilities of the role, nurse faculty, nurse administrators, and clinical agency personnel need to identify and select preceptors who have appropriate characteristics. Characteristics identified as important can be clustered into three distinct groups: clinical nursing characteristics, professional characteristics, and personality characteristics. Clinical nursing characteristics consist of at least one year of clinical experience, interest in professional growth, and mastery of clinical skills. Professional characteristics are excellent leadership skills, outstanding communication skills, good decision-making ability, advocacy for the learner, and an ability to effectively use resources. Personality characteristics include patience and enthusiasm; a nonthreatening and nonjudgmental attitude toward others; a flexible, open-minded, trustworthy attitude; a sense of humor; self-confidence; willingness to share knowledge and skills; and willingness to commit the time involved in being a preceptor.

Each person involved in the preceptorial experience must understand his or her respective role and how this role relates to others involved in the experience.[6] Specifically, the role of each of the key participants is as follows.

### Preceptor

The three primary roles for the preceptor are teacher/role-model, workplace socializer, and co-evaluator. *Thus the activities of the preceptor tend to include the following:*

- orienting and socializing the student to the health care agency,
- assisting with the development of teaching/learning objectives for the preceptorial experience,
- planning, delegating, and facilitating daily student clinical experiences that are guided by the course and student teaching/learning objectives,
- supervising and teaching the student in the clinical arena,
- communicating with the faculty on the progress of the student, and
- working with the faculty member to evaluate the student's progress.

### Student

The primary roles for the student are learner and collaborator. *Thus the activities of the student tend to include the following:*

- developing personal teaching/learning objectives based on course objectives in collaboration with the preceptor and the faculty,
- being accountable to both the preceptor and the faculty,
- informing the preceptor of personal goals and learning needs,
- creating, with the preceptor, a work schedule (days and hours involved) and the most effective mode of communication,
- notifying the preceptor if ill or of any schedule change prior to the start of the specific clinical experience,
- informing the preceptor if asked to do a procedure never before performed so that appropriate supervision can occur,
- communicating concerns and questions about patients to the preceptor,
- respecting confidentiality of patients, and
- applying appropriate leadership and management strategies in the clinical arena.

### Faculty

The primary roles for the faculty are consultant and co-evaluator. *Thus the activities of the faculty tend to include the following:*

- orienting the preceptor and the student to the preceptorial experience,
- meeting with the preceptor and the student on a regular basis to appraise and approve student learning needs and progress,
- providing consultation to the preceptor, and
- working with the preceptor to evaluate the student's performance.

### POTENTIAL PROBLEMS

Most problems involved in the preceptorial experience can be avoided with proper planning. An extensive orientation for all participants, careful selection of preceptors, and appropriate assessment of the student's suitability for the experience are measures that can assist in facilitating a successful preceptorial experience. On occasion, faculty members may encounter some difficulty relinquishing the traditional clinical teaching role. This, however, can be resolved by encouraging faculty to focus on the objectives of the experience and the assets of the teaching modality.

Another difficulty that may arise is the existence of a strained relationship between the student and the preceptor. This may be brought about by a difference in perceptions and/or expectations for performance on the part of the preceptor and/or the student. The student also may report the existence of a "personality conflict" with the preceptor as a maneuver to keep from working evenings or nights should that become the preceptor's schedule. In either case, the faculty member needs to assess the situation and determine if an unmanageable and unworkable preceptor/student relationship exists.

The expected outcomes of the student's individual preceptorial experience need to be based on sound educational principles. These principles should, in turn, be used by the faculty in making a final determination as to whether or not the student needs to be placed with a different preceptor. If the conflict cannot be resolved in a timely fashion, then the student needs to be reassigned to another preceptor and possibly to another agency. The faculty member, however, should use caution when assessing whether a personality conflict truly exists between the preceptor and the students. Students have been known to cite personality conflicts with a preceptor when, in fact, the real problem is the student's poor clinical performance as evaluated by the preceptor.

---

## EXAMPLE
## Preceptorial Experience in the Senior Year of a Baccalaureate Program

The preceptorial experience, a 15-week (one-semester) course consisting of 270 hours of clinical experience, was designed for senior nursing students who were in the last semester of their baccalaureate program. This teaching strategy was selected because it provided for professional role socialization, independent problem solving in the clinical arena, and exposure to aspects of health care delivery in the health care setting of the students' choice. For example, students were placed in a variety of rural and urban acute or chronic care facilities, the statewide prison health care system, and extended or home health care agencies. Students were free to select a health care facility anywhere within the state or within contiguous counties in bordering states, as long as the School of Nursing held a current contract with the facility.

Once health care facilities were selected, then a preceptor was identified and matched with each student. In turn, each preceptor/student team was assigned to a specific faculty member. No faculty member monitored more than 10 preceptor/student teams. Prior to the start of the preceptorial experience, faculty at the School of Nursing conducted an orientation for preceptors and students. The orientation included:

- the goals of the preceptorial experience,
- the role of the health care agency in which the preceptorial experience was being held,
- the responsibilities of the preceptor, the faculty, and the student,
- the objectives of the preceptorial experience,
- the evaluation process,
- the communication channels to be used, and
- a discussion of common preceptor concerns.

In addition, written materials were provided to all attendees that contained information on all of the issues addressed during the formal orientation; the syllabus for the preceptorial experience; the goals of the preceptorial experience; the evaluation tools; role descriptions; common preceptor questions and their answers; and the names and phone numbers of the preceptors, faculty, and students. The exhibits below provide information on the goals of the preceptorial experience (Exhibit 19–1); the preceptor qualifications (Exhibit 19–2); and the responsibilities of the health care agency, the preceptor, the faculty, and the student (Exhibits 19–3 to 19–6). Following the exhibits, a short situation is provided that demonstrates one possible problem that can occur during the preceptorial experience.

---

**Exhibit 19–1** Goals of the Preceptorial Experience

**The goals of the preceptorial experience are**
1. to provide professional role socialization,
2. to allow for independent problem solving in a specific clinical area, and
3. to provide for exposure to aspects of health care delivery in a setting of the student's choice.

**Exhibit 19–2** Preceptor Qualifications

**Required**
1. current registered nurse license,
2. at least one year of clinical work experience with education at the same or higher level than that of the student,
3. ability to interact with faculty and student and to clarify the preceptor role and the student's learning activities, and
4. maintenance of a student/preceptor ratio of not more than two students per preceptor.

**Highly Recommended**
1. interest in teaching,
2. ability to facilitate the student's role transition from nursing student to staff nurse, and
3. ability to share professional experiences and clinical expertise.

**Exhibit 19–3** Health Care Agency Responsibilities

**The health care agency will**
1. provide the preceptor, an RN, with at least one year of experience, to work with a student throughout the preceptorial experience,
2. ensure that the preceptor and student work within agency guidelines and State Board of Nursing Rules and Regulations,
3. facilitate the accomplishment of student objectives by allowing student access to various health care agency services, and
4. complete all required paperwork, including the State Board of Nursing Preceptor Qualification Record, the agency evaluation form, and a photocopy of each preceptor's nursing license.

**Exhibit 19–4** Preceptor Responsibilities

**The preceptor will**
1. complete the preceptor orientation,
2. orient and socialize the student within the unit and the health care agency (including parking regulations and security measures),
3. collaborate with the student and faculty to develop student learning activities,
4. plan, delegate, and facilitate the student's daily clinical experiences, guided by the objectives of the preceptorial experience,
5. supervise and instruct the student in the clinical area,
6. consult with faculty as needed or desired, and

*continues*

**Exhibit 19–4** continued

> 7. evaluate the student's practice by reviewing the student's objectives, providing ongoing feedback to the student on his or her performance, completing the required course evaluation in collaboration with the faculty and student, discussing the student's progress with the faculty during the weekly visits (or more often if needed), and notifying the faculty of any serious problems or incidents involving the student.

**Exhibit 19–5** Faculty Responsibilities

> **The faculty will**
> 1. initiate a meeting with the student before the preceptorial experience begins for the purpose of information giving and clarification,
> 2. meet with preceptor and student to appraise and approve student objectives and learning activities,
> 3. assist the preceptor by helping to identify learning experiences needed for the individual student, communicating with the preceptor on a weekly basis to discuss student progress, being available by phone or beeper for consulting during the student's clinical time, participating in the evaluation process, being a resource and support person, and guiding the preceptor in his or her role, and
> 4. evaluate the experiences of the preceptorial experience.

**Exhibit 19–6** Student Responsibilities

> **The student will**
> 1. engage in the preceptorial experience during the work hours of the preceptor,
> 2. be on time for clinical, wearing appropriate attire,
> 3. write personal enabling objectives in collaboration with the faculty and preceptor, revising them as needed,
> 4. show flexibility and willingness to learn,
> 5. discuss own strengths and limitations with preceptor and faculty,
> 6. accept responsibility for own learning in the clinical agency,
> 7. assume increasing responsibility for clinical activities on the selected unit under the supervision of the preceptor,
> 8. seek assistance from preceptor with skills as needed, and
> 9. maintain a daily log for evaluation of objectives.

**Situation**

A faculty member, Dr. J. Lane, visits a senior nursing student, Ms. Brown, in a rural hospital. The faculty member spends 30 minutes conversing with the student on her progress but fails to validate the student's assessment with the preceptor. The preceptor becomes upset and believes that the faculty member does not appropriately acknowledge her role.

*Problem:* Lack of understanding of role responsibilities of the preceptor on the part of the faculty.

*Expected outcome:* Role clarification of the preceptor role on the part of the faculty.

## NOTES

1. J. Nordgren et al., A Collaborative Preceptor Model for Clinical Teaching of Beginning Nursing Students, *Nurse Educator* 23, no. 3 (1998):27–32.

2. V. Lambert and C. Lambert, Role Theory and Effective Role Acquisition in the Health Care System, in *Nursing Issues in Leading and Managing Change*, ed. J. Lancaster (St. Louis: Mosby, 1999), 171–191.

3. L. Ferguson, Preceptors Enhance Students' Self-Confidence, *Nursing Connections* 9, no. 1 (1996):49–61.

4. O. Yonge, Assessing and Preparing Students for Distance Preceptorship Placement, *Journal of Advanced Nursing* 25, no. 4 (1997):812–816.

5. A. Mundy, Motivating Staff Nurses To Serve As Clinical Preceptors, *Nursing Management* 28, no. 6 (1997):66.

6. M. Oermann, A Study of Preceptor Roles in Clinical Teaching, *Nursing Connections* 9, no. 1 (1996):49–61.

## SUGGESTED READING

Barrett, C., and F. Myrick. 1998. Job satisfaction in preceptorship and its effect on the clinical performance of the preceptee. *Journal of Advanced Nursing* 27, no. 2:364–399.

Byrd, C. et al. 1997. Student and preceptor perceptions of factors in a successful learning partnership. *Journal of Professional Nursing* 13, no. 6:344–351.

Lambert, V., and C. Lambert. Role theory and effective role acquisition in the health care system. In *Nursing Issues in Leading and Managing Change*, ed. J. Lancaster (St. Louis: Mosby, 1999):171–191.

LeGris, J. et al. 1997. Collaborative partners in nursing education: A preceptorship model for BScN students. *Nursing Connections* 10, no. 1:55–70.

Nehls, N. et al. 1997. The preceptor model of clinical instruction: The lived experiences of students, preceptors, and faculty-of-record. *Journal of Nursing Education* 36, no. 5:220–227.

Schoener, L. et al. 1996. Faculty: The driving force in preceptorship. *Nursing Connections* 9, no. 3: 37–42.

# CHAPTER 20

# Mentorship

*Laurie Jowers Taylor*

## DEFINITION AND PURPOSES

Mentorship is a form of socialization for professional roles. It entails a relationship in which the mentor works closely with the protégé for purposes of teaching, guiding, supporting, and developing that individual. It is a "teaching strategy in which competencies of a scientific nature are promoted."[1] It is a supportive and nurturing relationship between an expert and a novice.[2] Over time, the relationship between the mentor and the protégé becomes mutually supportive and may evolve into a peer relationship. It is important to note that mentoring is not a panacea, but rather a method for promoting professional development.[3] Mentorship is different from preceptorship because it goes beyond teaching and role modeling. It is a dynamic, noncompetitive, nurturing relationship that promotes independence, autonomy, and self-actualization.[4]

A *mentor* is an individual who takes a personal interest in assisting an individual over a period of time to develop the knowledge and skills needed to realize the protégé's full potential and major life goals. The mentor guides the protégé through both formal and informal structures of the organization. Belcher and Sibbald coined the term *co-mentor*—a peer usually the same age and with similar experience but with expertise in a different area.[5] They also discuss the term *team mentoring*, where two people work together for the purpose of achieving a common goal. Each person has unique expertise in an area that contributes to accomplishment of the common goal. A *protégé* is an individual who willingly enters into a relationship with a mentor and accepts the help and support offered by the mentor.

Mentor behaviors are those engaged in by the mentor, which may include some or all of the following: (1) teaching new skills and promoting intellectual development; (2) serving as a guide to acquaint the junior individual with the values, customs, and resources of the profession; (3) being an exemplar for the junior individual to emulate; (4) providing counseling and moral support during times of stress; (5) fostering personal development by believing in the junior person; (6) supporting and facilitating the junior person's life dreams and goals; and (7) sponsoring the person for advancement.[6] In addition to filling roles of protector, advisor, and guide, the mentor serves subroles such as teacher, sponsor, host/ guide, counselor, and exemplar providing a standard of excellence.

In essence, mentors socialize the neophyte nurses to the norms and expectations of their own role. The mentoring relationship has been referred to as "the gray gorilla syndrome."[7] Gray gorilla refers to characteristics of the silverback primate, who serves as a leader-teacher-preceptor-role-model for his group.

The richness and value of mentoring relationships are important in the development of young professionals. For example, as the gray gorilla teaches and advises, the neophyte gains knowledge and assessment skills; as the gray gorilla models, the neophyte gains competency and confidence; as the gray gorilla coaches and guides, the neophyte gains problem-solving and decision-making skills; as the gray gorilla facilitates and counsels additionally, the neophyte gains communication and collaborative skills; as the gray gorilla inspires and influences, the neophyte gains humanistic values and creative ideas; and as the gray gorilla motivates and leads, the neophyte gains leadership skills and becomes a gray gorilla.

The quality of patient care is generally improved in settings with mentors. Units with a mentor are usually observed to be quieter and more efficiently organized and to provide a more therapeutic environment than those without a gray gorilla. In addition, nurses who had the support and guidance of mentors report greater self-actualization, more job satisfaction, better peer relationships, and less stress than those without mentors.[8]

## THEORETICAL RATIONALE

Role theory, including socialization, provides the framework for predicting how individuals will perform in given roles—in this case, the mentor and protégé roles. "Role theory represents a collection of concepts and a variety of hypothetical formulations that predict how actors will perform in a given role, or under what circumstances certain types of behaviors can be expected."[9] Role is viewed as stemming from interaction with actors in a social system. Roles are ongoing processes and are dynamic rather than static.

Roles are learned through the socialization process. Socialization may be viewed as "an interactional and reciprocal process in which the socializee (protégé) and socializer (mentor) are mutually influenced."[10] Socialization is defined by Brim as a "process by which persons acquire the knowledge, skills, and dispositions that make them more or less able members of their society." According to Brim, one learns role expectations and role behavior through the process of socialization.[11] As a primary agent of socialization and as a member of the protégé's support system, the mentor contributes to successful role development.

## CONDITIONS

The mentoring system is appropriate in any setting where individuals are exposed to new role expectations. It is also appropriate as a steppingstone for new graduates who have had the opportunity to participate in a preceptorship or internship experience. The mentorship model differs from the preceptorship or internship model primarily in intensity, duration, and purpose. Although a preceptorship experience may last for a specified length of time (such as an orientation to a particular unit), the mentor-protégé relationship may span several years or even a lifetime. In addition, the mentor-protégé relationship may be more intense than a preceptorship experience. Mentorship is more than guidance; it is a relationship in which the mentor helps the protégé set goals and standards and develop skills; protects the protégé from others in such a way that allows room for risk and failure; facilitates the protégé's successful entry into academic and professional circles; and affords the protégé an opportunity to reach self-actualization in a leadership role.[12] Mentorship varies depending on the stage of career development, the organization and the setting, and the profession.[13]

## TYPES OF LEARNERS

This strategy is most appropriate for those individuals assuming new role responsibilities or for those who are interested in facilitating their professional growth and development.

## RESOURCES

Mentoring may occur at any time or in any setting. It may involve time spent in the actual work setting or it may involve collaboration on a project such as a research study or a committee assignment. No specific equipment is necessary. The only requirements are human resources—two individuals committed to working together for the purpose of advancing the development of the protégé. Both the mentor and the protégé must actively participate and contribute in order to ensure a successful relationship. Additionally, institutional and collegial support is necessary to promote a positive, productive relationship between the mentor and protégé. Stachura and Hoff maintain that a formal mentoring program requires active participation and equal responsibility shared by the mentor and protégé, as well as institutional and collegial support.[14]

## USING THE METHOD

A mentor-protégé relationship often may evolve from a close working relationship with another individual; however, this situation is not always the case. It is certainly appropriate to ask an individual to serve as a mentor. This request may be difficult for people who fear rejection. It is important, however, to remember that most people will be highly flattered to be asked to serve as a mentor.

When considering a mentor, criteria should be used as a guideline for selection. Findings from research studies indicate that the ability to master concepts and ideas, as well as possessing integrity, professional values, and trustworthiness, are important qualities of the mentor.[15] Mentors are usually selected by the protégé, although the reverse may occur. Only a few individuals are lucky enough to fall into a mentor-protégé relationship. Therefore, it is vital that one intentionally seek a mentor who can contribute to one's professional development. It is a voluntary relationship based on trust, compatibility, mutuality, and personal attraction.

In describing the mentor, Bova and Phillips note that: "Mentors are those who practice most of the following principles: try to understand, shape and encourage the dreams of their protégés; often give their blessing on the dreams and goals of their protégés; provide opportunities for their protégés to observe and participate in their work by inviting their protégés to work with them; and teach their protégés the policies of 'getting ahead' in the organization."[16] Vance explored mentor relationships among nursing leaders. Specific help provided by the mentors included career advice, guidance, promotion, professional role modeling, intellectual and scholarly stimulation, inspiration and idealism, teaching, advising, and tutoring.[17]

Madison conducted a descriptive study to explore the general characteristics of mentoring relationships and their effects on professional lives as perceived by nurse administrators.[18] Ninety-seven percent attributed changes in their professional/personal lives to the mentoring relationship. Seventy-four percent noted a change in self-confidence as a result of the relationship, and fifty-six percent attributed self-actualization to the mentoring relationship. The following positive outcomes of the relationship were reported: enhanced global thinking, being treated as a human being, development of risk-taking behaviors, increased self-esteem, professional skill development, job enrichment and expansion, a check and balance of ideas, role-modeling, research expertise, human relationship knowledge and skills, recognition in the organization, goal changes, power, political awareness, and improved performance as managers.

Three major responsibilities of the protégé are (1) initiating—seeking and asking for advice/assistance, (2) sharing—openly sharing goals and needs, and (3) listening.[19] When looking for a mentor, it is vital to make one's goals known and to seek high visibility. Asking others for advice or help will let them know that their opinions are valued. A potential mentor will respond by commenting on one's work and being appreciative of one's efforts. One can test this potential mentor-protégé relationship by following up with a dialogue with this person. A major consideration when choosing a mentor is to make sure that the mentor fits with one's sense of self. Hall and Sandler offer some helpful suggestions when seeking a mentor:

- Introduce yourself and make the first contact with a professional subject.
- Ask for help regarding the strengths and weaknesses of your work.
- Try to become a research or teaching assistant, junior collaborator, proposal writer, intern, or other type of apprentice; this will provide the opportunity to demonstrate your abilities and commitment.
- Ask a colleague to mention you or your work to a potential mentor.
- Volunteer to serve on a task force, committee, or project where your potential mentor is also a member.
- Invite your potential mentor to be a guest lecturer in your class or before a campus group.[20]

The optimal situation is that the mentor-protégé relationship be (1) mutually established (i.e., both individuals volunteer to participate), (2) consist of career functions such as coaching, sponsorship, and exposure, (3) consist of psychosocial functions such as promotion of sense of competence and clarity of identity, and (4) consist of phases of the relationship and exist for a significant period.[21] Many times, however, all of these attributes may not be present. For example, in some settings, mentors are assigned. This does not mean that a significant relationship with positive outcomes cannot occur. A mentor-protégé relationship may not meet all of the criteria noted previously, especially when considering the necessity of a voluntary commitment by both parties and length of the relationship. An assigned relationship, however, can easily develop into a more intense mentor-protégé relationship.

## POTENTIAL PROBLEMS

The mentor-protégé relationship provides the opportunity for both personal and professional growth. As Rogers has noted: "The degree to which I can create relationships which facilitate the growth of others as separate persons is a measure of the growth I have achieved myself."[22]

Although mentoring is perceived as a very positive concept, it has the potential to be deleterious. For example, the mentor may be overprotective or too controlling, stifling the protégé's creativity and innovation. Exploitation is another potential problem related to the mentor-protégé relationship. The mentor may only want a protégé for self-serving reasons. Holloran investigated leadership experience of 274 nursing executives in hospitals throughout the United States.[23] When the mentor-protégé relationship did not work, the three most frequently occurring themes reported were overpossessive behavior, rejection of the protégé, and misuse of power.

The mentorship example that follows shows the status of mentorship among nursing faculty and a faculty member's personal encounter with mentorship.

# EXAMPLE
# A Mentoring Relationship

*Barbara Fuszard*

Every mentor-protégé dyad is unique. This relationship began at the end of the future protege's master's program in nursing administration. The director of the program made herself available to all students, took a personal interest in them, and had the background to serve as a mentor in many roles. She had been an educator, had published extensively, and had held a variety of administrative roles, so she understood well the positions into which her students were moving.

The protégé accepted a position as nurse administrator in a complex situation and soon called on the mentor to offer staff development workshops and personal consultation to her in this new situation. The assistance was given readily, and although no words of mentor-protégé commitment were spoken, a bond began to form.

The protégé returned to school for doctoral study, and the mentor become co-advisor for her doctoral study and dissertation. During the doctoral study, the mentor offered the protégé an opportunity to be graduate teaching assistant, teaching master's students in nursing administration through the case method. The protégé was introduced to group and committee work of graduate faculty, an experience she had not yet had. On occasion, both mentor and protégé attended national conventions together. At a meeting of the Council on Graduate Education for Administration in Nursing (CGEAN), the protégé "rubbed elbows" with educators from all over the country who taught nursing administration at the graduate level. A lifelong interest in nursing administration education began to germinate.

Both protégé and mentor had strong personalities. The relationship had bumpy times when the protégé felt dominated or the mentor felt that the protégé was not using her talents. One of the sensitive areas was related to progress on the dissertation. The mentor remembered her own experience of completing her doctorate after age 60 and was determined that this situation would not occur with the protégé.

Trust was established during a National League for Nursing convention. During a meeting of the House of Delegates, the protégé sat reading handouts she had obtained from salespersons at the exhibits. Her mentor scolded abruptly, saying she should be paying attention to the debates she came to hear. The protégé, normally schooled to respect authority, burst out angrily, "I have heard this debate three times in the last three days and nothing has changed. Their discussion is circular." The mentor was silent for a short time, and then said, "You're right." After this incident, the mentor would ask the protégé why she made a decision before she challenged it, and the protégé felt more comfortable about asking and discussing issues with the mentor.

The mentor-protégé relationship became collegial and friendly over the years. Discussions could be heated, but the protégé always felt support from her mentor. Positions in service and in education continued over the years for the protégé, and the mentor retired from her formal job. The mentor never stopped caring for or assisting her graduates. She continued her round of consultations and workshops for the benefit of all of them, including this protégé.

The mentor introduced the protégé to the discipline of writing. The mentor was editor of a national newsletter and permitted the protégé to write a regular column, an activity that continued for eight years. This activity eventually led to the protégé becoming editor of that newsletter.

After 20 years of the relationship, the mentor permitted the protégé also to become a gray gorilla, mentoring her own graduate students. A typical behavior of the mentor occurred when the protégé was faced with a difficult decision about whether to move to another position. The mentor, although on a fixed income, flew across the country "to be with you and support you while you make your decision." The new gray gorilla has yet to make such a self-sacrificing action for her protégés, but she plans to do so.

---

## NOTES

1. J.J. Fitzpatrick and I.L. Abraham, Toward the Socialization of Scholars and Scientists, *Nurse Educator* 12, no. 3 (May/June 1987):23–25.

2. B.H. Owens, C.A. Herrick, and J.A. Kelley, A Prearranged Mentorship Program: Can It Work Long Distance? *Journal of Professional Nursing* 14, no. 2 (1998):78–84.

3. C.O. Presholdt, Modern Mentoring: Strategies for Developing Contemporary Nursing Leadership (review), *Nursing Administration Quarterly* 15, no. 1 (1990):20–27.

4. Presholdt, Modern Mentoring.

5. A. Belcher and G. Sibbald, Mentoring: The Ultimate Professional Relationships, *Ostomy Wound Management* 44, no. 4 (1998):76–88.

6. D.J. Levison, *The Seasons of a Man's Life* (New York: Ballantine Books, 1978).

7. S.H. Pyles and P.N. Stern, Discovery of Nursing Gestalt in Critical Care Nursing: The Importance of the Gray Gorilla Syndrome, *Image: The Journal of Nursing Scholarship* 15, no. 2 (1983):51–57.

8. Pyles and Stern, Gray Gorilla Syndrome.

9. M.E. Conway, Theoretical Approaches to the Study of Roles, in *Role Theory: Perspectives for Health Professionals*, eds. M.E. Hardy and M.E. Conway (Norwalk, CT: Appleton & Lange, 1988), 63–72.

10. B.A. Hurley, Socialization for Roles, in *Role Theory: Perspectives for Health Professionals*, eds. M.E. Hardy and M.E. Conway (New York: Appleton-Century-Crofts, 1988), 29–72.

11. O.G. Brim, Jr., Socialization through the Life Cycle, in *Socialization after Childhood: Two Essays*, eds. O.G. Brim and S. Wheeler (New York: John Wiley & Sons, 1966), 3–49.

12. A.M. Valadez and C.A. Lund, Mentorship, Maslow and Me, *Journal of Continuing Education in Nursing* 24, no. 6 (1993):259–263.

13. E.A. Rankin, Mentor, Mentee, Mentoring: Building Career Development Relationships, *Nursing Connections* 4, no. 4 (1991):49–57.

14. L.M. Stachura and J. Hoff, Toward Achievement of Mentoring for Nurses, *Nursing Administration* 15, no. 1 (1990): 56-62.

15. L.J. Taylor, A Survey of Mentor Relationships in Academe, *Journal of Professional Nursing* 8, no. 1 (1992):48–55.

16. B.M. Bova and R.R. Phillips, The Mentoring Relationship as an Educational Experience, ERIC Doc. 2249: 224–244.

17. C. Vance, The Mentor Connection, *The Journal of Nursing Education* 12, no. 4 (1973):7–13.

18. J. Madison, The Value of Mentoring in Nursing Leadership: A Descriptive Study, *Nursing Forum* 29, no. 4 (1994):16–22.

19. R. Klaus, Formalized Mentor Relationships for Management and Executive Development Programs in the Federal Government, *Public Administration Review* 41, no. 4 (1981):489–496.

20. R.M. Hall and B.R. Sandler, Academic Mentoring for Women Students and Faculty: A New Look at an Old Way To Get Ahead, ERIC Doc. 240891 (1983):240–291.

21. L. Yoder, Mentoring: A Concept Analysis, *Nursing Administration Quarterly* 15, no. 1 (1990):9–19.

22. C. Rogers, The Characteristics of a Helping Relationship, *Personnel and Guidance Journal* 37 (1958):6–16.

23. S.D. Holloran, Mentoring: The Experience of Nursing Service Executives, *Journal of Nursing Administration* 23, no. 2 (1993):49–54.

## SUGGESTED READING

Alvarez, A., and K. Abriam-Yago. 1993. Mentoring undergraduate ethnic-minority students: A strategy for retention. *Journal of Nursing Education* 32, no. 5:230–232.

Arnoldussen, B. 1990. The mentor perspective. *Nursing Administration Quarterly* 15, no. 1:28–31.

Atkins, S., and A. Williams. 1995. Registered nurses' experiences of mentoring, undergraduate nursing students. *Journal of Advanced Nursing* 21:1006–1015.

Baldwin, D., and J. Wold. 1993. Students from disadvantaged backgrounds: Satisfaction with a mentor-protégé relationship. *Journal of Nursing Education* 32, no. 5:225–226.

Banoub-Baddour, S., and L.T. Gien. 1991. Student-faculty joint authorship: Mentorship in publication. *Canadian Journal of Nursing Research* 23, no. 1:5–14.

Belcher, A.E. 1997. Beyond preceptorships: Internships, apprenticeships, mentorships. In *The role of the preceptor. A guide to nurse educators and clinicians,* ed. J. Flynn, 119–137. New York: Springer Publishing.

Boyle, C., and S.K. James. 1994. Nursing leaders as mentors: How are we doing? *Nursing Administration Quarterly* 15, no. 1:44–48.

Cahill, H. 1996. A qualitative analysis of student nurses' experiences of mentorship. *Journal of Advanced Nursing* 24:791–799.

Caine, R.M. 1994. Empowering nurses through mentoring. *MedSurg Nursing* 3, no. 1:59–61.

Caine, R.M. 1990. Mentoring: Nurturing the critical care nurse. *Focus on Critical Care* 17, no. 6:452–456.

Campbell, G. 1998. Mentorship—a life long learning commitment: Standing on a firm foundation. *AACN News* 15, no.2:2.

Carey, S.J., and S.T. Campbell. 1994. Preceptor, mentor, and sponsor roles. Creative strategies for nurse retention. *Journal of Nursing Administration* 24, no.12:39–48.

Carlson, K. 1993. Evolutions: Open doors. *Journal of Post Anesthesia Nursing* 8, no. 6:435–436.

Chandler, G.E. 1993. The RN mentor program: An exercise in leadership. *NLN Publications* (14-2511):339–354.

Colling K., T. Grabo, M. Rowe, and J. Straneva. 1998. How To Develop and Sustain a Peer Mentored Work Group. *Journal of Professional Nursing* 14, no. 5:298–304.

Cooper, M.D. 1990. Mentorship: The key to the future of professionalism in nursing. *Journal of Perinatal and Neonatal Nursing* 4, no. 3:71–77.

Davidhizer, R. 1993a. Mentoring nursing students to write. *Journal of Nursing Education* 32, no. 6:280–282.

Davidhizer, R. 1993b. Self-care and mentors to reduce stress and enhance administrative ability. *Geriatric Nursing* 14, no. 3:146–149.

Davies, E. 1993. Clinical role modeling: Uncovering hidden knowledge. *Journal of Advanced Nursing* 18, no. 4:627–636.

DeMarco, R. 1993. Mentorship: A feminist critique of current research. *Journal of Advanced Nursing* 18, no. 8:1242–1250.

deTournyay, R. 1990. Setting limits (editorial). *Journal of Nursing Education* 29, no. 3:101.

Ellis, H. 1993. Teaching roles in critical care—The mentor and preceptor. *Intensive and Critical Care Nursing* 9, no. 3:152–156.

Fields, W.L. 1991. Mentoring in nursing: A historical approach. *Nursing Outlook* 39, no. 6:257–261.

Fox, W.J. et al. 1992. The mentoring relationship. *AORN Journal* 56, no. 5:858–867.

Grossman, M. 1993. Mentorship: Bonds that strengthen professions (editorial). *Canadian Journal of Nursing Research* 25, no. 3:7–13.

Haas, S.A. 1992. Coaching: Developing key players. *Journal of Nursing Administration* 22, no. 6:54–58.

Hockenberry-Eaton, M. 1992. Nursing research—Moving forward through networking, collaboration and mentorship. *Journal of Pediatric Oncology Nursing* 9, no. 3:132–135.

Joel, L.A. 1997. Charged to mentor (editorial). *American Journal of Nursing* 97, no. 2:7.

Jowers, L.T., and K. Herr. 1992. A review of literature on mentor-protégé relationships (review). *NLN Publications* (15-2339):49–77.

Lenkman, S. 1992. Mentoring in nursing administration. *Aspen's Advisor for Nurse Executives* 7, no. 11:5–8.

Levi, P.C., and A. Marriner-Tomey. 1991. Visiting professor mentorship. *Nurse Educator* 16, no. 3:11, 22, 30.

Maggs, E. 1994. Mentorship in nursing and midwifery education: Issues for research. *Nurse Education Today*. 14:22–29.

Mansour, M. 1991. Multiple mentoring strategy in the academic preparation of quality assurance directors. *Nursing Connections* 4, no. 2:53–61.

Marshall, C. 1993. Mentorship in critical care. *British Journal of Theatre Nursing* 2, no. 11:22–23.

Mills, J. 1991. The nurse manager as mentor. *Pediatric Nursing* 17, no. 5:493.

Orth, C.D. et al. 1990. The manager's role as coach and mentor. *Journal of Nursing Administration* 20, no. 9:11–15.

Parker, D. 1992. Mentoring concepts applied to clinical practice (review). *Gastroenterology Nursing* 15, no. 1:35–39.

Phippen, M.L. 1993. My orthopedic mentor (editorial). *Seminars in Perioperative Nursing* 2, no. 2:vi–viii.

Rawl, S.M., and L.M. Peterson. 1992. Nursing education administrators: Level of career development and mentoring. *Journal of Professional Nursing* 8, no. 3:161–169.

Rempusheski, V.F. 1992. A researcher as resource, mentor, and preceptor. *Applied Nursing Research* 5, no. 2:105–107.

Ryan, D., and K. Brewer. 1997. Mentorship and professional role development in undergraduate nursing education. *Nurse Educator* 22, no. 6:20–24.

Shaw, L.A. 1997. Mentoring APRN Students. *Nursing Spectrum* (Washington, D.C./Baltimore Metro edition) 7, no. 23:12.

Sidani, S. 1991. Mentoring the novice nurse researcher. *Journal of Pediatric Nursing* 6, no. 1:57–59.

Simpson, R.L. 1990. Contemporary leadership begins with mentoring (editorial). *Nursing Administration Quarterly* 15, no. 1:ix–xi.

Sorrell, J.M. 1992. Ethics of writing in nursing: Responsible mentorship. *Nursing Connections* 5, no. 4:67–71.

Sorrell, J.M., and H.N. Brown. 1991. Mentoring students in writing: "Gourmet express" versus "fast food service." *Journal of Nursing Education* 30, no. 6:284–286.

Stachura, L.M., and J. Hoff. 1990. Toward achievement of mentoring for nurses. *Nursing Administration Quarterly* 15, no. 1:56–62.

Sundwick, K. 1993. It could make a difference. *Gastroenterology Nursing* 16, no. 3:97–98.

Vance, C., and R.K. Olson. 1998. *The mentor connection in nursing.* New York: Springer Publishing.

White, L.M. 1990. The mentee perspective. *Nursing Administration Quarterly* 15, no. 1:32–35.

Woodron, P. 1994. Mentorship: Perceptions and pitfalls for nursing practice. *Journal of Advanced Nursing* 19:812–818.

Yates, P., J. Cunningham., W. Moyle, and J. Wollin. 1957. Peer mentorship in clinical education: Outcomes of a pilot program for first year students. *Nurse Education Today* 17, 6:508–514.

# PART VI

# Clinical Teaching

Clinical teaching is one of the most significant features of nursing education. Chapters in Part VI are introduced by philosophical underpinnings that should guide each instructor, and then are concluded by issues and cautionary suggestions for faculty. The clinical teaching chapters evolve through introductory skills lab and address complex situations such as literacy and the fluid community environment. Critical thinking and the development of higher-order thinking are key components of the chapter on concept mapping.

# CHAPTER 21

# Philosophical Approaches to Clinical Instruction

*Martha J. Bradshaw*

## INTRODUCTION

The purpose of clinical instruction is to give the student opportunities to bridge didactic information with the realities of nursing practice. In guided situations, students blend theoretical knowledge with experiential learning, in order to effect a synthesis and understanding of those endeavors known collectively as *nursing*. Clinical learning is directed by a nurse educator who operationalizes his or her practical knowledge about teaching. Through use of this practical knowledge, the instructor translates a formal curriculum into active engagement with students.[1] Clinical instruction has become more challenging because of changes in the health care environment and the need for health professionals to fulfill increasingly diverse roles. Instructors need to examine their personal philosophy (underlying beliefs) about teaching, especially considering the changes in traditional models of clinical learning. Managed care, change in patient acuity, and the transition from hospital-based to community-based care have impacted on the way we need to prepare nurses for future practice.[2]

## ROLE OF THE CLINICAL INSTRUCTOR

In the clinical setting, the teacher guides the students in applying theory to patient care. The faculty role in clinical instruction is as diverse and demanding as are the settings. The instructor is expected to be competent, experienced, knowledgable, flexible, patient, and energetic. The instructor should be capable of balancing structure with spontaneity. Paterson[3] describes two approaches to clinical instruction: *task mastery* and *professional-identity mentoring*. Task mastery instruction is based on the instructor's decisions about what behaviors and ways of thinking are important for nurses and, therefore, need to be reproduced in students. In essence, nursing instructors are gatekeepers, allowing students to enter the profession once they have demonstrated their ability. With the professional-identity approach, the instructor serves as a mentor, guiding students in decision making and inculcation of hallmarks of professional practice. Whereas no one perspective is "right" or ideal, the perspective used by the instructor determines approaches to teaching and clinical supervision and, therefore, affects student outcomes.

The successful student clinical experience—measured in terms of learning outcomes and an internalized sense of fulfillment—is largely influenced by the types of assignments the instructor provides. The planning and selection of these assignments, as well as actual teaching, are value-laden and reflect the faculty member's philosophical approach to clinical learning. Furthermore, the role or roles the instructor chooses to fulfill influence selection of student activities. The roles in which individual instructors see themselves may include interaction with students, serving as a role model, or functioning as an expert reference. Roles that students see as important for clinical instructors to hold have been identified as resource, evaluator, encourager, promoter of patient care, and benevolent presence.[4] Once this self-image is determined, teachers consciously or subconsciously shape situations that enable them to enact their various roles. This action enhances teacher effectiveness because the instructor is most comfortable in fulfilling preselected roles.

In addition to self-image, other personal attributes influence the instructor's thinking regarding student assignments. There is some indication that background knowledge and preferences for orientation to practice strongly influence planning and decision making by teachers.[5] Therefore, an instructor with a concrete, structured practice background (such as surgical nursing) may select or plan patient assignments that are more structured than those selected by an instructor from a less structured background (such as psychiatric nursing). The potential conflict exists between teacher and student regarding learning and practice preferences. With careful planning and collaboration with the students, the clinical instructor can best shape the learning situations to meet students' needs.[6]

## FOUNDATIONS FOR SELECTION OF CLINICAL ACTIVITIES

Another philosophical perspective that governs clinical learning is the instructor's view of the *purpose* of the clinical learning experience. The three most common purposes are for students to (1) apply theoretical concepts, (2) experience actual patient situations, and (3) see and implement professional roles. Based on the chosen perspective, the instructor selects the agency or unit and plans the type of clinical assignment that is best suited for the identified purpose. The realism of clinical activities brings added benefit to any of the three types of experiences.

The planning and supervising of clinical learning call for the instructor's own philosophical stance to be blended with the selected goal(s) of the clinical experience. Student assignments may have one of the following goals:

- Learn the **patient**: provide one-to-one total care
- Learn the **content area**: practice a variety of care activities in one setting
- Learn **role(s)**: function as a staff or team member, as a practitioner, administrator, or other selected roles

Assignments can be based on theories of action:

- **People-centered**: interpersonal interaction systems
- **Health**: promotion, maintenance, functioning
- **Nature of practice milieu**: decision making, leadership, collaboration[7]

The instructor who selects a student focus for clinical assignments may value empowerment as part of his or her philosophical approach to teaching. The aims of this approach are the cultivation of responsibility, authority, and accountability in novice practitioners.[8] Selected clinical activities directed toward empowerment could include:

- **Analytic nursing**: use of actual experiences (instructor or student based) to define and solve problems
- **Change activities**: develop planned change and identify resources to effect this change
- **Collegiality**: professional interactions (instructor-student, student-student, student-staff) to solve problems and promote optimal care
- **Sponsorship**: Collaboration and interaction with preceptors, administration; analysis of bureaucratic system[9]

Within the framework of the assignment, the instructor then makes decisions about which activities will enhance learning outcomes. This process again reflects the teacher's values, beliefs about how learning should take place, and how teacher role fulfillment will influence this learning. For example, the instructor who values participatory learning and role-modeling will be actively involved in many aspects of the student's activities, and his or her presence will be felt by the student—at the bedside or interacting with staff members. Purdon points out that such role-modeling has positive benefits for students, such as reducing fears and seeing effective communications.[10] The instructor who wishes to foster independence in students may take on the role of resource person and become centrally available to students as needed. The instructor who places emphasis on organization and task accomplishment will oversee numerous student activities and facilitate completion of the assignments within a designated period. Many instructors value all of these activities as a part of student learning. To accomplish all of these activities calls for a great deal of diversity and planning by the teacher.

Some philosophical approaches to teaching and role assumption by educators are more subtle, yet promote more complex, higher-order learning. More specifically, the teacher who values empowerment and accountability in students will take on a less directive role and assume one that is more enabling. The instructor who wishes to promote independence in students must be willing to release a certain amount of control, in order to give freedom for students to learn and grow.

Periodic, timely feedback is essential. Students can only recognize strengths and areas for improvement when they are given objective, constructive feedback. Feedback should be not only evaluative but also encouraging to bolster confidence and independence. Augustine[11] investigated feedback by clinical instructors and discovered that, in addition to group feedback, such as in conferences or orientation, students felt the need for personal feedback from the instructor until they were certain what the instructor wanted from them. This need indicates not only the value of the instructor as a guide but also the emphasis students place on feedback for clinical success or failure.

Dimensions of feedback given by instructors reflect the instructor's philosophy and teaching style. Augustine[12] found that instructors are less likely to give positive feedback in the patient's room than elsewhere, and instructors give a high amount of cautionary or negative feedback during procedures. These findings exemplify the gatekeeping role of the instructor, with a more negative quality to feedback.

## CLINICAL ACTIVITIES AND PROBLEM SOLVING

The instructor who promotes problem-solving abilities in students fashions clinical activities to meet this goal. Discovery learning is one way in which student autonomy and problem solving can be enhanced. Students can have experiences where they can realize, or discover, patient responses to certain aspects of care, or how structuring an activity differently is more time-saving. These discoveries boost self-esteem when students see what they have learned on their own, or that they have the ability to resolve certain problematic situations. Discovery learning also has been found to increase student motivation, interest, and retention of learned material.[13] The instructor then is rewarded by seeing growth take place in the students.

Another approach to promoting problem-solving abilities is by placing emphasis on the clinical, or patient, problem, rather than on the clinical setting. Student assignments that take place in familiar, repetitive settings enable students to deal with patients *in that setting*. As Reilly and Oermann point out, nursing practice settings are moving away from acute care environments, and students should be equipped to work with clinical problems in diverse settings. In addition to learning how to deal with clinical problems, students also experience professional socialization through role discontinuity. In making the transition from instructor-directed, structured, familiar assignments to empowering, unstructured, undefined patient problems, students experience new ways of defining their own roles and responsibilities as practitioners.[14]

## STUDENT DEVELOPMENT

The strategy of reciprocal learning not only meets clinical learning needs but promotes collegiality as well.[15] Reciprocal learning usually takes the form of peer teaching, or student-to-student instruction. This learning informally occurs within most clinical groups and can become more purposeful and goal-directed through instructor planning. By pairing students for specific learning activities, the student learner gains information, experience, and insight in new ways. Learners receive individualized, empathetic instruction and may feel more relaxed with a peer than with a faculty teacher. The student teacher also learns about instruction, helping, and working with others. Student teachers also assume the responsibility of role-models and collaborators.[16]

## FACULTY DEVELOPMENT

The powerful influence of the instructor as a person should not be overlooked. Development of an effective clinical instructor and the evolution of a meaningful, positive clinical learning experience are based on insight, planning, and implementation by the faculty member. Therefore, individual teachers need to cultivate an appropriate self-image as a teacher. In addition, the clinical instructor should indulge in periodic self-reflection: Is my own clinical competence being maintained? Are my own views on nursing and the teaching-learning process congruent with student perspectives and needs? Should teaching strategies, types of assignments, or communication skills be revised? The effective faculty member may need to reshape his or her own teaching perspectives to better blend with those perspectives held by the clinical students.

## CONCLUSION

The philosophical approach to teaching is the foundation by which the instructor operationalizes his or her own practical knowledge. The responsibilities for the instructor are great, calling for clinical expertise, role-modeling, and understanding of teaching and learning principles for a variety of students, settings, and clinical experiences.

Carlson-Catalano pointed out that much of the instruction that takes place is related to how the instructor has internalized professional values and developed a self-image as a practitioner and role-model.[17] The clinical instructor is a pivotal person for developing positive or negative self-concepts in students.[18] The instructor who wishes to promote empowerment in students must see himself or herself as empowered to do so. Only then can needed socialization and empowerment take place. The empowered instructor is able to visualize the potential learning opportunities in the clinical environment.[19] The nature of clinical practice has been redefined, as so must the nature of clinical learning experiences.

Faculty members need to adapt to these changes and be willing to give up their "comfort zone" of familiar, yet limited, clinical settings and methods of instruction.[20] Effective clinical instruction emerges from conscious efforts by the instructor. These efforts should be based on background knowledge, strongly formed values, and a well-defined self-image as a nurse teacher. Applying these personal resources enables the teacher to bring about effective clinical instruction. Formal and personal learning outcomes then are achieved.

**NOTES**

1. M. Johnson, Review of Teacher Thinking: A Study of Practical Knowledge, *Curriculum Inquiry* 14, no. 4 (1984):465–468.

2. M.H. Mundt, A Model for Clinical Learning Experiences in Integrated Health Care Networks, *Journal of Nursing Education* 36, no. 7 (1997):309–316.

3. B. Paterson, The View from Within: Perspectives of Clinical Teaching, *International Journal of Nursing Studies* 31, no. 4 (1994):349–360.

4. S. Flagler, S. Loper-Powers, and A. Spitzer, Clinical Teaching Is More Than Evaluation Alone! *Journal of Nursing Education* 27, no. 8 (1988):342–348.

5. D. Yaakobi and S. Sharan, Teacher Beliefs and Practices: The Discipline Carries the Message, *Journal of Education for Teaching* 11, no. 2 (1985):187–199.

6. L. Sutcliffe, An Investigation into Whether Nurses Change Their Learning Style According to Subject Area Studied, *Journal of Advanced Nursing* 18, no. 7 (1993):647–658.

7. D.E. Reilly and M.H. Oermann, *The Clinical Field: Its Use in Nursing Education* (Norwalk, CT: Appleton-Century-Crofts, 1985).

8. M. Manthey, Empowerment for Teachers and Students, *Nurse Educator* 17, no. 1 (1992):6–7.

9. J. Carlson-Catalano, Empowering Nurses for Professional Practice, *Nursing Outlook* 40, no. 3 (1992):139–142.

10. J.E. Purdon, Fear of Persons with HIV Infection: Teaching Strategies for Helping Students Cope, *Journal of Nursing Education* 31, no. 13 (1992):138–139.

11. C.J. Augustine, Dimensions of Feedback in Clinical Nursing Education, *Dissertation Abstracts International*, 54-02A (1992):0433.

12. Augustine, Dimensions of Feedback.

13. S. DeYoung, *Teaching Nursing* (Redwood City, CA: Addison-Wesley, 1990).

14. Reilly and Oermann, *The Clinical Field.*

15. D. Goldenberg and C. Iwasiw, Reciprocal Learning among Students in the Clinical Area, *Nursing Outlook* 17, no. 1 (1992):27–29.

16. Goldenberg and Iwasiw, Reciprocal Learning, 28.

17. Carlson-Catalano, Empowering Nurses, 139.

18. B. Kelly, The Professional Self-Concepts of Nursing Undergraduates and Their Perceptions of Influential Forces, *Journal of Nursing Education* 31, no. 3 (1992):121–125.

19. P.S. Chally, Empowerment through Teaching, *Journal of Nursing Education* 31, no. 3 (1992):117–120.

20. Mundt, A Model for Clinical Learning, 315.

# CHAPTER 22

# Refocusing the Nursing Skills Laboratory

*Glenda F. Hanson*

## DEFINITION AND PURPOSES

Theory-based practice has long been recognized as a key element in the development of nursing science.[1,2,3] Yet, in searching for ways to establish the connections between theory and practice for the undergraduate nursing student, the educator has been both challenged and frustrated.[4] Beginning students are generally given an introductory overview of nursing and its theories; however, application of these theories in clinical practice is often neglected because of emphasis on communication, patient comfort, patient safety, and other areas of immediate concern during early clinical experiences. This situation may lead to the belief that theory is abstract and disconnected from reality and not essential to nursing practice.[5] Additionally, like most forms of learning, the meaningfulness of the theoretical information is diminished as the time between introduction and application is prolonged. The purpose of this chapter is to explore one way to facilitate an early foundation of theory-based practice in the nursing curriculum.

## THEORETICAL RATIONALE

Knowles'[6] model for adult learning provides a framework for education that incorporates principles that value the individual's life experiences. The model promotes a climate that requires openness, collaboration, competence, creativity, and success. Kolb's[7] experiential learning model bases learning on the premise that humans move from concrete experience to abstract conceptualization by a process of experience and experimentation. These educational premises are judged by this author to have elements that are common and compatible with the Science of Unitary Human Beings, as first described by Martha E. Rogers.[8,9] Rogers' theory will be used to provide an example later in this discussion.

While providing learning opportunities, nurse educators are responsible for structuring the environment to provide students with experiences that move them to increasingly higher levels of cognition. By grounding these experiences in nursing theory, the educator is able to promote the concept of theory-based practice.

## CONDITIONS

A theory-based education derives from a theory-based curriculum. The first step in curriculum development is to define and articulate the faculty's beliefs. Nursing theories such as Martha Rogers' Science of Unitary Human Beings provide a basis by which this process may unfold. The beliefs (or concepts) gleaned from the theory provide faculty with the basis from which the curriculum is constructed.[10] Once this basis is established, the curriculum specifics should unfold from this perspective.

Many schools of nursing provide nursing skills laboratory experiences early in the curriculum. Infante[11] states that the purpose of a nursing skills laboratory is to provide a simulation of reality so that "the reality can be better understood, controlled, and practiced." The laboratory allows the student to rehearse the wide range of psychomotor activities used to engage in nursing practice. The contained setting of the campus laboratory thus provides the teacher and learner with early opportunities to apply the ideals of the nursing theories in a low-risk, custom-designed environment. The faculty is responsible for examining the curriculum content and searching for specific strategies to illustrate the flow of practice from its conceptual systems.

## TYPES OF LEARNERS

The typical undergraduate nursing student in skills laboratory experience is beginning or about to begin the first clinical sequence. The student at this point has usually had some exposure to nursing theory but little or no opportunity to apply the theory to nursing practice activities. The focused laboratory allows for the atmosphere to be ordered so that the student understands the focus and objectives of the experience and is able to relate the experience to the overall curriculum objectives. The student should be given the freedom and motivation to set his or her own goals and to assume responsibility for moving from concrete knowledge to the more abstract applications of the knowledge. Structure, guidance, and direction are provided by the educator and accepted by the learner in the spirit of collaboration.

## RESOURCES

The practice of skills in the nursing laboratory often focuses on subjects such as comfort, safety, management of personal hygiene, administration of medications, or health assessment. Skills are practiced in a controlled, simulated setting that allows the student the opportunity to focus on learning without the environmental distractions or constraints of a clinical setting. Available resources are used to provide a sense of realism because the more the experience approximates the practice setting, the more likely it is to bridge the gap between classroom and clinical. Environment is a key concept in nursing practice, and its importance is demonstrated in the educational setting. The laboratory environment may be as simple or as sophisticated as the budget allows.

Laboratory faculty must be grounded in the theory they are seeking to apply. They must be committed to promoting the beliefs and values of the framework in the students and to providing opportunities for developing or patterning students toward the identified objectives. Strategies may include allowing the student to set individual goals, experimenting with various techniques, working in groups, imitating the performance of others, assembling and handling applicable equipment, questioning freely, and/or practicing for proficiency.

## USING THE METHOD

Once the decision is made to use the skills lab as a focal point for nursing theory, the educator begins by examining the environment of congruency with the theoretical framework. For example, self-directed learning is not well represented in a lecture hall with a podium and rows of desks. Neither is holistic nursing care reflected by the use of plastic body parts such as pelvic models to demonstrate urinary catheterization. Attention is given to such aspects as general atmosphere, colors, lighting, ventilation, sounds, sights, teacher-learner ratio, and flow of movement.

Next, the overall structure of the laboratory experience is examined. Freedom and self-direction are impaired by activities that are overly structured and tightly monitored. Strict adherence to checklist criteria and emphasis on testing hamper learners from experimentation, creativity, and setting of individual goals. Although standards of patient comfort and safety must be maintained, students and educators realize that a variety of methods and circumstances may lead to the accomplishment of the stated objectives. One need only examine several nursing textbooks to realize the range of options and interpretations that make up nursing practice.

All lab activities must be framed within the theoretical perspective. Interventions may remain constant between theories, but perspectives will vary. Patient immobility, for example, may be perceived as a self-care deficit or an impairment of human field motion, depending on the view and circumstances. Students must constantly be encouraged to explore and articulate these connections to theory as they move through lab experiences.

## POTENTIAL PROBLEMS

The methods described in this chapter work only when students and faculty collaborate together toward the common goal of excellence in nursing practice.

Some students are ready to flourish in an atmosphere of openness and collaboration. Other students may be more comfortable with structure and rigidly fixed criteria. Likewise, some faculty members may find it difficult to relinquish some of their control over the student experience. The educator remains sensitive and responsive to the differences in readiness that participants bring to the laboratory setting. Faculty members often report that teaching in a nontraditional atmosphere often requires more rather than less energy on their part. Included in the choices available to the students may be the choice of more structure and more prescribed learning. This structure may be in forms such as optional computer activities, additional laboratory time, individual appointments with faculty, supplemental projects, or structured group activities.

## DISCUSSION

The nursing skills laboratory is an environment that is rich with potential. In this setting, educators may find an early focus point to model and articulate theoretical applications through their teaching styles and strategies. Likewise, students may take risks and experiment in ways that might not be appropriate in the clinical setting. Implications are plentiful for any and all activities taking place in the lab, including leadership/management role-playing research, problem solving, critical-thinking exercises, computer-assisted instruction activities, and specifics of care for patients in various stages of living and dying. Limitations exist only in the minds of the participants.

The visionary nurse educator has a responsibility to facilitate the student's transition to the role of professional nurse. Education may be conceptualized as the bridge between the science and the practice of nursing. The professional nurse whose practice flows naturally from a theoretical perspective will be better prepared to meet the challenges of twenty-first-century nursing and beyond. Preparing this professional is the challenge facing the nurse educators of today. The following example illustrates how theory-based practice can be used as a basis for nursing skills laboratory activities.

---

# EXAMPLE
## Toward Theory-Based Practice

*Glenda F. Hanson*

The Science of Unitary Human Beings, as developed by Martha Rogers and others, is used to illustrate how the nursing skills laboratory can facilitate the transfer of theory to practice. A nursing curriculum based on

Rogers' theoretical framework would include an emphasis on the following elements of nursing practice: "the whole person, continuous innovative pattern changes, increasing complexity and diversity, continuous mutual process with the environment, complex and diverse evolution, (and) manifestations of change" (M.E. Rogers, personal communication, 1989). The school using this framework would be philosophically committed to promoting these beliefs and values in students, to providing opportunities for developing or patterning the student toward increasing complexity and diversity, and to fulfilling the role of the professionally educated nurse.

Ways of changing or modifying the environment to meet specific situations have been investigated by researchers within the Rogerian conceptual system. Environmental factors such as motion,[12] color,[13] sound,[14] lighting,[15] and activities[16] have been investigated by Rogerian researchers and have been shown to be associated with a positive direction of human energy flow. It follows that the Rogerian-based laboratory would use this information to create a learning environment that is a pleasant, dynamic, and creative activity center. Research within the framework dictates that the surroundings be colorful, with a predominance of hues from the high end of the color spectrum (blues and violets). Freedom of choice is the hallmark of the system, with students being allowed to select from and move through a variety of activities that would promote their achievement of perceived goals. Guidance from faculty is an available option, and learning in groups is encouraged. Faculty members should consciously maintain their own high-energy level, using mutual process to promote student empowerment. Students are encouraged by verbal and nonverbal cues to develop their own creative and diverse characteristics.

Management of alteration in respiratory pattern manifestations, such as airway obstruction, is a skill that is often taught in nursing laboratories. The following section uses this focus to provide a specific example of applying Rogers' theory in the nursing skills laboratory. The nursing process approach is used to structure the discussion, and terminology is congruent with the theory.

### Assessment

Although "true Rogerian scholars would view physical assessment techniques as particulate and not holistic" (M.C. Rogers, personal communication, 1989), it is maintained that professional nurses should be able to gather information regarding the health of the patient in any way possible, including the use of health assessment skills, tools, and techniques. The focus on assessment provides the educator with an opportunity to articulate the concept of holism, leading into a discussion of the Rogerian concept of the human environmental field. This strategy can be applied to all body systems, but assessment of the respiratory system is selected to provide an example for illustration.

Students focusing on the respiratory system may be led in a discussion of the ways in which data collected are manifestations of the irreducible human being and not just a physiological function of the lung tissue. The meaninglessness of examining a single lung, separate from the human organism, illustrates this point. When led in discussion, students commonly describe how changes in respiratory patterns may reflect agitation or biochemical changes stemming from processes in other body systems, such as diabetes mellitus. Integrality (oneness with the environment) is a key principle within the Rogerian framework, which may be illustrated by providing audio reproduction or peer stimulation of various lung sound. Invariably, students report personal discomfort when listening to sounds of respiratory distress, such as wheezes or stridor, thus allowing the educator to point out the students' own continuous mutual process with the environment.

In addition to typical assessment techniques such as inspection, palpation, percussion, and auscultation, the Rogerian educator may add other manifestations of health such as language patterns, posturing, narrative, photo-disclosure,[17] or sleep patterns.[18] Fragmentation of the assessment process is rejected in favor of a holistic and intuitive exchange with the patient in a continuous mutual process. Students should be reminded often that knowledge of the parts cannot predict the state of the whole.

### Planning

Students who have been led to identify the patient with an alteration in respiratory pattern may be led in conceptualizing the situation in terms of an obstruction of typical motion and energy flow. Information gathered from the assessment process is used to formulate nursing plans for creative and therapeutic interventions. Goals are articulated to reflect the movement of the patient toward increasing diversity and actualization. Short-term goals focus on immediate needs, and long-term goals seek to maximize the potential for restoration of health. The patient with an impaired airway will be expected to have short-term needs for a sense of well-being, healing or optimal functioning, actualization, and creative adjustments to change.

### Intervention

Interventions are selected to meet the appropriately stated, desired outcome of transforming the patient's presentation of blocked motion (air movement). The student caring for this simulated patient should consider interventions designed to pattern or change the patient's environment in a way promoting normal airflow. Techniques considered may include imposed motion, positioning, or altering the environmental field with the strategic introduction of humidity, coolness, sounds, touch, and so forth. It should be pointed out that none of these interventions involve direct manipulation of the anatomically defined respiratory system.

The art of nursing may be presented in case study performance based on patient perceptions, with attention to the stated goals. The student, as an appropriate helping intervention under a given set of circumstances, may select suctioning of the respiratory passages by introduction of a catheter. In this case, the performance of the procedure would be guided by the scientific principles of motion, sterility, anatomy and physiology, pathophysiology, and physics. The technical aspects of the procedure and the care of the (simulated) patient with a respiratory obstruction should evolve naturally and logically, with faculty guidance offered as necessary. The patient's comfort and relaxation would be emphasized through the awareness that the procedure involves the unitary human field, and not just the respiratory tree. Therapeutic touch, imagery, and other techniques to promote patient relaxation should be incorporated into the study of this and other appropriately selected nursing skills.

## Evaluation

Continuous evaluation is vital to both nursing and educational processes. Within the Rogerian framework, evaluation is emphasized in the context of the continuous process of change and diversity. Similar to assessment, evaluation is directed toward the whole or unitary human being. Using the goals as a guide, the nurse focuses on the process of patterning the human and environmental fields. Subjectively, the patient's report of greater comfort, awareness, sense of well-being, and harmony with the environmental field would indicate new pattern development. Objectively, additional data may be gathered by again using the techniques of human environmental field assessment.

Evaluation of student learning performance should be a mutual process between student and faculty, and based on the student's goals. Faculty members are guided by the principles of the selected nursing theory, educational principles, the individual's own expertise, and the standards of practice in nursing. Students completing the process should report feeling secure in their technical clinical preparation, educational growth, and ability to apply nursing theory in the patient setting.

## NOTES

1. A.I. Meleis, *Theoretical Nursing: Development and Progress* (Philadelphia: J.B. Lippincott, 1997).

2. S. Pryjmachuk, A Nursing Perspective on the Interrelationships between Theory, Research, and Practice, in *Philosophical and Theoretical Perspectives for Advanced Nursing Practice*, ed. J.W. Kenney (Boston: Jones & Bartlett, 1999), 289–296.

3. P.H. Walker and R. Redman, Theory-Guided, Evidence-Based Reflective Practice, *Nursing Science Quarterly* 12 (1999):298–303.

4. B.E. Smith, Linking Theory and Practice in Teaching Basic Nursing Skills, *Journal of Nursing Education* 31 (1992):16–23.

5. R.B. Harris, Introduction of a Conceptual Nursing Model into a Fundamental Baccalaureate Course, *Journal of Nursing Education* 2 (1986):66–69.

6. M.S. Knowles, *The Modern Practice of Adult Education* (New York: John Wiley, 1980).

7. D.A. Kolb, *Experiential Learning: Experience as the Source of Learning and Development* (Englewood Cliffs, NJ: Prentice Hall, 1984).

8. M.E. Rogers, Nursing Science and Art: A Prospective, *Nursing Science Quarterly* 1 (1988):99–102.

9. M.E. Rogers, Nursing Science and the Space Age, *Nursing Science Quarterly* 5 (1992):27–34.

10. J.S. Creasia, Theories and Frameworks for Professional Nursing Practice, in *Conceptual Foundations for Professional Nursing Practice*, eds. J.S. Creasia and B. Parker (St. Louis: Mosby, 1996), 140–167.

11. M.S. Infante, *The Clinical Laboratory* (New York: John Wiley, 1985).

12. H.M. Ferrence, The Relationship of Time Experience, Creativity Traits, Differentiation, and Human Field Motion, in *Explorations on Martha Rogers' Science of Unitary Human Beings*, ed. V. Malinski (Norwalk, CT: Appleton-Century-Crofts, 1986), 95–104.

13. B. Ludomirski-Kalmanson, *The Relationship between the Environmental Energy Wave Frequency Pattern Manifest in Red and Blue Light and Human Field Motion in Adults with Visual Sensory Perception and Total Blindness* (Unpublished dissertation, New York University, 1984).

14. M.J. Smith, Human Environment Process: A Test of Rogers' Principle of Integrality, *Advances in Nursing Science* 9 (1986):21–28.

15. S. Thomas, Modeling the Human Environment Encounter (Paper presented at the meeting of the Society for Rogerian Scholars, Southeast Region, Augusta, Georgia, August 17, 1989).

16. S.H. Gueldner, The Relationship between Imposed Motion and Human Field Motion in Elderly Individuals Living in Nursing Homes, in *Explorations on Martha Rogers' Science of Unitary Human Beings*, ed. V. Malinski (Norwalk, CT: Appleton-Century-Crofts, 1986), 161–172.

17. K. Bultemeier, Photo-Disclosure: A Research Methodology for Investigating Unitary Human Beings, in *Patterns of Rogerian Knowing*, ed. M. Madrid (New York: National League for Nursing Press, 1997).

18. J. Watson, Measuring Dreaming as a Beyond Waking Experience in Rogers's Conceptual Model, *Nursing Science Quarterly* 12 (1999):245–250.

## SUGGESTED READING

Madrid, M., ed. 1997. *Patterns of Rogerian knowing.* New York: National League for Nursing Press.

Miracle, D.J. 1999. Teaching psychomotor nursing skills in simulated learning labs: A critical review of the literature. In *Evidence-based teaching: Current research in nursing education*, eds. K.R. Steves and V.R. Cassidy, 71–103. New York: National League for Nursing.

# CHAPTER 23

# Teaching Patients with Low Literacy Skills

*Connie F. Cowan*

## DEFINITION AND PURPOSES

America's literacy problems have been a concern for years, prompting many communities to institute literacy programs and classes for their citizens. In the 1980s, 20 percent—or one out of five—of adults were estimated as being functionally illiterate and having difficulty reading at or below a fifth-grade level or low-literacy level.[1] A more recent study by the National Center for Educational Statistics, however, indicates that approximately 50 percent of America's adults fall in the lowest two levels (out of five levels) of literacy when tested, which categorizes them as being functionally illiterate.[2] A reading level this low negatively influences one's ability to function effectively in society. Everyday skills such as reading a menu, filling out a job application, or properly addressing an envelope become matters of difficulty for the person with low literacy skills (LLS). Understandably, difficulties evolve when trying to teach these people about complex health care matters. As the primary patient educators for health care matters, these statistics affect nurses greatly. The high percentage of the population with LLS requires us to plan and implement our patient education strategically and to choose carefully the written materials utilized.

Several national accrediting agencies now require health care professionals to ensure that patients understand the medical information which they are given. The 1995 National Committee for Quality Assurance (NCQA) guidelines include provisions which focus on reading levels of written materials provided to clientele of managed care organizations. The Joint Commission on Accreditation of Health Care Organizations (JCAHO) requires that hospitals establish a mechanism to determine if their informed consent procedures, medication and discharge instructions, and other communications can be understood by patients (p. 170).[3]

Multiple studies have evaluated low literacy levels as they relate to patient education and written materials. Doak et al. studied 100 common patient education materials (i.e., diet instructions, patient Bill of Rights, etc.) and found that the mean reading level needed to comprehend them was the tenth grade.[4] They studied a corresponding patient population and found their reading ability to be at a seventh-grade level despite most being high school graduates. This study was replicated by the South Carolina Diabetes Control Project in 1984, resulting in similar data. An expansion of the Doak study tested 300 common patient education materials from around the United States and found that the reading level needed for these materials was 11th grade.[5] Grimm evaluated the reading levels of 100 diabetic patients in a large teaching hospital.[6] Of this population, 60 percent read at a fifth-grade level or below (42 percent of this group were reading at a third-grade level). Grimm also evaluated the reading level of 40 of the most commonly used national diabetes educational materials. The average readability level of these materials was tenth grade.

Meade and Byrd studied 258 subjects from a primary care clinic in Milwaukee as part of a smoking cessation program.[7] Their study revealed a median reading level of sixth grade and a median educational level completion of tenth grade. Most of the patient education booklets that they evaluated for their study were written above the ninth-grade level.

Dixon and Park studied the reading difficulty and overall comprehensibility of various booklets and consent forms utilized in an 830-bed, private, Midwest hospital. The materials all scored at reading levels between grades 9.5 and 13.8.[8] Streiff reported similar results when she studied 28 patient education materials and 106 patients in an ambulatory care setting. The mean readability level for the materials was the 11th grade. Five of the pamphlets specific to the topic of contraception required a reading level of grade 13.2. The patients had a mean completed grade level of 9.9 but a reading skill level of grade 6.8.[9]

In recent years, many more low literacy studies have been conducted relating to patients' understanding of medical directions and instructions. These studies represent multiple fields of health care, such as emergency departments, oncology, and diabetes.[10–15]

A review of the literature also reveals that most written patient education materials, relating to a variety of health topics, require at least a tenth-grade reading level.[16–19] Yet a person's reading level does not necessarily correlate with the number of years he or she has attended school. Several studies have revealed a two- to four-grade level disparity between the level of schooling completed and one's reading level.[20–25] In Grimm's study, however, the statistics were more disturbing. The mean of one-half of the study population completed the tenth grade, yet read at a sixth-grade level, whereas the mean of the other half completed the 11th grade, and read at a fourth-grade level![26] This disparity between the reading level of educational materials and the patients' reading level suggests that much of the written patient education information is being poorly understood or misunderstood. Ultimately, the use of high-level written materials as the primary method of patient education negatively affects learning, comprehension, and adherence. "In addition, the legal implications of this situation are cause for alarm" (p. 126).[27]

## THEORETICAL RATIONALE

Orem's theory of self-care is utilized as the framework for the integration of self-care concepts into patient education and adherence. Self-care as explained by Orem is the behavior from life situations that persons direct to themselves or their environment to regulate factors affecting their own development, health, or well-being.[28] She further describes self-care concepts as learned and goal-oriented activities.

Hill and Smith add to Orem's theory by describing specific conditions that they deem essential for meeting self-care needs:[29]

- specific knowledge, skills, and the responsibility for health care needs
- motivation and energy to initiate and persevere in the self-care process
- a high value on health
- the belief that the health behaviors involved in self-care will reduce vulnerability to illness

Hill and Smith also relate that in Orem's theory, education is the primary means used to correct self-care deficits or problems in providing for one's own health care needs.[30] Inherent in Orem's theory is the premise that when a self-care need is not met, a self-care demand is present. Self-care deficits exist when people are unable to meet their self-care demands. Education/learning is extremely important in influencing one's self-care practices and ultimately the motivation to comply with health regimens. Education (formal and informal) can influence how patients may utilize specific information to direct or improve their lives. Patients cannot be expected to follow treatment instructions when they lack a basic understanding of the rationale, procedures, and requirements of their regimen.[31] If a self-care deficit evolves, then patient education may be required as an intervention. Thus, a nurse or other provider may be involved in an educative or consultative relationship to help alleviate or correct the self-care deficit.[32]

Spees emphasizes that possessing knowledge and understanding instructions is a necessary step in fostering patient compliance and adherence.[33] According to Hussey and Gilliland, low literacy and illiteracy are major contributing factors to nonadherence.[34] Although a person may possess adequate reading skills, understanding and interpretation are not guaranteed. The authors believe that the idea of being able to function or act on content, after reading it, has led to the development of functional literacy. They define this concept as "anything and everything connected with basic skills education for adults" (p. 607). In other words, in order for people to function or act on content they have read, they must be able to read well enough to understand and interpret it, plus use that information as it was intended. Thus, a person with poor reading skills may not be able to demonstrate correct or intended interpretation and thus would be considered to have impaired functional literacy. Poor reading skills have an impact not only on understanding and interpretation of meaning but also on the patient's organization of thought, perception, and vocabulary development. All of these factors can cause confusion and misunderstanding, so that instructions may become misinterpreted.[35] Without comprehension, adherence is by chance rather than by choice.[36]

## CONDITIONS

In order to teach people with LLS, we must first understand the difficulties and obstacles these people may encounter. Doak et al. explain that people with LLS experience several areas of difficulty in addition to reading: reading ability, comprehension, process, organization of perceptions or thoughts, and problem-solving skills.[37]

*Reading ability* relates to a person's actual ability and level of reading; it involves letter and word recognition. Persons with LLS often read letter by letter to derive each word, and thus read in a slow, halting manner. This method also negatively affects comprehension. These persons recognize typed or printed words more easily than handwritten, cursive words.

*Comprehension* involves understanding the meaning of what is read, not just recognizing the words; it includes listening comprehension (understanding what is being read or verbally instructed). Comprehension is usually lower and less complete for people with LLS, often because of reading as well as language deficits. Thus, poor vocabulary and listening skills make it more difficult for persons with LLS to express themselves or to fully understand others who have greater fluency; however, Grimm notes that this is not always the case. In that study, many patients were found to be articulate and able to communicate quite effectively, yet had LLS when tested. Grimm states that often these patients have dealt with their deficit for many years and have learned to cope with and conceal their deficits.[38]

*Process* is a person's ability to utilize reading, language, and comprehension skills to develop a whole picture—being able to utilize resources, internal and external (i.e., life experiences) to derive a logical connection (comprehension) of a concept, situation, or instructions. It involves the *organization of perceptions or thoughts,* which is a person's ability to formulate a logical sequence to thoughts, ideas, events, and so on, which in turn helps to organize data into a whole, logical, sequential picture. This sophisticated cognitive process often causes difficulty for patients with low literacy skills. It requires that information be taught in small increments for better understanding and for the sequence to be remembered. *Problem-solving skills* are often delayed for persons with LLS. Because of a deficit in this area, directions (verbal or written) are often taken quite literally, with no understanding as to why, and with no room for adaptation of thoughts or actions based on circumstances.

Parker et al. relate that the patient's ability to recognize and utilize numbers (numeracy literacy) is also an important condition for functional health literacy. This skill is especially important in pharmaceutical instructions. Hence, they developed a literacy tool, the Test of Functional Health Literacy in Adults (TOFHLA), to capture people's numeracy literacy abilities as well as their reading abilities.[39]

Thus, considering all of the aforementioned possible obstacles, the physical conditions for learning may now be addressed. These conditions include time for demonstration, questions, repeat demonstration, and further questions. The environment should be quiet, structured, and conducive to learning, as for any adult learner. Teaching patients with LLS requires patience on the part of the teacher, as well as astuteness in determining whether the patient is really understanding the instructions.

## TYPES OF LEARNERS

Low literacy applies to adolescents and adults who have deficits in reading abilities, process, and comprehension. Low literacy affects people of all races. Socioeconomic status does not determine illiteracy because illiteracy is found in all levels of society.[40] The point must be made here that although a person may not be able to read or to read well enough to understand or interpret meaning does not mean that he or she is lacking intelligence. Illiteracy does not equate to low IQ or low intelligence.[41] As stated previously, the number of years a person has completed in school does not necessarily predict his or her literacy abilities. Unskilled and poorly skilled readers have several characteristics in common:

- They usually agree with everything. If you ask whether they understand, the answer will usually be "yes".
- They are well defended. They are not easy to distinguish, and they try hard to maintain their dignity.
- They tend to be literal and concrete. This approach causes them difficulty with conceptualization because their databases are limited (normally, data are usually acquired through reading). Comprehension is slow and usually incomplete. They also have difficulty in classifying information.
- They may not view words or pictures from left to right and may not be good at sounding out words. They also may not be able to recognize signs, symbols, abbreviations, or synonyms.
- Their perspective is usually limited to direct personal experiences; thus they operate on a more restricted information base.
- They are usually restless in teaching-learning environments because of the threat of exposing their poor literacy or illiteracy.
- They usually will not volunteer to answer questions when in a group setting.

## RESOURCES

Multiple resources are available to assist people with LLS and the professionals trying to teach these people. National, regional, and local literacy programs have been designed to assist people with LLS. The professional may consult with the National Institutes of Health Literacy Program in Bethesda, Maryland; Patient Learning Associates, Inc. (Cecelia and Leonard Doak) in Potomac, Maryland; regional, statewide, or local literacy programs; teaching facilities in local or regional colleges; health education institutions/hospitals; libraries; and local audiovisual services. National societies such as the National Cancer Institute, the American Cancer Society, and the American Heart Association can offer resources for teaching patients with LLS. If local resources are limited, then the development of in-house materials may be warranted. Several references listed at the end of this chapter can assist in the creation of materials.[42–46]

## USING THE METHOD

First, before teaching patients with LLS, an assessment of the patient's reading and numeracy abilities should be established. Brez and Taylor state that, although consensus on word recognition tools for screening patients with LLS varies, their use is supported.[47] Experts accept this strategy for screening purposes when the intended outcome is the appropriate selection of teaching materials and interventions, rather than for diagnostic labeling (Brez and Taylor, 1997). Although it is important to mention a couple of new assessment tools (REALM and TOFHLA)[48,49] are available for determining patient's reading and/or numeracy abilities, this chapter will focus on teaching methodology.

Successful methods of teaching patients with LLS include verbal instruction, repetition or review of the instructions, demonstration and return demonstration, and teaching in small increments to allow for process and comprehension. Focus the instruction on the desired patient behavior(s), eliminating information that is extraneous or not directly relevant to achieving those behaviors.[50] Repeatedly reviewing the information and procedures is important.[51] The nurse/educator should seek consensual validation by having the patient repeat the instructions as they were interpreted. Verbal instructions should include the patient's own terminology, and key instructions should be concise, ordered, and as vivid and explicit as possible. Each idea or topic should be taught one step at a time, and information and teaching sessions should be limited. Instructions being given should be broken down into segments or components. Breaks should be provided at the end of each segment/component to provide time for review, feedback, and questions.[52] Brez and Taylor recommended using audiovisual presentations to augment the written instructions, when possible.[53] They also recommend presenting patients with a wide range of learning options and allowing them to select the option that best suits their learning style, thus possibly eliminating the need for literacy screening.[54]

Written materials should be used only if they are written at a level that correlates with (or near) the patient's reading level. These materials should be printed or typed with lowercase and uppercase letters, and not handwritten, especially not in cursive writing. The type size should be large, for ease in distinguishing letters.[55-58] The use of all capitalized letters should be avoided because it is harder to read. Educational materials should include a few key points and graphics or pictures, which add to the understanding of the concept being taught.[59-61] The utilization of subheadings assists patients in sifting through information to find the topic of interest or need.[62,63] "Chunking" words or ideas together in a meaningful context assists patients in understanding and remembering the intended educational message.[64] Only one idea should be conveyed in each sentence or paragraph.[65,66] The use of active voice (conversational style) makes materials easier to read and comprehend and makes it more personal.[67-69]

## POTENTIAL PROBLEMS

The term *simplified* should not be misinterpreted to mean simplistic or intended for a simpleton. When this perspective occurs, materials for patients with LLS end up being childlike, or childlike associations are made. Pictures may be "silly" or cartoonlike despite trying to convey adult concepts. This approach is insulting and demeaning to the patient. "Talking down" to the patient defeats the collaborative educator/learner role and places the learner in a more subservient role.

Careful attention must be paid to the patient's actual capabilities and understanding; otherwise, incorrect assumptions may ensue. There is a danger in making assumptions because the actual problem may be that patients are quiet in normal circumstances or that they have already received education related to the topic you are trying to teach. When low literacy is suspected, the nurse must use extreme caution and avoid any hint of disapproval, impatience, or judgment.

## CONCLUSION

Many people in the United States today have LLS. The condition is cross-cultural and is not dependent on social class. Adherence is often a problem for these patients because written instructions on their level are not readily available for reference and because they often will not ask questions.

Patients with LLS usually learn best from verbal and demonstrative teaching, supplemented with written materials tailored to their level. The educator is responsible for ensuring that the patient has every opportunity to learn by whatever means necessary. A person's educational level does not necessarily correlate with his or her reading level or abilities. Therefore, to maximize comprehensibility, foster self-care practices, and facilitate adherence, the level of written materials must be properly matched to the intended target audience.[70] Teaching in increments works well with patients with low literacy because their ability to comprehend and process information is delayed. Therefore, the nurse educator must tailor patient education to the patient's actual needs and abilities rather than the nurse's perceptions of such. This task requires an accurate and ongoing assessment of each individual and of all materials utilized for patient education.

---

# EXAMPLE
# Teaching Reflux

The following example is a portion of a patient instruction handout that was formerly utilized in a clinic in a large Southeastern teaching hospital. It was revised, following the principles in this chapter, for use with patients with LLS. A section from those instructions is used here to illustrate how written instructions may be revised for use with these patients.

**Example #1**
**(ORIGINAL TEXT):**
**"Reflux"**

Many children and adults have regurgitation of food, liquids, and/or acid from the stomach back into the esophagus and throat. Sometimes it causes no problems, but it may cause heartburn, chest pains, vomiting, wheezing, coughing, or even pneumonia or sinusitis. Some respiratory symptoms may be related to or precipitated by gastroesophageal reflux. When this is the case, our recommended approach to treatment is as follows: AVOID high acid foods such as licorice, mint, tea, coffee, cokes, chocolate, ketchup, and alcoholic beverages. Smoking may worsen the condition, and thus patients must be encouraged to ELIMINATE smoking behaviors. Elevation of the head of the bed approximately 2–4 inches on a brick or block assists in reducing reflux by means of gravity.

(7 sentences; 118 words; 22 polysyllabic words; written in passive voice; 10-point print; uses capital letters for emphasis; no order to the instructions). Using the SMOG[71] method of evaluating written materials for literacy levels, the original text, in its entirety, scored at an 11th-grade reading level.

## Example #2
## (REVISED, SIMPLIFIED TEXT VERSION):
## "Reflux"

Reflux is when food, liquid, or acid backs up from your stomach into your throat. It may cause "heartburn," chest pains, vomiting (throwing up), wheezing in your lungs, or coughing. It may even cause infections in your lungs or sinuses. If your doctor thinks reflux is causing some of your lung problems, here are some things that may help you.

1. <u>Do not</u> eat licorice, mint, chocolate, or ketchup.
2. <u>Do not drink</u> tea, coffee, cokes, or sodas.
3. <u>Do not drink</u> beer, wine, or liquor.
4. <u>Stop Smoking!!</u>
5. Raise up the head of your bed on a brick or block (about 2–4 inches)

(9 sentences; 99 words; 5 polysyllabic words; written in active voice; 14-point print; title is enlarged and points are underlined for emphasis; instructions are ordered; print is block letters for ease in distinguishing letters). Using the SMOG[72] method of evaluating written materials for literacy levels, the revised text, in its entirety, scored at an eighth-grade reading level.

Note: This example includes only the revisions made to the text portion of the handout. Illustrations have since been added to further improve the readability and comprehension of this handout.

---

**NOTES**

1. C.C. Doak et al., *Teaching Patients with Low Literacy Skills,* 2nd ed. (Philadelphia: J.B. Lippincott, 1996).

2. Educational Testing Service and National Center for Educational Statistics, *Adult Literacy in America: National Adult Literacy Survey* (Washington, DC: Office of Education Research and Improvement, U.S. Department of Education, 1993).

3. B.D. Weiss et al., Communicating with Patients Who Have Limited Literacy Skills: Report of the National Work Group on Literacy and Health, *Journal of Family Practice* 46, no. 2 (1998):168–176.

4. Doak et al., *Teaching Patients with Low Literacy Skills.*

5. L.G. Doak and C.C. Doak, Lowering the Silent Barriers to Compliance for Patients with Low Literacy Skills, *Promoting Health* 8 (1987):6–8.

6. J. Grimm, The Development of Diabetes Footcare Pamphlets for Patients with Low Literacy Skills (Master's Thesis, Medical College of Georgia, 1990).

7. C.D. Meade and J.C. Byrd, Patient Literacy and Readability of Smoking Education Literature, *American Journal of Public Health* 79, no. 2 (1989):204–206.

8. E. Dixon and R. Park, Do Patients Understand Written Health Information? *Nursing Outlook* 38, no. 6 (1990):278–281.

9. L.D. Streiff, Can Clients Understand Our Instructions? *Image: Journal of Nursing Scholarship* 18 (1986):48–52.

10. D.A. Brooks, Techniques for Teaching ED Patients with Low Literacy Skills, *Journal of Emergency Nursing* 24, no. 6 (1998):601–603.

11. R.D. Powers, Emergency Department Patient Literacy and Readability of Patient-Directed Materials, *Annals of Emergency Medicine* 17, no. 2 (1998):124–126.

12. D.M. Williams et al., Emergency Department Discharge Instructions and Patient Literacy: A Problem of Disparity, *American Journal of Emergency Medicine* 14, no. 1 (1996):19–22.

13. M. Hearth-Holmes et al., Literacy in Patients with a Chronic Disease: Systemic Lupus Erythematosus and the Reading Level of Patient Education Materials, *Journal of Rheumatology* 24, no. 12 (1997):2335–2339.

14. M.E. Cooley et al., Patient Literacy and the Readability of Written Cancer Educational Materials, *Oncology Nursing Forum* 22, no. 9 (1995):1345–1351.

15. F.L. Wilson et al., Patient Literacy Levels: A Consideration When Designing Patient Education Programs, *Rehabilitation Nursing* 22, no. 6 (1997):311–317.

16. Doak et al., *Teaching Patients with Low Literacy Skills.*

17. Doak and Doak, Lowering the Silent Barriers.

18. Dixon and Park, Do Patients Understand Written Health Information?

19. Streiff, Can Clients Understand?

20. Doak et al., *Teaching Patients with Low Literacy Skills.*

21. Grimm, The Development of Diabetes Footcare Pamphlets.

22. Meade and Byrd, Patient Literacy and Readability.

23. Streiff, Can Clients Understand?

24. M.D. Boyd and R.H.L. Feldman, Health Information Seeking and Reading and Comprehension Abilities of Cardiac Rehabilitation Patients, *Journal of Cardiac Rehabilitation* 4, no. 8 (1984):343–347.

25. J.M. Swanson et al., Readability of Commercial and Generic Contraceptive Instructions, *Image: Journal of Nursing Scholarship* 22, no. 2 (1990):96–100.

26. Grimm, The Development of Diabetes Footcare Pamphlets.

27. Powers, Emergency Department Patient Literacy.

28. D.E. Orem, *Nursing: Concepts of Practice,* 4th ed. (St. Louis: Mosby-Year Book, 1991).

29. L. Hill and N. Smith, *Self-Care Nursing: Promotion of Health,* 2nd ed. (Norwalk, CT: Appleton & Lange, 1990).

30. Hill and Smith, *Self-Care Nursing.*

31. A.G. Taylor et al., Do Patients Understand Patient Education Brochures? *Nursing & Health Care* 3, no. 6 (1982):305–310.

32. Hill and Smith, *Self-Care Nursing.*

33. C. Spees, Knowledge of Medical Terminology among Clients and Families, *Image* 23, no. 4 (1991):225–229.

34. L.C. Hussey and K. Gilliland, Compliance, Low Literacy and Locus of Control, *Nursing Clinics of North America* 24, no. 3 (1989):605–611.

35. Hussey and Gilliland, Compliance, Low Literacy and Locus of Control.

36. Doak and Doak, Lowering the Silent Barriers.

37. Doak et al., *Teaching Patients with Low Literacy Skills.*

38. Grimm, The Development of Diabetes Footcare Pamphlets.
39. R.M. Parker et al., The Test of Functional Health Literacy in Adults: A New Instrument for Measuring Patients' Literacy Skills, *Journal of General Internal Medicine* 10, no. 10 (1995):537–541.
40. A. Haggard, *Handbook of Patient Education* (Gaithersburg, MD: Aspen Publishers, 1989).
41. Haggard, *Handbook of Patient Education.*
42. Doak et al., *Teaching Patients with Low Literacy Skills.*
43. United States Department of Health and Human Services, *Clear and Simple: Developing Effective Print Materials for Low Literacy Readers*, NIH Publication #95-3594 (Bethesda, MD: National Cancer Institute Office of Cancer Communications, 1995).
44. J.E. Shield and M.C. Mullen, *Developing Health Education Materials for Special Audiences: Low Literacy Adults,* American Dietetic Association Publication #1312 (Chicago: American Dietetic Association, 1992).
45. Grimm, The Development of Diabetes Footcare Pamphlets.
46. Meade and Byrd, Patient Literacy and Readability.
47. S.M. Brez and M. Taylor, Assessing Literacy for Patient Teaching: Perspectives of Adults with Low Literacy Skills, *Journal of Advanced Nursing* 25, no. 5 (1997):1040–1047.
48. Parker et al., The Test of Functional Health Literacy in Adults.
49. T.C. Davis, Rapid Estimate of Adult Literacy in Medicine: A Shortened Screening Instrument, *Family Medicine* 25, no. 6 (1993):391–395.
50. Doak and Doak, Lowering the Silent Barriers.
51. A. Walker, Teaching the Illiterate Patient, *Journal of Enterostomal Therapy* 14, no. 2 (1987):85.
52. Doak and Doak, Lowering the Silent Barriers.
53. Brez and Taylor, Assessing Literacy for Patient Teaching.
54. Brez and Taylor, Assessing Literacy for Patient Teaching.
55. Doak et al., *Teaching Patients with Low Literacy Skills.*
56. Doak and Doak, Lowering the Silent Barriers.
57. P. Farrell-Miller and P. Gentry, How Effective Are Your Patient Education Materials? Guidelines for Development and Evaluation of Written Educational Materials, *The Diabetes Educator* 15, no. 5 (1989):418–422.
58. M.D. Boyd, A Guide to Writing Effective Patient Education Materials, *Nursing Management* 18, no. 7 (1987):56–57.
59. Doak et al., *Teaching Patients with Low Literacy Skills.*
60. Doak and Doak, Lowering the Silent Barriers.
61. Farrell-Miller and Gentry, How Effective Are Your Patient Education Materials?
62. Dixon and Park, Do Patients Understand Written Health Information?
63. Boyd, A Guide to Writing Effective Patient Education Materials.
64. Doak et al., *Teaching Patients with Low Literacy Skills.*
65. Boyd, A Guide to Writing Effective Patient Education Materials.
66. C.D. Meade and D.M. Howser, Consent Forms: How To Determine and Improve Their Readability, *Oncology Nursing Forum* 19, no. 10 (1992):1523–1528.
67. Doak et al., *Teaching Patients with Low Literacy Skills.*

68. Farrell-Miller and Gentry, How Effective Are Your Patient Education Materials?

69. Boyd, A Guide to Writing Effective Patient Education Materials.

70. Taylor et al., Do Patients Understand?

71. H.G. McLaughlin, SMOG-Grading: A New Readability Formula, *Journal of Reading* 12 (1969):639–646.

72. McLaughlin, SMOG-Grading.

# CHAPTER 24

# A Community-Based Practicum Experience

*Betty G. Davis and Pat Christensen*

## DEFINITION AND PURPOSES

Health screening involves the identification of unrecognized problems or potential problems in individuals or populations. Health screenings can also provide opportunities for unique partnerships between schools of nursing and agencies that provide services to patients. These partnerships can be mutually beneficial. The screening experience contributes to student learning while providing invaluable health professional services to the community.

In the experience described in this chapter, the health screenings involve the assessment of head and neck, hearing, vision, development, skin integrity, height and weight, and nutritional status of groups of high-risk, school-aged children in an after-school program sponsored by the Salvation Army Boys' and Girls' Clubs and other community agencies. The purpose of the practicum experience is twofold: (1) to provide an opportunity for nursing students to learn about children's health, and (2) to provide the children with skilled observations about their health status. In anticipation of the practicum experience, the students complete extensive reading in child physical, social, and cognitive development. The groups of children screened consist mainly of children who, by virtue of their low socioeconomic status, are considered to be at high risk for unidentified and untreated problems that could impair their health and learning.

## THEORETICAL RATIONALE

The theoretical framework for this experience is a synthesis of the primary care model of prevention and learning theory. The relationships among poor health, delayed childhood development, learning problems, inadequate academic achievement, and socially inappropriate coping skills have been well documented.[1-3] Health care has moved increasingly from acute care to community-based settings, and nursing faculty members need to provide a wider range of community-based experiences for students. Nursing education needs to be patient-centered and take place where the population is available, in order to provide opportunities for students to learn the necessary skills and to meet the needs of patients. In addition, service-oriented learning has gained more attention and is valued as a partnership of education and service.[4] Child health activities, in particular, are increasingly community-based in schools, day-care settings, after-school programs, and family homes. Some of the greatest problems of delivering primary care to children are that a large percentage of children are not covered by health insurance, and many parents work and cannot transport their children to a doctor or clinic.[5]

An essential component of primary health care is participation of communities and health care organizations. The relationships forged by these partnerships can be reciprocal and mutually beneficial. Community agencies can identify needs, and health professionals can help deliver necessary services to meet those needs. Thus, the screening of vulnerable populations by nursing students is an expression of a mutually supportive relationship, whereby the students can learn and can serve the community.

## CONDITIONS

Health screenings can be used in a wide variety of settings with diverse populations. In the example discussed here, the population is school-aged children. The screenings are promoted as "Healthy Kids Programs." Other situations could include screenings of the elderly for hypertension, stress, medication effects, cholesterol, and so forth. College students could be screened for hearing, vision, scoliosis, nutritional status, height, weight, knowledge of birth control methods, and a myriad of other age-appropriate data. Almost any group of individuals could be utilized for health screenings. The settings for the screenings can vary from schools, senior citizen centers, stores, and shopping malls to churches, homeless shelters, and anywhere that groups of people frequent.

Because the objectives for each group screened are different, the learning opportunities for the students are diverse. The careful planning, implementation, and evaluation of the screenings provide a full spectrum of learning experiences for nursing students. Students are expected to explore human development thoroughly, to communicate effectively with diverse groups, to utilize observational and health assessment skills, and to evaluate essential patient data. The reporting and follow-up activities of those persons with identified problems provide invaluable links to health care providers for the patients and students alike.

## Planning

The screening activities require a great deal of advance planning, which can involve students as well as faculty and community agencies. The degree of student involvement in planning varies depending on the time frame for the practicum and the focus of the learning objectives. Where the time frame is short and the focus for student learning is primarily implementation and evaluation, students' involvement in planning may be limited to individual preparation; however, students' participation in planning may be extensive. At the onset of the course, students can identify the population and settings as part of the clinical experience.

After contacting the agency (school, community center, and so forth), the faculty members provide the students with the opportunity to write the objectives, identify resources, provide the materials, publicize the event, and implement and evaluate the experience. This clinical practicum can be offered on a select basis (one time) or can be a major project that spans several weeks or a whole semester. The whole class is divided into work groups, each of which is assigned a certain responsibility for the activity. After the assignment of groups, students can work independently of each other (with consultation and assistance from faculty) to accomplish their particular objectives. The hours spent in planning are counted as part of the required clinical time.

It has been gratifying to observe that, given an explanation of the screening and its value to children and students, business organizations and other community agencies often donate materials and resources to help defray any expenses. The cooperation and support of these organizations further promote the community/school partnership.

## Modifying

It may be necessary for faculty members to do some of the advanced planning, especially when agency contracts for student experiences are negotiated several months in advance. In addition, permissions from school officials, community agencies, and parents can likewise be time consuming. The system for these permissions must be put in place before students can begin the screening activities. Although the authors have not had problems with parental permissions, it is advisable to plan well ahead for any eventualities. A careful explanation of the screening activities (including statements that the students will not be undressed) may forestall any hesitation on the parents' part to grant permission. Additionally, the permissions should identify a contact person (the nursing faculty member supervising the clinical) in the event that parents want further information.

Another outcome of the screening process may be a continuing relationship between the school and the community agency, based on patients' needs. Faculty and students need to anticipate the need for follow-up sessions and plan for them.

For example, when screening school-aged children, the students have often identified children with nutritional deficiencies. As a follow-up activity, the students present a teaching/learning project on healthy snacks. Other such activities have included brushing and flossing teeth and safety issues.

## TYPES OF LEARNERS

Health screenings are appropriate learning activities for undergraduate and graduate students. Screening activities can be simple (only assessing height and weight) or quite complex (multisystem assessments) and can include various groups in a wide range of settings. The amount of faculty supervision can vary, depending on the skill level of the student. Obviously, graduate students and senior nursing students would be able to perform more independently and to participate in more extensive planning.

The health screening described in this chapter is placed in the junior-level, parent-child course; however, other screenings have been part of the senior-level community health course. Regardless of the level of student, health screenings can provide an enriching clinical experience. The objectives can be adjusted to the skill level of the students and advanced as the students become more proficient.

## RESOURCES

The use of health screenings is an excellent teaching strategy for child health community-based practicums because screenings can be performed in a variety of settings, and most schools of nursing already have the needed resources and personnel for implementation. The type and amount of room space and the equipment needed are determined by the particular health assessment components to be performed and numbers of children or other patients to be screened.

The community agency programs used as examples in this chapter are excellent settings for child health screenings because approximately 75 to 100 children participate in each of the after-school programs utilized. Child health assessments are performed in a general-purpose room or classroom, separate from the recreational area, which provides for privacy. Tables and chairs are located in the screening rooms and in most settings, and sinks for handwashing are located nearby.

Different types of screenings are performed depending on the time frame and number of participants. In some situations, selected screenings are performed on two different days. The first screening may include patient history and physical assessment relative to height and weight; blood pressure, pulse, and respiration; skin and nails; vision and hearing; and developmental assessment—for example, the Goodenough Draw-a-Man Test, Draw-A-Person Test[6]—or a more general assessment based on observations and patient history reported during the interview. A second screening may include physical assessment relative to head and neck, eyes, ears, nose, sinuses, mouth and throat, musculoskeletal system, nutritional status, and level of exercise. At other times, a more comprehensive assessment is performed for each child within the one screening. These assessments are typical of screenings for the school-age population.[7–9]

A comprehensive assessment form has been developed for use in any of the health screenings. For screenings with a narrow assessment focus (for example, blood pressure or vision), a more concise assessment form can be easily created from the comprehensive document. The comprehensive assessment form includes both patient history and physical assessment data. A checklist format for selected review of systems data, normal findings, and variations provides for increased efficiency in documentation. Assessment components listed on the comprehensive form are found in Exhibit 24–1.

Eight to ten students and one faculty member are present for each screening. All equipment and assessment materials are provided by the school of nursing: vision charts (Snellen alphabet and Snellen E), portable scales, a measuring tape (for measuring distance from the eye chart and for use as a height measurement), sphygmomanometers, stethoscopes, tuning forks, audiometer, penlights, tongue blades, alcohol swabs, fragrant substances (flavored gum, chocolate candy, etc.) for assessing Cranial Nerve I, white paper and pencils for developmental assessment, ink pens for documentation, and assessment forms.

Rewards (prizes) are offered as incentives for the children to participate in the screenings and follow-up sessions, rescreening, and health teaching as needed. These rewards are donated by faculty, students, and outside sources such as dentists, businesses, and church groups. The reward items include pencils, erasers, notepads, folders, toothbrushes, toothpaste, sample-size soaps, stickers, sugarless gum, raisins, and apples. An effort is made to give rewards that are useful, safe, and appealing to the

---

**Exhibit 24–1**  Example of Assessment Components

- Height and Weight (measurements and percentiles)
- Vital Signs (pulse, respiration, blood pressure, and occasionally temperature)
- Skin and Nails
- Head, Face, and Neck
- Eyes (external appearance, ophthalmoscopic exam, and vision)
- Ears (external appearance, otoscopic exam, and hearing)
- Nose, Sinuses, Mouth, and Throat
- Musculoskeletal System (gait, muscle tone and strength, range of motion)
- Dietary History (24-hour recall, food preferences or dislikes, food allergies and intolerances, and appetite)
- Exercise (types and frequency)
- Developmental Assessment

school-age group. Rewards might also include items such as coloring sheets, crossword puzzles, health-related booklets, and so forth. Many of these items are available at no cost through community agencies such as health departments, law enforcement agencies, fire departments, and American Red Cross chapters.

The costs for some screening materials and reward items may be appropriated in the school of nursing budget provided funds are available for service-oriented learning experiences and advance planning is made. Additionally, seeking sponsorship from businesses and organizations in the community can be an effective strategy for promoting community and school partnerships. The community agency partner may have funds to help with some selected items. With increasing economic concerns of academic institutions and community agencies, faculty members may need to seek grants to cover the expenditures.

## USING THE METHOD

The success of health screening in a community setting as a teaching strategy depends largely on planning and collaboration with the community agency personnel. Extensive planning and collaboration are used in the example described in this chapter. In an initial meeting, agency administrators and faculty identify: (1) probable unmet health care needs of the high-risk school-age population to be served, (2) experiences needed for student learning (practice of assessment skills and related follow-up care, including rescreening and referrals for abnormal findings and mini-teaching sessions based on identified needs), and (3) services to be provided by school of nursing faculty and students as well as dates and times for the screenings and follow-up care. Faculty members elicit information about the children who attend the after-school program, including a general description, special needs of any of the children (handicaps, allergies, and so forth), and the schedule of a typical day's activities at the facility.

During this initial meeting, there is discussion and agreement concerning specific resources to be provided by the community agency and those to be provided by the school of nursing. Also, there has been agreement that the children's participation will be voluntary. Faculty members agree to provide promotional materials such as a poster for the agency's bulletin board and fliers for distribution to children and families. The agency staff agrees to promote the screenings by verbally supporting the screenings in their communications with children and their families, listing the screening activities on their printed calendar of events, displaying the poster on a prominent bulletin board, and distributing the promotional fliers. Meeting at the community agency facility provides faculty members with the opportunity to observe the physical environment and anticipate needs relative to setup and implementation.

Accreditation criteria and liability concerns dictate the need for establishment of formal contracts between the school of nursing and the agency, as well as the need for signed parental permission forms prior to implementation of screenings. Faculty members provide the parental permission forms, and the agency staff distribute and collect the forms.

The faculty's role in physical preparation for the screenings is critical for successful implementation of screenings and enhancement of student learning. For the practicum described in this chapter, students are not usually involved in the planning and physical preparation because of a limited time frame and focus for the students. Faculty responsibilities are as follows:

- developing specific student learning objectives (Exhibit 24–2)
- developing clinical preparatory assignments for students (Exhibit 24–3)
- developing the various forms: assessment form, parental permission form, and summary/referral form for parents
- obtaining outside sources and funding for promotional materials and incentive rewards, as well as purchasing or collecting the items to be used as rewards
- creating, printing, and distributing promotional materials that clearly delineate the screenings and incentive awards

---

**Exhibit 24–2** Health Screening for High-Risk School-Age Children

**Learning Objectives**
During the health screening practicum, the student will:
1. Perform selected aspects of physical, nutritional, and developmental assessment, including patient history and physical exam components. (Instructor will designate selected aspects. Students should be prepared to perform comprehensive assessments.)
2. Document assessment findings on child health assessment forms.
3. Identify normal findings for physical, nutritional, and developmental assessment of the school-age child.
4. Utilize effective techniques in communicating with children.
5. Identify techniques that can be utilized to encourage cooperation and participation of children.
6. Identify characteristics of high-risk school-age children.
7. Analyze assessment findings, including comparison of actual findings for individual children to normal findings.
8. Identify specific needs for follow-up care (rescreening, referrals) for individual children.
9. Complete a summary form of assessment findings and recommendations regarding rescreening or referrals to give to parents of the children.
10. Identify an action plan for a mini-health teaching session based on a common health need of high-risk children.

**Exhibit 24–3** Clinical Preparation

1. Required Readings in Wong, D.L. 1999. *Whaley & Wong's Nursing Care of Infants and Children,* 6th ed. St. Louis: Mosby, Chapters 2, 6, 7, and 17.
2. Review of Content:
   a. Information covered in prior and current courses relative to physical assessment, nutrition, and sociocultural influences for school-age children.
   b. Information covered in campus lab relative to developmental assessment and communication strategies for children.

- determining the number of assessments to be performed during each screening
- reserving equipment and supplies from the learning resource center in the school of nursing
- transporting equipment and supplies to and from the screening site
- identifying resources for referrals

Although students come to the course with prior knowledge and competency in performance of physical assessment skills, including an overview of physical assessment skills for children, they are expected to prepare extensively for the screenings. Their preparation includes review of physical, developmental, and nutritional assessment, and child health textbooks. Also, prior to the screenings, students participate in a campus laboratory exercise that addresses developmental assessment and communication strategies for children.

During a preconference, the faculty member serves as a facilitator for student discussion of general expectations, the physical setup, and operations of the screening. Faculty members review and clarify procedures, skills, normal findings for school-age children, assessment form content, and documentation based on student questions and input. Other topics discussed are characteristics of high-risk populations, sociocultural values and practices, the impact of socioeconomics on health practices, and the importance of confidentiality. Faculty members guide students through a brainstorming session to identify ways to encourage children to participate in the screenings—for example, interacting with children in recreational areas, explaining and demonstrating equipment and procedures, giving compliments and praise to the children, and thanking the children for their cooperation and participation. Faculty members assist students to identify informal teaching opportunities within the screenings, such as the purpose of equipment, hygiene measures, the proper way to cleanse the ear canal, and healthy habits (e.g., nutritional snacks and exercise). Students are directed by faculty members to observe for and document any unusual findings or outstanding characteristics (signs of abuse, hyperactivity, etc.) and to observe social interactions (what children talk about—their fears, interests, likes, and dislikes).

There are several ways to operationalize health screenings. For the afterschool health screenings, two different methods have been used, with only one method in operation on a given day. In the first type of screening, the participants move from one station to another, in sequence. This method is especially beneficial when screening large numbers of children and when equipment is limited (for example, scales, sphygmomanometers, and eye charts). Students organize themselves into several small groups, with two or three students per group and one group at each station. With faculty guidance, students establish a rotation schedule that provides opportunities for all students to perform each type of assessment. An advantage of this method is that student learning is enhanced through the active participation in organization and team efforts.

In the second type of screening, each student completes the total assessment for one child at a given time. One advantage of this one-on-one approach is increased rapport and communication with the child. Another advantage is student acquisition of a more holistic, comprehensive assessment of a child's health status, which enhances the analysis of assessment findings.

With both types of screenings, children receive incentive rewards at several intervals or at the end of the screening. Throughout the screenings, the faculty member facilitates student learning by being available for consultation, demonstrating assessment techniques as needed, assisting with students' performance of skills, and role-modeling effective communication and assessment techniques.

## EVALUATION

The evaluation component of health screenings has multidimensional importance as a teaching-learning strategy. The evaluation process for the example cited here includes (1) an analysis of assessment findings and identification of any needed follow-up measures, (2) an evaluation of the screening process and identification of areas for change, and (3) an evaluation of students' learning.

Much of the evaluation occurs during a postconference, which immediately follows the screening. Students begin to compare assessment findings for each child to normal findings, using their textbook as a reference. Abnormal findings and potential health problems are highlighted and discussed by the entire group of students, with the faculty member serving as a facilitator. Students compare their actual observations of growth and development as well as the characteristics and behaviors of high-risk children to expected findings. Specific plans are made for follow-up, as needed, based on three action plans:

1. rescreening—for example, blood pressure, vision, hearing
2. referral of parents to other health care sources—for example, school nurses, free medical clinics, health departments (If a school of nursing has a nursing practice center, this would be an ideal place for referral.)

3. mini-teaching sessions based on an overall need of the high-risk children in the after-school program

Following the screening and postconference, students finalize the analysis of data and plans for follow-up care. In addition, students write a summary of assessment findings and recommendations for parents. Faculty members review all summaries for accuracy and completeness.

To maintain confidentiality, faculty members place all assessment forms in school of nursing files. Assessment findings for individual children are not shared with community agency staff unless parental permission to do so has been given; however, the staff assists faculty and students in scheduling rescreenings for children who had abnormal findings and in communicating with parents regarding assessment findings and the need for follow-up.

Evaluation of the health screening by students, faculty, and agency staff involves stating an overall impression of the effectiveness of the screening, as well as specific identification of the positive aspects and areas for change. The faculty member initiates a request for an oral evaluation by students in postconference discussions. Discussion provides valuable insight into problems, feelings, frustrations, enthusiasm, and successes experienced during the screenings. Students and faculty evaluate the screening in relation to types and sequence of assessments performed; the organization, time frame, and clinical site (physical environment and cooperation of agency staff); adequacy of equipment and supplies; use of incentive rewards; availability of faculty; and workability of the assessment forms. Discussion of these factors provides valuable information for future screenings, especially delineation of components that might need to be changed. The faculty members ask questions and share personal observations to guide the discussion.

The most commonly identified areas for change relate to the short time frame for students to organize themselves at the assessment stations, improvements for traffic flow, and ways to decrease the noise level for selected assessments, such as blood pressure and hearing. Students occasionally report feeling overwhelmed by the large number of students who wanted to participate and, thus, feeling rushed to complete the screenings. Feedback from staff members at each of the community agencies indicates that the screenings definitely have been viewed as a service to the agency, to the children in the after-school program, and to the community. In addition, agencies report that the children enjoy the individual attention and look forward to subsequent visits of the students and faculty. Consistently, agencies have expressed a desire to continue the collaborative partnership to offer "Healthy Kids Programs" for children served by the agencies.

Evaluation of students' learning is based on stated learning objectives for the health screening experience. Discussion in postconference, students' comments on a written self-evaluation of clinical performance, faculty observations of student performance during pre- and postconferences and the screenings, and course evaluations are the vehicles for evaluation. All evaluation data indicate that health screening is a positive teaching strategy for educating students about child health because it provides an opportunity for students to:

- practice child health assessment (hands-on experience) for multiple patients
- practice communication skills with school-age children
- assess growth and development
- provide informal health teaching for children
- develop professionalism through accountability and service to the community
- introduce and/or reinforce the importance of healthy behaviors
- increase personal awareness of the impact of cultural and socioeconomic factors on health status
- assess the characteristics and health needs of a high-risk population
- plan strategies for health promotion and illness prevention
- participate in critical thinking through analysis of data and planning strategies for follow-up care

## POTENTIAL PROBLEMS

Several potential problems may impact the effectiveness of health screening as a teaching-learning strategy. A primary concern is that inadequate planning and preparation may result in insufficient resources, lack of organization, and ineffective implementation. Another concern is uncertainty of patient numbers in a setting where patients are strictly volunteers. Having either too many or too few volunteer participants could prevent achievement of students' learning objectives. Guidelines are established for limiting the number of volunteers in the after-school programs but are sometimes difficult to implement because of the desire to accommodate the many children who want to participate. Limiting the number of participants is necessary but frustrating to students, faculty, agency staff, parents who have given permission, and the children themselves.

Another potential problem is limiting the number of community partnerships established. Faculty members may have difficulty juggling the requests of multiple community agencies for free child health services, the increased emphasis of the academic institution to serve the community and to provide experiential learning for students, and personal desires to meet the needs of underserved children. Limitation is necessary, however, to maintain the quality of the health screenings as teaching-learning experiences.

Professional liability is another significant concern. A formal, written contract with the agency and a parental consent form should be used. Questions of liability relative to referrals should also be explored. Should there be a mechanism to determine whether parents follow up on suggested referrals? Should the school of nursing seek formal contracts with other health care providers for follow-up care? These questions and others will need to be considered in the planning phase. Consultation with legal professionals or the state board of nursing may be indicated.

With increased clinical practice in community settings, student safety has become a major challenge for faculty. In the practicums described here, students have reported some initial concerns, but no problems have been encountered. The parent of one student was concerned and followed the student to the setting in a separate car to make sure the student arrived safely. Faculty members' initial identification of clinical settings must include assessment for safety, including mapping out the safest route for travel. Also, faculty members should provide specific written directions to the setting. The use of beepers and cell phones, as well as encouraging students to travel in groups, promotes safety and reduces student anxieties. It is important to explore students' perceived threats to safety, to increase their awareness of potential concerns for safety, and to identify safety measures that must be followed. Exploration of perceived threats may be accomplished through group discussion or through the use of a standardized instrument.

Carroll, Morin, Hayes, and Carter have found the Environmental Comfort Scale III to be a valid and reliable instrument for assessing students' perceived threats, and they suggest that the instrument can be used to stimulate discussion about community safety. Further, their suggestions for preparation of students include the institution of a community awareness project, implementation of an environmental safety workshop, a treasure hunt for safe and unsafe features of the community setting, and the development of instructional materials such as case studies and CD-ROMs.[10]

## CONCLUSION

Health screenings can be excellent opportunities to form and maintain mutually beneficial partnerships between schools of nursing and agencies that provide services to patients. The screening experience contributes to student learning while providing invaluable professional health services to the community. Students have the opportunity to observe the benefits of collaboration and partnerships in health care delivery.

In the practicum experience described in this chapter, the health screenings involve school-age children. The groups of children screened consist mainly of children who, by virtue of their low socioeconomic status, are considered to be at high risk for unidentified and untreated problems that could impair their health and learning. It is hoped that the screening activities can contribute significantly to the well-being of these vulnerable children.

**NOTES**

1. D.L. Wong, M. Hockenberry-Eaton, D. Wilson, M.L. Winkelstein, E. Ahmann, and P.A. DiVito-Thomas, *Nursing Care of Infants and Children*, 6th ed. (St. Louis: Mosby, 1999), 12–25.

2. J. Brooks-Gunn and G.J. Duncan, The Effects of Poverty on Children, *Children and Poverty* 7, no. 2 (Summer/Fall, 1997):55–71.

3. J.B. Kotch, ed., *Maternal and Child Health: Programs, Problems, and Policy in Public Health* (Gaithersburg, MD: Aspen Publishers, 1997).

4. A. Hale, Service-Learning within the Nursing Curriculum. *Nurse Educator* 22, no. 2 (March/April, 1997):15–18.

5. M.E. Edmunds and M.J. Coye, *America's Children: Health Insurance and Access to Care* (Washington, DC: National Academy Press, 1998), 11–20.

6. Wong et al., *Nursing Care of Infants and Children*, 297–298.

7. M. Green, ed., *Bright Futures: Guidelines for Health Supervision of Infants, Children, and Adolescents* (Arlington, VA: National Center for Education in Maternal and Child Health, 1994), 79–219.

8. C.R. Uphold and M.V. Graham, *Clinical Guidelines in Family Practice*, 3rd ed. (Gainesville, FL: Barmarrae Books, 1998), 1–46.

9. Wong et al., *Nursing Care of Infants and Children*, 215–231, 234–299.

10. M.C. Carroll, K.H. Morin, E.R. Hayes, and S.V. Carter, Assessing Students' Perceived Threats to Safety in the Community: Instrument Refinement, *Nurse Educator* 24, no. 1 (January/February 1999):31–35.

---

## SUGGESTED READING

Brooks-Gunn, J., and G.J. Duncan. 1997. The effects of poverty on children. *The Future of Children* 7, no. 2:55–71.

Carroll, M.C., K.H. Morin, E.R. Hayes, and S.V. Carter. 1999. Assessing students' perceived threats to safety in the community. *Nurse Educator* 24, no. 1:31–35.

Ciaccio, J., and G.C. Walker. 1998. Nursing and service learning: The Kobayashi Maru. *Nursing and Health Care Perspectives* 19, no. 4:175–177. [CINAHL Link]

Green, M., ed. 1994. *Bright futures: Guidelines for health supervision of infants, children, and adolescents.* Arlington, VA: National Center for Education in Maternal and Child Health.

Hales, A. 1997. Service-learning within the nursing curriculum. *Nurse Educator* 22, no. 2:15–18.

Kotch, J.B. 1997. *Maternal and child health: Programs, problems, and policy in public health.* Gaithersburg, MD: Aspen Publishers.

Mellon, S., and P. Nelson. 1998. Leadership experiences in the community for nursing students: Redesigning education for the 21st century. *Nursing and Health Care Perspectives* 19, no. 3:120–123. [CINAHL Link]

Ryan, S.A., R.F. D'Aoust, S. Groth, K. McGee, and L. Small. 1997. A faculty on the move into the community. *Nursing and Health Care Perspectives* 18, no. 3:138–141.

Uphold, C.R., and M.V. Graham. 1998. *Clinical guidelines in family practice*, 3rd ed. Gainesville, FL: Barmarrae Books.

Williams, A., and J.L. Wold. 1996. Healthcare for the future: Caring for populations in alternative settings. *Nurse Educator* 21, no. 2:23–26.

Wong, D.L., M. Hockenberry-Eaton, D. Wilson, M.L. Winkelstein, E. Ahmann, and P.A. DiVito-Thomas. 1999. *Nursing care of infants and children*, 6th ed. St. Louis: Mosby.

# CHAPTER 25

# Nursing Process Mapping Replaces Nursing Care Plans

*Charlotte James Koehler*

## DEFINITION AND PURPOSES

The *nursing process mapping* format is a tool to assist nursing students to organize their thoughts and actions and to communicate these to their clinical instructor. It can be used in conjunction with an in-depth assessment database and is used instead of a traditional nursing care plan.

Mapping is defined as a graphic or pictorial tool used to arrange key concepts. In nursing education, the key concepts are assessment data that students collect either through case studies or their clinical assignments. The map develops as students diagram schematically the relationships among various clinical data. This process assists the students to visualize complex relationships and to apply theory to the clinical area.

Traditional nursing care plans have been with us for a long time and have served a much-needed purpose, but with the growth of nursing knowledge and the continuous reassessment of the role of the nurse comes evaluation of tools and ways of accomplishing tasks. In evaluating the traditional nursing care plan, as used by students, several problems come to mind. To begin with, it is rarely used as a plan but is frequently used in retrospect and developed almost completely after the care has taken place. To call it a care plan is a misnomer. Format rather than substance is often emphasized. For example, we spend many hours ensuring that the student knows what column the information goes in and how to phrase the information correctly, rather than focusing on the thought processes that the student used in developing the "plan."

Another problem with the traditional nursing care plan is the use of documenting rationale, which often becomes an all-consuming task. In the early stages of nursing care plans, this task was important. The profession was building a scientific base, and nursing textbooks provided very little nursing care documentation. Today, nursing care is included in all textbooks and is covered thoroughly in nursing education programs. Students know to use ice to reduce swelling of an incision—it is common knowledge—but they spend time finding the correct page and line when this time could be spent thinking about what is happening with the patient, selecting important information, and relating the material. Another situation that often occurs with students is the ready access of care plans from texts and hospital computers. It is not unusual for students to select a few appropriate aspects and then use them with very little thought.

The purpose of mapping nursing practice in nursing education is to have students develop critical thinking skills; that is, assess the patient, gather information from the literature, select relevant points, relate all of this information to the care of the patient, and illustrate the information graphically. This process helps the students establish priorities, seek relationships among information, and build on previous knowledge.[1]

## THEORETICAL RATIONALE

Concept mapping is well documented in education literature, especially in the fields of math and science. It has been used to analyze changes in the development of concept understanding held by students and to promote meaningful learning.[2] Mapping has been given various labels, depending on the intended use. It has been called cognitive mapping, idea mapping, patterned mapping, patterned note taking, and flow charting.[3] Jones and Sims state that mapping facilitates creativity; students are able to access their own thinking and experiences, find new associations, and generate a new set of ideas.[4]

Miccinati states that to create a map the student must think, select important points, relate the information, and then illustrate the information graphically, all of which require the student to think critically.[5] In the literature, concept mapping is defined as a method of organizing information in graphic form.[6] Heinz-Frye and Novak define concept mapping as a tool to enhance meaningful learning.[7]

Several authors have discussed using concept mapping as a tool to link nursing theory and clinical practice. Baugh and Mellott used concept mapping with case studies in small groups during an advanced medical-surgical course. These maps were updated as students continued to increase their theoretical knowledge and clinical experience.[8] Beitz discussed concept mapping in relationship to classroom nursing education and as preparation for examinations. Maps can show content inadequacies as well as illogical associations presented. They can also help decipher what concepts are most important.[9]

Irvine states that the need to promote meaningful learning in education must be supported by appropriate teaching and learning strategies, and that research evidence indicates that the technique of concept mapping improves all levels of student performance.[10]

Kathol et al. state that using mapping provides students with an ability to visualize components of the nursing assessment and to help them to visualize the interrelatedness of the multiple aspects of patient care. In this study, the maps were used for clinical preparation, and students developed a map from a case study as part of the final exam.[11]

## CONDITIONS

Mapping is a versatile technique that can be used in a variety of situations. The process requires instructor flexibility and students whose anxiety level is low enough to be introduced to something new and different. Because mapping is a process, it can be used in a variety of ways and can be simplistic or developed to a complex format. Because this process is so adaptable, it can be used with a learner of almost any age and in a variety of situations. The application is limited only by the imagination of the user.

### Planning and Modifying

Teachers who are new to this technique can become more familiar and comfortable with it by using it in lecture. Mapping can be used to represent a concept or idea in lecture, such as the relationships among information, psychomotor skills, cognitive skills, and attitude as they relate to competence in giving nursing care (see Figure 25–1).[12] It can also be used more informally to organize thoughts for a classroom presentation. Teachers can also devise interesting but familiar ideas for students to map as a classroom activity to introduce the mapping process.

Mapping can also be a successful tool in leading and guiding discussions during post conference. This approach is especially appropriate with a complex patient where many students have been involved. The greater the number of students that can participate in the mapping process, the more meaningful the discussion. Students can assist each other to draw relationships among large amounts of data and to eliminate that material that is irrelevant.

The mapping of clinical concepts also assists beginning nursing students to assign priorities to assessment data and to develop meaningful and relevant nursing diagnoses.

## TYPES OF LEARNERS

Mapping is appropriate for undergraduate and graduate students. Students can use it as an independent process; it can be used for small group work or in a very large classroom situation. It is especially useful in assisting students to think critically about the interrelatedness of new information, as well as to look at old information and relate it in different ways. Mapping can be simple or complex and can

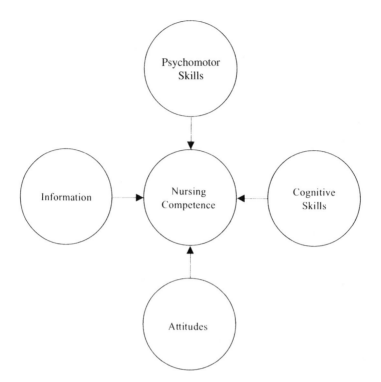

**Figure 25–1** Development of Nursing Competency. *Source:* Adapted with permission from Wager, W., Teaching/Learning Process, paper presented at Teaching Skills for Health Professions Educators, St. Simons Island, GA, August 1994.

be varied widely to suit many learning situations. It is important to introduce this process in a way that students with a variety of experiences and knowledge can relate to it and see its usefulness.

Many theorists have described various learning styles and learning preferences that would fit well with the use of concept mapping. Gardner and Hatch's visual/spatial form of intelligence emphasizes the ability to visualize and create mental images.[13] Students who have strength in the visual/spatial form of intelligence find mapping to be an easy and fulfilling method to relate their understanding of clinical situations. The ability to spatially describe the clinical situation helps them to better comprehend all aspects of patient care.

Dickenson noted that nursing emphasizes connectedness.[14] Using mapping encourages students to connect and interconnect patient problems in the clinical area. For example, in using mapping, the student has the opportunity to connect hypertension and pregnancy. The use of the nursing care plan does not allow for the ability to relate two separate problems into a unified whole.

Schon discusses reflection, which he relates to problem solving and synthesis.[15] Concept mapping allows students the opportunity to synthesize supposedly unrelated information and to develop a holistic picture of the patient situation.

Kelly and Young noted that a connection between experiences brings about meaningful learning.[16] Only simplistic connectedness exists in nursing care plans, whereas the premise of mapping is to show the relationship of each part of the patient and to unify it into a whole.

Kolb's learning style of assimilator is described as a person who is able to connect diverse items into an integrated whole.[17] Assimilation is the essence of mapping. Students gather all of the available information about the patient and use it in creating their maps to assist them in thoroughly comprehending the clinical situation.

Svinecki's last operating principle states that learners need to be aware of their ideal learning strategy.[18] Nursing faculty, in turn, need to enable the students to become more aware of their own personal learning style and to offer varied experiences to facilitate different learning styles. Concept mapping is one avenue to learning that will assist with different types of learners as well as allow faculty and students to become more creative in teaching and learning.

## RESOURCES

Mapping can be used in almost any setting and requires few resources. A paper and pencil are the only necessary supplies. Wycoff states that color activates the brain and helps us think better; adding colored pens and paper could help the student be more creative and enjoy the exercise.[19] Wycoff also states that music increases right brain activity and helps turn on our thinking process, which assists the development of mapping. Using one or both of these strategies would be helpful if it is appropriate to the setting.

## USING THE METHOD

Becoming familiar with the process and planning how it can be used in individual situations is most important to overall effectiveness. Using mapping in visual aids in class and in handouts is an effective way to introduce the concept of mapping. This can be done without labeling it or calling attention to the method, but just as a way of graphically representing information that the educator wants the students to comprehend. Figure 25–1 is an example of mapping that could be used in an introductory nursing class to help the students understand how information, skills, and attitudes learned from life, prenursing courses, and nursing courses are all necessary and important in reaching the aspiration of nursing competence.

A way of further involving the students is to have them use the technique personally and in a nonthreatening way. Wycoff suggests that the students be provided selected background music, colored pens, and paper,[20] and then asked to write a specific word or draw a representation of the word on the center of the paper. Starting with something concrete such as "desk" or "chair" and moving to something more related to nursing, such as "injection" or "bed bath" can be easy for students to relate to. The students are to spend no more than five minutes on any one map. They should be instructed to write down all thoughts and words that come to mind and to write as fast as they can. These ideas should flow from the central word or picture with ideas that generally relate to each other on branches. Remind the students that this is a process and that whatever they put on their map is acceptable. There are no right or wrong answers.

Once students become familiar with the concept of mapping, they can be directed to specific uses for communicating nursing assessment, care, and evaluation. This process is creative, and giving the students a great deal of direction stifles this creativity; the process once again will become focused on form rather than substance. Giving this type of guidance without structure allows the students to think critically about the patient, focus on important assessment information, choose appropriate nursing interventions, and visualize the interrelatedness of the nursing care process.

Student examples of mapping (see Figures 25–2 through Figure 25–5) vary tremendously in format and terminology, but the thought and insight needed to care for patients is evident much more so than in traditional nursing care plans. These maps were used with a comprehensive database. On the reverse side, the students included a brief (two or three sentences) evaluation of the care that they gave during the clinical, a brief evaluation of how they are meeting course objectives, and a general reference statement (i.e., author or lecturer). They were also required to attach a copy of a nursing journal article. They were encouraged to use a nursing research article, but a clinical article was accepted. They underlined how their article helped them to better care for their patient.

## EVALUATION

When asked a few simple questions about this process, students were overwhelmingly positive. They stated that this process made them think through things on their own, and they didn't just copy out of the book. They felt that they were better able to see the interrelatedness of the entire process. It was easy for them to use and generally less time consuming.

Faculty members using the form assessed that it communicated more succinctly what care was given and what thought process was used by the student. It was easier to read and evaluate, as well as being interesting.

Any time something new is used, the potential for problems exists. Questions to ask those involved are: "Will all students be able to use and feel comfortable with a non-guided format?" "Will faculty members feel comfortable with the evalua-

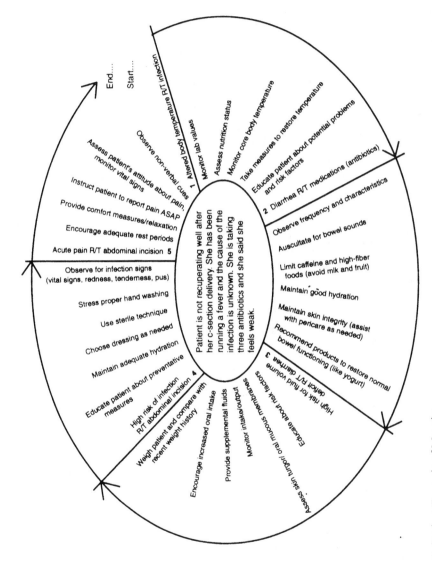

**Figure 25–2** Student Example of Mapping

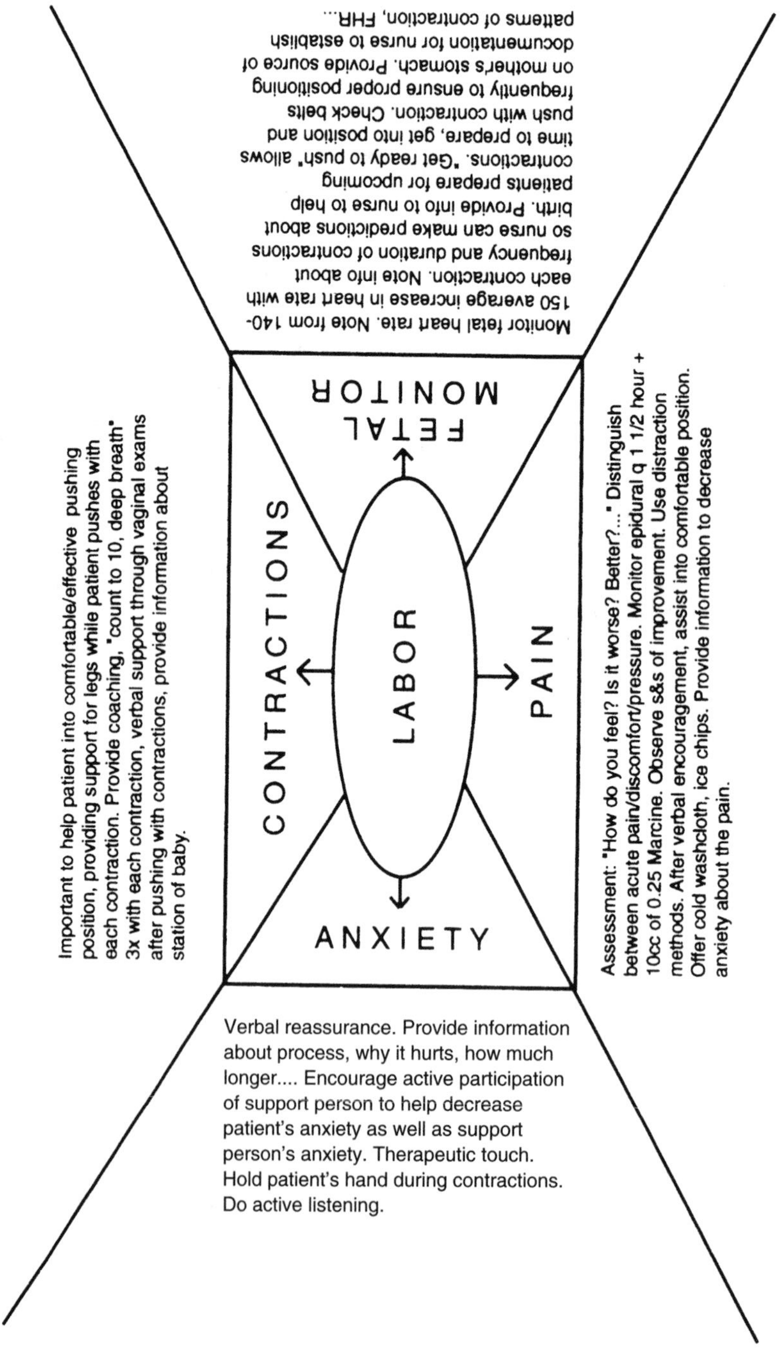

Monitor fetal heart rate. Note from 140-150 average increase in heart rate with each contraction. Note info about frequency and duration of contractions so nurse can make predictions about birth. Provide info to nurse to help patients prepare for upcoming contractions. "Get ready to push" allows time to prepare, get into position and push with contraction. Check belts frequently to ensure proper positioning on mother's stomach. Provide source of documentation for nurse to establish patterns of contraction, FHR...

Important to help patient into comfortable/effective pushing position, providing support for legs while patient pushes with each contraction. Provide coaching, "count to 10, deep breath" 3x with each contraction, verbal support through vaginal exams after pushing with contractions, provide information about station of baby.

FETAL MONITOR

CONTRACTIONS

LABOR

PAIN

ANXIETY

Assessment: "How do you feel? Is it worse? Better?..." Distinguish between acute pain/discomfort/pressure. Monitor epidural q 1 1/2 hour + 10cc of 0.25 Marcine. Observe s&s of improvement. Use distraction methods. After verbal encouragement, assist into comfortable position. Offer cold washcloth, ice chips. Provide information to decrease anxiety about the pain.

Verbal reassurance. Provide information about process, why it hurts, how much longer.... Encourage active participation of support person to help decrease patient's anxiety as well as support person's anxiety. Therapeutic touch. Hold patient's hand during contractions. Do active listening.

**Figure 25–3** Student Example of Mapping

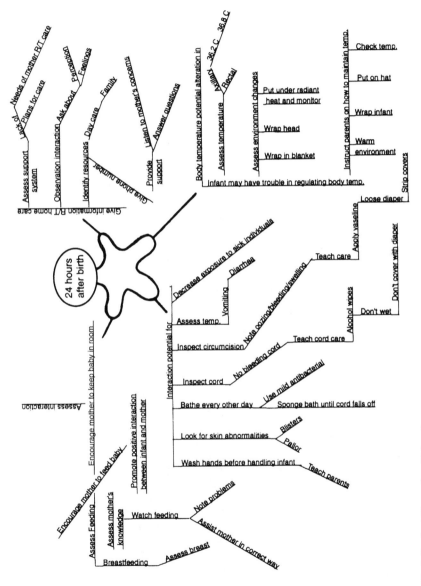

**Figure 25–4** Student Example of Mapping

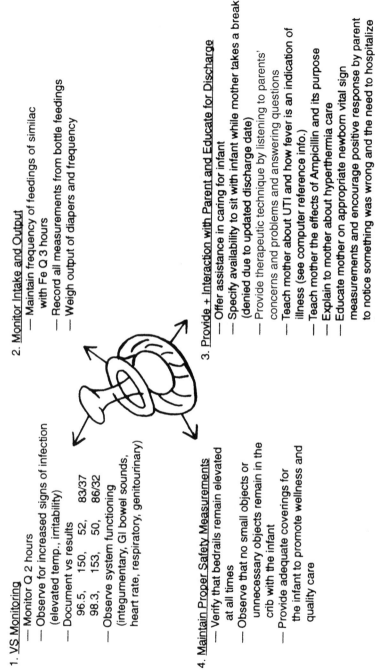

1. VS Monitoring
   — Monitor Q 2 hours
   — Observe for increased signs of infection
     (elevated temp., irritability)
   — Document vs results
       96.5,    150,    52,    83/37
       98.3,    153,    50,    86/32
   — Observe system functioning
     (integumentary, GI bowel sounds,
     heart rate, respiratory, genitourinary)

2. Monitor Intake and Output
   — Maintain frequency of feedings of similac
     with Fe Q 3 hours
   — Record all measurements from bottle feedings
   — Weigh output of diapers and frequency

3. Provide + Interaction with Parent and Educate for Discharge
   — Offer assistance in caring for infant
   — Specify availability to sit with infant while mother takes a break
     (denied due to updated discharge date)
   — Provide therapeutic technique by listening to parents'
     concerns and problems and answering questions
   — Teach mother about UTI and how fever is an indication of
     illness (see computer reference info.)
   — Teach mother the effects of Ampicillin and its purpose
   — Explain to mother about hyperthermia care
   — Educate mother on appropriate newborn vital sign
     measurements and encourage positive response by parent
     to notice something was wrong and the need to hospitalize
   — Answer any questions

4. Maintain Proper Safety Measurements
   — Verify that bedrails remain elevated
     at all times
   — Observe that no small objects or
     unnecessary objects remain in the
     crib with the infant
   — Provide adequate coverings for
     the infant to promote wellness and
     quality care

**Figure 25–5**  Student Example of Mapping

tion?" The most important question to ask about mapping is: "Will mapping facilitate the learning process?" These questions will be answered as the mapping process is used. Perhaps the most important question of all is: "Does our current method facilitate learning?"

---

## NOTES

1. J. Miccinati, Mapping the Terrain: Connecting Reading with Academic Writing, *Journal of Reading,* March (1988):542–552.

2. P. Horton, An Investigation of the Effectiveness of Concept Mapping as an Instructional Tool, *Science Education* 77, no. 1 (1991):95–111.

3. Miccinati, Mapping the Terrain.

4. S. Jones and D. Sims, Mapping as an Aid to Creativity, *Journal of Management Development* 4, no. 1 (1985):47–60.

5. Miccinati, Mapping the Terrain.

6. P. Gold, Cognitive Mapping, *Academic Therapy* 19, no. 3 (1984):277–284.

7. J. Heinz-Frye and J. Novak, Concept Mapping Brings Long-Term Movement toward Meaningful Learning, *Science Education* 74, no. 4 (1990):461–472.

8. N. Baugh and K. Mellott, Clinical Concept Mapping as Preparation for Student Nurses' Clinical Experiences, *Journal of Nursing Education* 37, no. 6 (1998):253–256.

9. J. Beitz, Concept Mapping: Navigating the Learning Process, *Nurse Educator* 23, no. 5 (1998):35–41.

10. L. Irvine, Can Concept Mapping Be Used To Promote Meaningful Learning in Nursing Education? *Journal of Advanced Nursing* 21 (1995):1175–1179.

11. D. Kathol, M. Geiger, and J. Hartig, Clinical Correlation Map: A Tool for Linking Theory and Practice, *Nurse Educator* 23, no. 4 (1998):31–34.

12. W. Wager, Teaching/Learning Process (Paper presented at Teaching Skills for Health Professions Educators, St. Simons Island, GA, August 1994).

13. H. Gardner and T. Hatch, Multiple Intelligencies Go to School: Educational Implications of the Theory of Multiple Intelligencies, Technical Report No. 4 (New York: Center for Technology in Education, 1990).

14. G.L. Dickenson, The Unintended Consequences of Male Professional Ideology for the Development of Nursing Education, *Advances in Nursing Science,* March (1993):67–83.

15. D.A. Schon, *The Reflective Practitioner: How Professionals Think in Action* (New York: Basic Books, 1983).

16. E. Kelly and A. Young, Models of Nursing Education for the 21st Century, *Review of Nursing Research in Nursing Education,* vol. vii (1996):1–39.

17. D.A. Kolb, *Experiential Learning Theory* (Englewood Cliffs, NJ: Prentice Hall, 1984).

18. M.D. Svinicki and N.M. Dixon, The Kolb Model Modified for Classroom Activities, *College Teaching* 35, no. 4:141–146.

19. J. Wycoff, *Mindmapping: Your Personal Guide to Exploring Creativity and Problem Solving* (New York: Berkeley Books, 1991).

20. J. Wycoff, *Mindmapping.*

# CHAPTER 26

# Issues in Clinical Teaching: Cautionary Tales for Nursing Faculty

*Pat Christensen*

## INTRODUCTION

"My patient doesn't have an apical pulse!" declared the sophomore nursing student to her instructor. "Really?" the wary instructor asked as she and the student headed toward the patient's room. Once at the bedside of a smiling, very alert elderly woman, the student indicated to her clinical professor the spot where she was attempting to auscultate the heartbeat at approximately the level of the small intestine. "You said we should listen one inch below the nipple line," she said, as she indicated the area of the sagging breasts.

This situation is just one of the hilarious anecdotes reported by a nursing faculty member in the *Journal of Nursing Jocularity.* "I could write a book" can be heard around the tables in the faculty lounge at most nursing schools. Nursing students are nowhere a greater challenge than when they attempt to demonstrate their newfound knowledge in the clinical area on real, live patients. Thankfully, most of the students' mistakes do not have dire consequences, but the supervision of students raises issues that are of concern. Long gone are the days when a doctor told a patient—and the patient bought the story—that her shaved head was "part of her treatment," this after a horrified student nurse discovered that she had prepped the wrong patient for a craniotomy! This true story illustrates how far accountability for mistakes has evolved. Patients today would not accept that story—nor should they.

In the dynamic environment of clinical teaching, issues and events occur unexpectedly. Although one cannot accurately know all eventualities, it is wise for nursing faculty members to be aware of, and plan for, student clinical errors and problems. Presented here are vignettes of clinical situations—all true—that may be useful to faculty members to explore as they venture forth with neophyte nurses-to-be.

## CASE HISTORY 1: PROTECTION OF PATIENT SAFETY

Approximately three hours into a busy clinical day on an obstetrics unit, Rhonda, a junior nursing student, approached her clinical instructor. "I don't feel so good," Rhonda said. "I have this fever and my neck is all swollen." "What?" her instructor exclaimed. "What are you doing here with a fever?" "I didn't want to miss a clinical day. You said we should make sure to meet all our clinical objectives," the student responded. The student was immediately sent home and the patient was reassigned to a staff nurse. The clinical instructor reported the incident to the nurse manager and finished the clinical day. The faculty member had practically forgotten the incident when, two days later, the student called and reported, "Guess what? I have the German measles." The faculty member thought back on the patient this student had cared for on that day. With a sickening feeling, she remembered that the student had cared for the only antepartal patient on the unit— a patient in early pregnancy with hyperemesis gravidarum. What if the student had infected the pregnant woman? Immediately, the faculty member called the patient's doctor and reported the ghastly coincidence. After a quick check of the patient's file, it was established that the patient had already been immunized for rubella, so there was no further cause for concern.

Today, with students required to show proof of immunizations, this particular case probably would not occur. Students can still report to the clinical area with a wide array of possible infectious processes, however. For example, a common cold sore can infect a newborn with the herpes virus, which can prove deadly to the baby. With clinical time at a premium in most facilities, the students are frequently warned not to be absent for clinical days. Clinical absences can mean the loss of valuable experiences and faculty scrambling to make up labs at semester's end. Although no faculty member would suggest that a student come to clinical sick, faculty members can send a message that clinical days are so valuable that students had better not miss them. Students, often conscientious and not wanting to miss valuable clinical time, may underreport or minimize an illness.

## CASE HISTORY 2: THE STUDENT NURSE UNCOVERS A SCANDAL

Helen, a senior nursing student in her last semester before graduation, was attempting to complete the assignments for the nursing management practice. As part of her requirements, she had to assess an organizational unit independently, including leadership style, structure, strengths and weaknesses of the unit, and so forth. She had been assigned to a community long-term care facility, where she also worked as a patient care technician. The student was having difficulty completing the assessment because she had become aware of some very disturbing incidents that were occurring at the nursing home, and she was unclear how to handle them. Serious suspected problems such as patient abuse, employees reporting to work inebriated, and inadequate supervision of unlicensed personnel were among the student's concerns. In her clinical conference, the instructor cautioned the student to report only her observations and not to draw conclusions, but nevertheless, the instructor was concerned. When the student submitted her final report on the facility, the instructor was aghast to read what the student had reported. Although the student had, in some instances, reported naive conclusions, the student had also undoubtedly made some astute observations of real problems—suspicious bruises on elderly patients' arms, the smell of alcohol on an employee's breath, and the absence of licensed personnel at certain times.

Armed with this information, the faculty member requested a conference with the dean of the nursing school to discuss the legal and ethical responsibilities of the student, the instructor, and the school in this case. Likewise, the dean was alarmed and deemed it imperative to include the university's attorney in the conference. After careful consideration, the attorney determined that most of the damning information in this case had been obtained while the student was an employee of the institution, not as a student. Therefore, the school's responsibility lay in urging the student employee to report her suspicions to her supervisor. The student did this with very unsatisfactory results—denial by the supervisor of any trouble and an accusation that the student was mistaken. The student subsequently resigned from that nursing home; no further attention was given to her suspicions. The nagging doubt remained, however, in the minds of the student, the instructor, and the dean—were patients in that facility at risk, and what should have been done?

This case illustrates the real dilemma faced by nursing faculty members when students observe reportable conditions—things such as child abuse and neglect—but that the nursing instructor does not witness. Do the faculty member and the school of nursing have a responsibility to report these cases? All states have laws that govern reportable incidents by health professionals, and it is incumbent upon faculty members to explore these issues. Consultation with the state board of nursing, the state department of social services, and the university attorney may be indicated in these cases.

## CASE HISTORY 3: SAFEGUARDING OF NURSING STUDENTS

In the community health course, junior nursing students were assigned to various agencies within the health department and assigned as well to visit homes of families in the community. Many of the homes were in poor, neglected, crime-ridden areas. (All students had been cautioned about safety concerns while in dangerous neighborhoods and were encouraged to go in pairs on their home visits.) The instructor took turns going with each student, but for most of the semester, the students had to make their home visits without the instructor.

Nursing student Rebecca was assigned to a new, single mother and her infant in a government housing project. On the scheduled home visit day, Rebecca was unable to arrange to visit with another student and so proceeded to the client's home alone. While walking toward the new mother's apartment, the student's progress was impeded by a group of young men who were loitering around the project. As Rebecca attempted to make her way down the walkway, the five young men made lewd and suggestive remarks to her. Eventually, the men surrounded the student but did not touch her. The remarks included, "Hi, baby, whatchoo doin' here?" "Can we help you?" "Man, you are some chick." The student attempted to retain her composure, but she later stated that she was very afraid. With as much confidence as she could muster, she told the group that she was a nurse and she came to take care of Ms. Wilson's baby. As she spoke, she continued to walk toward her client's home. She was able to reach the client's apartment and complete her assessment of the newborn, but she dreaded returning to her car. She wanted to call her instructor, but the young mother did not have a phone. Rebecca waited in the apartment until the young men moved on and then made a quick walk to her car and sped away. She was unhurt, but the episode was very unsettling for her, and later for her instructor, whom she told about the incident at the clinical conference.

This encounter was reported to the program director and the dean, and a committee was formed to study the issue of student safety in the community health course and to formulate policies and procedures to deal with these potential problems. Among the recommendations were that students were never to make home visits alone. At least one other student, public health nurse, or the instructor must accompany each student. Additionally, students and faculty members were issued beepers so that their whereabouts could always be determined.

Student safety is a major issue on college campuses today. Families have the right to expect that their son or daughter will be safe while at that school. Nursing students, especially in community health courses, are often exposed to environments such as the one described previously. The schools of nursing must take extra precautions while students are out on clinical experiences. Not only are students sent to unsafe neighborhoods, but they are also often en route in other students' cars and vans. Insurance coverage must be adequate to cover all eventualities. A system must be put in place to ensure that students and the school are adequately served in the area of student safety.

## CASE HISTORIES 4 AND 5: STUDENTS AS POLICE

Nursing professionals, including students, are often confronted with situations where liability for reporting to authorities is unclear. For example, where is the line between child abuse and discipline as understood by parents and nurses? Is a smack on a child's face by a parent, in the presence of a nurse, child abuse or the parent's usual mode of discipline? Situations like this can and do arise in the course of clinical experiences. The following two vignettes illustrate some examples.

## Case History 4

Betty, a senior nursing student, was assigned to a welfare mother and her two children for home visits as part of the requirements for the child health course. She was supposed to make a series of visits to assess the children's growth and development, their immunization status, and other aspects of primary care.

In the state where Betty practiced, it was unlawful for women to receive welfare benefits if they were living with, or being supported by, a man in the house. Welfare fraud had become a major issue in the state, and all abuse of the system was to be reported. On several of her visits, Betty observed a young man, who the mother stated was the father of her children, playing with and caring for the children. Betty also observed that the father kept his clothes and personal effects in the trailer he shared with the young family. The dilemma that confronted Betty was, should she report this case? Betty consulted with her clinical instructor and together they attempted to analyze as many aspects of this case as possible, with the overriding question being, what was best for these children?

On the numerous occasions that Betty had been at the home, she had observed the father interacting lovingly with his children and providing much-needed help with their care. Betty did not ask directly, nor was it ever mentioned by the parents, the exact circumstances of the man living with the family. The two small children appeared to be benefiting from the relationship, and it appeared that the family badly needed the consistent financial support of welfare. A central question appeared to be, should nurses be part of law enforcement? Was this a case of fraud or a matter of client confidentiality? After careful consideration, Betty and her instructor decided to just leave well enough alone and not report that the children's father probably lived in the home. This was a case where the nurse did not feel it to be her responsibility to report a suspected violation of policy or law. Would the situation have been different if the children were not being cared for as well? Another case of a student nurse in a difficult clinical situation shows a different perspective.

## Case History 5

Philip, a senior nursing student, was assigned to a single-parent family in his community health course. In the home lived a 22-year-old mother, a three-year-old girl, and an infant boy six months of age. Also, it appeared that different men lived with the mother occasionally. Philip found the public housing apartment to be extremely dirty and untidy on all occasions when he made home visits. The children were often hungry and poorly dressed, but no one had observed the mother or the various men abusing the children, nor were they left alone. Frequently, however, no one would answer the door when the student knocked. One Sunday morning, the clinical instructor read in the paper that the woman who was Philip's client had been arrested for prostitution and was suspected in the death of a man who had come to the apartment for sex. After verifying that, indeed, the woman reported in the paper was the children's mother, the question arose, was there an obligation to report possible child neglect? After careful consideration, the student and the clinical instructor decided that, in this case, it would be prudent to report to the social services authorities that the children needed further evaluation of the home to be safe from abuse and neglect.

Both of these cases illustrate the need for careful analysis of cases on an individual basis. Most families, especially poor ones, have very complex relationships that can either hinder or enhance the well-being of children. If nurses are seen as agents of law enforcement, then they may lose the confidence and rapport that has been fostered over many years of public health tradition. More important, if nurses are not trusted, poor, vulnerable families may lose the care that they so desperately need.

## CASE HISTORY 6: THE INCOMPETENT STUDENT

Eleanor, a second-semester junior student, was the daughter of a trustee of the university where she attended nursing school. She appeared to be an average student in her classwork, but her clinical skills were incompletely assessed. In her first two years of clinical courses, her final evaluations reflected that she had met the objectives, but lacked confidence and was reluctant to ask for assistance. Eleanor was very open about being the daughter of a trustee and made numerous remarks about her influential father and their discussions of her nursing school experiences.

One clinical day in her parent-child course, Eleanor was assigned to a young woman in labor. All students had been assigned readings and audiovisual aids to see before they attempted patient care in the hospital. The objectives for that clinical laboratory were to provide comfort measures, to assess the progress of labor, to provide psychological support, and to observe and report any possible signs of complications. Although a staff nurse was also assigned to the patient, that staff nurse was very busy that day and did not stay in the room with the patient at all times.

About four hours into labor, the fetal monitoring strip of the unborn baby began to show decelerations (slowing heart rate), and on several occasions the mother stated that she felt "faint and dizzy." Eleanor, who was in the room alone with the patient for approximately 20 minutes, did not assess the fetal monitoring strip, take the vital signs of the mother, or report to the nurse or her instructor what the patient stated. On entering the labor room, the instructor immediately observed the slow fetal heart rate and promptly turned the mother on her side and took her blood pressure. Within a few minutes, the fetal heart rate was within normal limits and the mother was comfortable. Her blood pressure, which had been 90/48 when the instructor entered the room, rose to her baseline reading of 128/78.

On interviewing the student about the situation, it became clear to the instructor that Eleanor lacked even basic judgment and knowledge about the relationship among vital signs, patient well-being, and indicated nursing actions. Somehow, through copying other students' and published care plans and being quiet and unobtrusive, Eleanor had progressed through two years of clinical courses with minimal clinical skills. The question lingered in the instructor's mind: had other clinical faculty been intimidated—perhaps unconsciously—by the student's father's influence in the university? On careful evaluation, the instructor determined that Eleanor would receive a failing grade for the clinical course.

When the student was informed of her grade, she stated that she thought it was unfair and said, "I'll tell my father." After several conferences with the program director and the dean, it was determined that because the student had passed other clinical courses and was allowed to progress in the program, she was entitled to extra tutoring and could not be failed at that time. Vast amounts of faculty time were spent in extra tutoring for Eleanor. After she graduated with her class, Eleanor took the NCLEX exam on two occasions and failed both times.

In subsequent faculty discussions, there was always the issue lurking: how had this student had been allowed to progress and graduate? In an effort to ensure that a similar situation did not occur, stricter and more objective clinical evaluation methods were instituted. These methods included objective clinical exams, as well as tests of performance. In addition, a policy was adopted that did not permit progress in the program after a clinical failure. Also, a warning system of identifying and reporting students at risk for failure was instituted.

**CASE HISTORY 7: THE PEANUT BUTTER SCARE**

As part of a family nursing course, students were enthusiastically planning for a teaching program on healthy snacks for a group of elementary school students. The nursing students worked diligently on a poster and handouts for the young children. They planned for an enthusiastic and interactive teaching project, which would involve the children. Among the planned activities was the serving of healthy snacks. There were many suggestions such as "ants on a log" (peanut butter in celery ribs with raisins as the "ants"), cheese crackers, carrots, apples, and other fruits and vegetables. The students made arrangements to buy the food and prepare the snacks.

The day of the teaching project, the students met at the school and assembled the snacks. The teaching project went well, with a lot of interaction occurring between the nursing students and the children. The children enthusiastically identified the cutout pictures of healthy snacks on the colorful poster. They outlined the coloring sheets with bright crayons. As the snacks of fruit, "ants on a log," and milk were put out, the children clamored for their healthy snack. Each of the children came forward and eagerly accepted the paper plates with the equal portions of fruit, celery sticks with peanut butter, and a small cup of milk. One child, a small eight-year-old girl, tugged on a student nurse's shirt and shyly asked if there were any other snacks she could have. The student said, "No, these are all we have. Don't you like fruit and peanut butter?" The little girl turned away with her plate and sat at her desk.

While the other children ate their food, this young girl just looked at her plate. Another one of the nursing students noticed this behavior and approached the child. "What's the matter? Aren't you hungry?" "My mommy won't let me eat peanut butter. It makes me sick," the little girl responded. Just then, the girl's teacher came to the class. "Oh, no!" she exclaimed. "Judy can't eat peanut butter. She is very allergic. She can go into shock." The nursing student realized with a sudden rush of anxiety that a major disaster was narrowly averted. She immediately took the plate away and apologized to the girl. As a substitute, she gave the child an extra helping of apple and orange slices on a clean plate.

During post conference with her instructor and the other students, the student relayed the scary experience. The nursing faculty member realized at once that somehow, in the planning and implementation of the learning experience, the risk of food allergy had not been adequately addressed.

Increasingly, there are reports of severe allergic reactions among all segments of the population, including children. Many of the culprits are well-loved and frequently consumed foods such as peanut butter. Other sensitivities that are of concern include latex products, including examining gloves, foods with dyes or other additives, and common household products. The list of possible antigens is long and diverse. What implications does this reality have for nursing education? Most nurses are mindful of allergies among hospitalized patients because these conditions are assessed and noted prominently on the patients' charts, but what about community clients? How can these risks be minimized in that population? The answer lies in two major strategies—assessment and informed consent.

As a result of the peanut butter episode, the faculty formulated and implemented a policy that all community clients must be assessed for allergies and sign an informed consent. In the case of children, permission forms are to be distributed to parents and returned to the school or other setting. The forms not only ask for allergies but also grant permission for the child to participate in a health project. Although it may be difficult to implement, *only those children whose parents have given permission will be allowed to participate in clinical experiences with nursing students.* Unfortunately, the risks to children and the financial liability of the school must limit the participation of children who do not obtain permissions in advance from parents and guardians.

## GUIDELINES FOR FACULTY

Although problems such as the ones reported here are unpredictable, clinical nursing faculty members would be wise to consider some contingency plans for the unexpected. One of the most important considerations in protecting the student, the patient, and the school is open communication. An ongoing and supportive relationship between the school of nursing and the respective state board of nursing is essential. Additionally, an open communication line with the university attorney (or an attorney consultant) can provide essential legal guidance. Paramount in these relationships is the need for immediacy in replies. Often, situations occur that demand an answer quickly. Relationships must be forged on a trusting basis that allows for on-the-spot consulting.

Another dimension of open communication centers on informing students of their rights and responsibilities while attending the school of nursing. A student handbook is often an avenue for distributing such information. A written account, such as a handbook, can serve as a contract for students. A student handbook should be specific enough to be useful, but not so specific as to limit the school in a changing environment. For example, it is not possible—or desirable—to attempt to list every eventuality that may occur. Pertinent information can be catalogued under headings such as "Uniform Policy," "Student Illness in the Clinical Area," and "Student Safety in the Clinical Area."

Another avenue of student information can be a complete and mandatory student orientation. There is often a need to convey information to students that is more fluid and changing than can be covered in a handbook—for example, the location of an agency, parking, contact persons in the clinical area, and so forth. In many cases, having students sign for written information can form a "contract of understanding." Under no circumstances can school officials assume that students have essential information upon entry into the program or course. A certain amount of redundancy in student expectations for each course is to be expected.

The National League for Nursing and program nurse consultants at all state boards of nursing can provide guidance to schools on the formation of student policies and handbooks. It is advisable to have policies and handbooks pilot-tested and read by students, faculty, and parent groups for clarity and meaning before officially disseminating them to students and faculty. This author also advises a legal opinion on policies.

In the dynamic environment of clinical teaching, events occur that are unpredictable and troublesome. Although no one can accurately know all eventualities, nursing faculty members should be aware of, and plan for, student clinical errors and problems. The careful and judicious formulation of student policies and handbooks and open and ongoing communication with students, faculty, state officials, and legal consultants will diminish the chances of dire consequences arising from student mishaps.

## SUGGESTED READING

Carroll, M.C., K.H. Morin, E.R. Hayes, and S.V. Carter. 1999. Assessing students' perceived threats to safety in the community. *Nurse Educator* 24, no. 1:31–35.

Kotch, J.B. 1997. *Maternal and child health, programs, problems, and policy in public health.* Gaithersburg, MD: Aspen Publishers.

Mellon, S., and P. Nelson. 1998. Leadership experiences in the community for nursing students: Redesigning education for the 21st century. *Nursing and Health Care Perspectives* 19, no. 3:120–123.

Noble, M.A., G.M. Redmond, J.K. Williams, and C. Langley. 1996. Education for the nurse of tomorrow: A community-focused curriculum. *Nursing and Health Care Perspectives* 17, no. 2:66–71.

Shoultz, J., and M.J. Amundson. 1998. Nurse educators' knowledge of primary health care: Implications for community-based education, practice, and research. *Nursing and Health Care Perspectives* 19, no. 3:115–119.

# PART VII

# Evaluation

The final section of this text presents a brief glimpse at a key aspect of any educational program: evaluation. Whereas the importance of evaluation is often overlooked, it is an essential part of the teaching-learning process. Educators predominantely think of evaluation either in the form of testing and grading or in clinical evaluation. Two chapters in this section describe innovative strategies by which the faculty can conduct student evaluation.

The final chapter is a fitting conclusion to this book. Evaluation of nursing education starts at the lower levels of evaluation of learning to indicate how well students are meeting outcomes of the course and the program. This information then feeds into total program evaluation and provides data on the curriculum, teaching effectiveness, and the use of learning activities. A thorough evaluation provides information for the future.

# CHAPTER 27

# Computer-Based Testing

*David J. Anna*

## DEFINITION AND PURPOSES

Computer-based testing (CBT) is the administration of test questions/examinations via a computer through the application of specialized computer software that has been commercially developed. CBT software is multifunctional and can be utilized to create and administer formal examinations, questionnaires, surveys, tutorials, and presentations. CBT has grown in importance to the process of evaluation and licensing in the United States with wide use and increasing acceptance. During the 1990s, it was extensively adopted for national medical and nonmedical licensing examinations, with more than 600 specialty areas transitioning to this format.[1] One of the earliest examinations to use CBT was the Graduate Record Examination (GRE), which has been offered in computerized format since 1992. More recent CBT conversions are the professional licensing examinations for registered nurses (NCLEX-RN), practical nurses (NCLEX-PN), architects, physical therapists, blood bank specialists, and radiologic technicians. The English proficiency test for international students (TOEFL) and Praxis I: Computer-Based Academic Skills Assessments (a national test for prospective teachers) have also changed to the CBT format.

The Educational Testing Service, which administers many of the examinations, notes multiple advantages: "It allows for new kinds of assessment that get away from strictly multiple choice; computerized testing can be adaptive, gearing questions toward the individual test-taker's performance level; and can be administered at conveniently located sites in an atmosphere more comfortable than at mass administrations of paper-and-pencil tests."[2] The exponential growth of computer testing software has been phenomenal in terms of diversity, complexity, and use.

From a historical perspective, CBT programs emerged during the mid-1980s, permitting educators to create and store banks of test items for the first time. Although rudimentary compared to current programs, they offered tremendous savings in test assembly time. Items could be easily copied and pasted between computer files and printed out as ready-to-go pencil-and-paper examinations. Textbook publishers subsequently began to provide test banks on computer disk as well as in printed form as part of their teaching-learning packages. Users could scan the questions, select those they wished to use, and print out the test on paper. Software development proceeded rapidly, and soon programs that could deliver and score tests via computer were appearing.

Initially, these programs operated from individual computers, but as networked systems emerged, the software grew to accommodate the technology. From these quite humble beginnings of only being able to deliver tests from an individual computer with a floppy disk, CBT has evolved to worldwide Internet-based testing capability with inclusion of sophisticated graphics and adaptive questioning strategies. Improved data analysis features provide educators with profiles of class and/or individual test results and how well test items performed.[3] Although not a "set-it-and-forget-it" technology, CBT is well suited to many testing requirements and a valuable addition to the educational process.

## THEORETICAL RATIONALE

Technology use in education has grown explosively over the past decade and with it the need to develop testing methods of equal sophistication. Higher education courses are moving from the traditional classroom to distance learning environments and "Web-based" via the Internet. Paper-and-pencil testing methods are not suitable for such wide dispersion of students who receive instruction totally or in part via electronic means. Gathering students together for mass testing, which has been the standard of testing for decades, is exceedingly more difficult and unlikely. Students often are trying to manage child care, family demands, and full- or part-time employment. Traditional paper-and-pencil tests do have benefits but always restrict examinations to predetermined days and times. Options to take an examination outside of these preset dates are scant to none. The need for evaluation still exists, however, and challenges educators to find suitable ways of administering tests when these are included as part of the course design. CBT may be a solution for these issues.

The use of CBT in a nursing curriculum provides students with exposure to computers for evaluative purposes and in doing so assists in reducing the element of computer anxiety that may accompany their NCLEX experience. Even at this time of computer penetration into almost every aspect of our lives, some people still have significant discomfort with the technology. Faculty should not underestimate this phenomenon and recognize that practice, familiarity, and comfort with CBT will aid these students to feel more at ease during the licensing exam.[4] Students are now expected to have some facility with regard to computer skills, but most have not previously experienced CBT. Many will have used a computer for word processing, personal communications, entertainment, and exploring the Internet but will not have encountered it for testing and evaluative purposes.

Although other interactions with computers do take place in a nursing curriculum (e.g., computer-assisted instruction and interactive videodiscs), they are primarily for presenting information, not testing, and do not affect course grades.[5] Anna additionally states that "Educators need to ask themselves whether students, somewhere in their nursing curriculum, experience the combination of sitting before a computer screen and having their keystrokes affect a meaningful outcome as it relates to grades? If the answer is, 'Well no', the question to be asked is 'Why not'?"[6] Preparing nursing students to take their licensing examination by computer through exposure to CBT is a valid rationale for its introduction into the nursing curricula.

The time that faculty members invest in the development, administration, and scoring of tests will be substantially reduced. This is a function of the ease with which questions/tests can be assembled and subsequently delivered over a computer/computer network. Analyzing the results of the student performance is markedly improved with the ability to examine individual or group results from a faculty member's office immediately following completion of a test. Students appreciate the flexibility that CBT provides in terms of offering expanded testing times, which may give them choices as to when to take a test. Giving students feedback at the end of a test for questions they have missed provides a method of reteaching the information at the most optimum moment.

## CONDITIONS

Faculty members should be able to adapt most, if not all, of their testable material to a CBT format unless essay responses are required. The software does not have the capability to grade this type of question. Examples of question types include traditional multiple choice with a flexible number of distractors; multiple response questions that allow more than one choice; questions that include a graphic and ask the respondent to place a marker over a requested position; numeric answer, text matching in which the typing in of a word or short answer is required; and selection questions that ask the student to match items to choices. Text-matching types of tests are challenging to use because they require the determination of all possible correct answers so a question would be graded correctly. Even misspelled words would result in the item being marked incorrect.

Testing can be accomplished any day of the week and any time of the day that a designated computer is available. Faculty members traditionally have restricted testing to weekdays, but with the use of CBT that can be expanded to weekends. The use of weekend days might seem to be encroaching on students' free time, but one study surprisingly found that the available time slots for Saturdays were almost always filled first.[7] Students commented that they felt less pressured by other commitments on a weekend day and that it gave them one more day to prepare.

A shorter test-taking time is a common finding with CBT, especially if students are permitted to proceed only in a forward direction and not allowed to go back to previously answered questions. They learn to analyze the question more thoroughly, apply a problem-solving approach, and arrive at an answer much quicker. A 50-item examination with a 50-minute time period set in a unidirectional structure will be completed in about 30 to 35 minutes.

Some CBT programs have an "adaptive-like" testing capability to mimic the style of the NCLEX licensing examination. The adaptive element refers to the testing structure being able to offer questions of varying degrees of difficulty based on previously answered items.[8] A much larger test item bank including content-similar questions with differing levels of difficulty is necessary to support the adaptive-like approach. Considerably more investment of time and proficiency with the CBT software would be necessary to set up the parameters of the examination to utilize this feature.

## TYPES OF LEARNERS

Students at any point in their nursing curriculum will benefit from exposure to CBT, but it is best introduced at the beginning. Early and continued exposure to the process will assist students in their question analysis and critical-thinking ability. Few will experience difficulty once they are familiarized with the software. For students with special learning needs who require additional time to take an examination, this process can be adjusted to accommodate those situations.

Student response to CBT will not be reflective of their learning styles or abilities but rather of their previous test-taking experience. Not all students will embrace computerized test taking as advantageous, even though they are aware that this is the format of the licensing exam. The majority will have come from an exclusively pencil-and-paper testing environment. Test-taking strategies will have been developed and internalized from years of personal experience and secondary school faculty guidance. This method has served them well until now but is not necessarily transferable to CBT. They are used to having several pieces of paper in front of them that they can quickly scan, doing the easiest questions first, and certainly looking for information in one question that provides an answer to another. When computer-based tests are structured so that students can only move forward and not revisit questions (thus emulating the NCLEX), they may experience a degree of frustration. Anna noted that the single most frequent disagreement that students had with CBT was with this "unidirectional" setting.[9] This issue will surely arise, and faculty need to have discussed it beforehand and be prepared to respond appropriately; however, do not be dissuaded from using this approach because it forces students to critically examine only the information presented on the screen and to decide which distractor is correct.

Orientation to the testing software before any examinations are administered is an absolute requirement.[10] Students must know how to navigate within the system, and a practice examination needs to be developed and in place prior to the actual course examinations. The goal should be to make this a no-stress, enjoyable experience. It can be accomplished by creating sample questions around a topic of interest to students (e.g., contemporary music, famous personalities, trivia regarding the institution, etc.). Everything about how this familiarization test appears before students on the computer monitor should mimic the actual course examinations. Having it accessible at all times and without restriction as to how many times it can be taken helps students' comfort and confidence level. A requirement should be established that all students practice with the familiarization exam before actual testing begins and that documentation of this activity occurs. Many students believe they are quite computer literate, but this is the exception, not the rule. Students who do not practice with the software may encounter difficulty navigating within it. "The software isn't running right" or "Something's wrong with my computer" are likely student responses, but the malfunction is not in the program but with the student's failure to follow faculty directions.

Because examination times are often spread over a day or more, signing up for a time that complements students' academic or personal needs is now possible. Everyone has a peak performance time during the day, and the flexible testing schedule may allow students to sign up for a time that complements that situation. The benefits for students far outweigh the adjustment to a CBT format.

Most test-takers like to know as soon as possible how they performed on a test, and CBT displays that result on the monitor promptly upon finishing. This instant performance feedback is received as a mixed blessing—great if they did well, not so if they did poorly—but the anxiety of waiting several days for grades to be posted is removed. One of the most appreciated features for students is the ability to receive feedback on all questions or just those missed, which can be displayed as they proceed through or complete a test, thus eliminating the need to go over them at a separate time.[11,12] Knowing what was missed and what answer is correct reinforces content presented in other learning activities. This feature is educationally sound, exceptionally well received by students, and almost totally obviates the need for test review and reteaching of material. As most nursing faculty can attest, test review in the classroom, in addition to taking time, can be a challenging experience because students wish to debate their point of view. Some CBT programs permit teacher-defined feedback in addition to showing the correct answer. An illustration of this might be: "The nursing care plan on page 177 of your textbook should have led you to the correct answer" or "Did you recall that urinary incontinence is a risk factor for impaired skin integrity?"

## RESOURCES

Resources necessary to implement CBT require an investment of time, personnel, computer hardware, space, and financial resources. Time will be needed to compare and preview software, select the most compatible program, and train persons in its use. Criteria for selection of CBT software should center around a short learning curve, ease of use, the key issue of network compatibility, and the features desired. Enormously easing the process of software review is the comparative examination by Kirkpatrick et al. of seven computerized test development programs.[13] These authors reviewed and categorized the features of each and offer suggestions on foundational aspects of implementation. They highly suggest that "nurse educators understand their goals for computerized test development and administration in the context of their own setting before purchasing a program."

Computer support personnel will be needed to assess current computer resources, the institution network configurations, and Internet access. Such consultations include determining the number of computer stations/classrooms linked together, how security of CBT operation files will be handled, and alternatives should technical problems arise during the administration of an exam. Faculty members can facilitate this assessment by determining how many courses would be adopting CBT, the number of students involved, and outlining other demands on existing computer resources. Introducing CBT into only one course at a time to develop a comfort level with the process and identify any technical or logistical problems is suggested as the most prudent approach. Administrative support personnel are necessary to keystroke the test questions into the software and make changes as required. They would need some training time to become familiar with the software functions.

Space in the form of computer classrooms/learning resource centers is a must. The ideal classroom could be reserved to ensure a quiet testing environment and would have computers spaced sufficiently far apart to dissuade test-takers from glancing at another student's monitor. The location of the classroom on the campus is not a critical issue. With network software, the test can be delivered to any connected computer. The numbers of available computers should be sufficient to ideally test all students within an 8- to 10-hour period. When this is not possible, expanded testing times would have to be considered.

Finally, a financial commitment is essential to procure not only the CBT program and associated site licenses but also any additional hardware on which to run and deliver the tests to the greatest number of students at one time as is feasible. These vital infrastructure elements must be in place if successful outcomes are to be achieved.

## USING THE METHOD

The underlying and fundamental principle to achieve success when using CBT is careful attention to detail. Computer software will do only what it is told, and if something is left out or a step is missed in setting up the examination, it will not run properly. Imbedded in this detail-orientation requirement is the need for someone to have a proficient understanding of the program. It may be the faculty member, administrative, or computer support person, but that individual is a vital link to the program's success. Previewing each test before the student takes it facilitates knowing that all is in readiness and that the student answer files are being saved in the designated area.

The actual assembly of tests will continue to be the largest consumer of faculty time. Keystroking questions into the software requires the bulk of the time, followed by setting the parameters of how the test will be delivered. One initial task is to decide if the questions in the test should be "grouped" into different content areas. This approach has a decided advantage when analyzing results. Once this task is accomplished, the next aspect is setting the structural parameters of how the test will be presented. Choices are made regarding: screen colors and fonts, the time limit of the exam, if answer files are to be saved or not (they almost always are), what information will be continually on the screen for students (e.g., countdown clock, question number, name of the exam, etc.), the order of question presentation, ability of students to freely move about the exam or proceed only in one direction, how many times a question may be attempted, type of question feedback to be given, and how the final score is reported. Other elements may need to be decided depending on the software program, but these choices are typically common to most programs.

Once testing dates are determined and reservations for the computer rooms made, student sign-up sheets are prepared. Competition for these rooms may occur and necessitate flexibility in setting the testing dates. Unlike other testing situations, students may be given choices as to when they will take the examinations or faculty can opt to assign them. Sign-up sheets with dates and times can be posted outside faculty offices or common areas. Students sign up for a time that complements their other commitments. No restrictions need to be imposed on the number of times students can change the date or time as long as the number of open spaces is not exceeded. Students can monitor the sign-up sheet themselves. Rarely will a student miss a graded activity. In developing sign-up sheets, faculty members should be sensitive to blocking out times when other colleagues' classes may be occurring. If this is not done, then students may take the test during someone else's class time, which could create animosity among faculty.

Administering the test is usually a joint function of the faculty member and computer support services. The support services personnel ensure that the program is in a secure place on the network, icons are created to start the test, the test is accessible on the dates required, answer files are delivered where they need to be, and a "test drive" confirms that all elements are working as programmed. Faculty absolutely must be able to depend on computer support for assistance in making CBT a success at their institution.

The scoring of tests is an automatic function of the software. As soon as the student has completed the test, the grade is calculated and presented on the monitor screen. Faculty members no longer need to hand-score or send optical scanning sheets off for processing. Posting of results outside faculty offices can be eliminated. Software options may permit faculty feedback to students on ranges of scores. If score bands that are linked to letter grades have been defined, then a message appropriate to each band could be developed (e.g., "93 percent That's a terrific score" or "76 percent I'm concerned about this low grade, please make an appointment to see me.") Structuring access to students' answer files from the faculty member's office computer can provide prompt processing of grades and analysis of student and class performance.

A difficulty encountered when using paper-and-pencil tests is how to easily and precisely determine what areas were most or least challenging for students. At least one CBT program addresses this need by incorporating the ability to group "like-content" questions together in a separate test item bank, which can be analyzed independent of others. To illustrate: if an examination focused on oxygenation issues and contained questions related to health promotion, disease entities, nursing interventions, etc., then the questions could be grouped and presented separately. Subsequently, student or class performance within each group could be determined when the answer files are analyzed. If each of the topics had been taught by a different faculty member, then feedback to them could be provided regarding student performance on their material. This information is valuable and can assist faculty members to determine if their presentation method achieved their desired outcomes. Features such as this one are also helpful to determine how to assist students at risk or who are not progressing well. Faculty members could examine the answer files of individuals or groups of students within certain score ranges and quickly see how the students performed on any of the grouped questions. Remedial instruction could then be pinpointed only to those content areas. Never before has information been available so easily and with such specificity.

The use of "situation"-style questions and their compatibility with the CBT format deserves some discussion. This type of question has long been used in nursing, and before the NCLEX-RN became computerized, they were included as a style on the licensing examination. Situation questions begin with the presentation of a scenario containing clinical information followed by several specific questions relating to it. They can be used in CBT but with certain adjustments. Because it would be confusing for a student to have to move backward to the question that first presented the "situation," this information needs to be presented on the monitor screen for each item in that series. Font size may need to be reduced to accommodate large amounts of text. These questions are best "grouped" together and their order not shuffled. Although situation-style questions as described are no longer included on the NCLEX examination, they may serve a valid purpose for an in-course test.

The first day of computerized testing is typically filled with excitement and a measure of anxiety for faculty. Several trial runs of the software are usually undertaken, but there is still the nagging uncertainty that an unanticipated problem will arise. As a precautionary measure, traditional paper-and-pencil exams may be prepared as a backup. Ideally, all students will have practiced with the familiarization test sufficiently to have achieved a comfort level with the software. Proctoring issues (see the following Potential Problems section) should have been ironed out, but for the first day of testing having faculty available for the occasional software navigation question is endorsed. If a course is being taught by distance learning or Web-based over the Internet, then CBT can still be used. Exams can be distributed via floppy disks, taken on an available computer, and mailed back to faculty. Some CBT programs have been specifically developed to be compatible with the Internet. Students could log on at home or wherever the Internet could be accessed, take the examination, and receive their score. Answer files would be generated and stored in the Web-based software, which faculty members can then retrieve.

One commonly perceived benefit of CBT is the freeing up of additional classroom time for instruction because examination scheduling is spread out instead of occurring during a designated class period. Because the assigned time for "in-class testing" is not used, faculty may perceive that this extra class period is available to present more content. Most academic institutions require that testing, except for final examinations, be accounted for in the total number of hours of available instruction in the course. CBT does not change that requirement, and faculty members need to be sensitive that this apparent "opportunity" for new teaching hours does not exceed academic guidelines.

## POTENTIAL PROBLEMS

A major issue with CBT is that of faculty comfort level with computers. Not every faculty member will see the integration of CBT into a nursing curriculum as "progress." Lewis and Watson noted that some faculty members do have concerns about the implementation of computer technology and that this "technology anxiety" can be reduced by attending computer workshops.[14] Other researchers found that some educators perceive technological change as a threat to their traditionally accepted role as instructor, believing that technology helps transfer power from instructor to student, with a resulting loss of status for the instructor.[15] With this in mind, it is important that individuals who can envision the benefits of CBT be recruited as leaders in the initiative to expand testing methods currently used.

Implementing computerized testing produces several issues for faculty that were not previous concerns when paper-and-pencil exams were in use. Among the most controversial is whether or not to proctor an examination. Proctoring by faculty has always served the purpose of minimizing the chances of cheating and being available to students who have questions. The expanded testing times, dates, and sometimes off-site locations challenge its use with CBT. The pros and cons of proctoring should be outlined and debated by the teaching team, but the factor that may become the most influential is the extended testing period. Full and even partial proctoring will increase the faculty time commitment to this activity enormously.

A concomitant and equally important issue is that of cheating. Without a proctor present, should student cheating be anticipated? How do faculty members prevent the sharing of information among students who take the exams at different times or days? How can one be sure that the student's name on the answer file is really that of the student who took the exam? Realistically, cheating (regardless of the testing modality) does occur, students do talk, and the likelihood that some test information will be shared is possible. Of all the debatable issues regarding CBT, how to address possible cheating will dominate the discussion. Unfortunately, there is no simple or all-inclusive answer to address this problem. The following options are offered as suggestions to consider:

1. Inserting the institution's student honor code into each examination as the first screen of text with a YES/NO selection required before any questions are presented could be a means to reinforce the issues of honesty and integrity. This presentation is a clear reminder that each student is expected to uphold the code. The answer file of each student would capture their responses and could be accessed if the need arose. Violations of the code need to be pursued and consequences assessed if there is to be any validity to having it presented in the first place.

2. Selecting the option to have the software shuffle the order presentation of the test questions greatly minimizes the likelihood of the same question being on adjacent computer monitor screens at the same time. This strategy is strongly endorsed and a benefit when electronic classroom configurations place monitors close together, which might tempt students to glance at another student's screen.

3. Developing a large test item bank and directing the software to randomly select questions for each student essentially generates a unique examination for each student. One complicated aspect of this strategy mandates that all test items in the bank need to be of equal difficulty to avoid the chance opportunity of one randomly selected set of questions being more or less challenging than another.

4. Assigning a password to each student without which he or she could not access the test helps to ensure security; however, this measure does not prevent the desperate student from arranging for a peer to take the test with his or her designated password. If the password is restricted to a single entry attempt, then several "escape" passwords (known only to the instructor) should be added to the authorized list. Without these additional access codes, reentry to the examination would not be possible should a student have exited the test prematurely.

5. Monitoring the grades as the testing times and dates proceed will allow for observation of any upward grade creep, which may be an indication that some information sharing about the contents of the examination has occurred. The efficacy of CBT analytical abilities will allow almost immediate examination of answer files for such determinations.

Maximizing test security is another area of great concern. How can one prevent students who are very computer literate from entering examinations at inappropriate times or tampering with the test or answer files? A separate, secure area on individual or networked computers, which is accessible only to those with appropriate clearance, absolutely must be identified. These locations would house the computer files that are necessary to actually initiate and run the examination. Without the main CBT program being available, these files cannot be opened, thus making tampering improbable. Student answer files that are generated by each test-taker ideally should be directed to the faculty member's office networked computer, which usually has personal password access. This step greatly assists faculty in reviewing testing results and determining the difficulty and discrimination indices of individual questions. Unauthorized excursions into these secure areas that could permit tampering with computer files have not been reported in the nursing literature.

When icons that initiate the examination are placed on the network desktop for extended periods, a concern that access to a test might occur before or after the designated examination times might arise. This situation is prevented by making a small change to a key file that starts the program (i.e., changing the file extension of the executable file from .exe to .xxx). Extensive computer knowledge is not necessary to accomplish this task. Faculty members should have access to these files from their office computer and thus be able to turn on and turn off the test as required.

Although CBT holds many benefits, some educators still criticize its use. The National Center for Fair and Open Testing notes a host of unresolved problems.[16] This is an advocacy organization working to end what it believes are the abuses, misuses, and flaws of standardized testing and to ensure that evaluation of students and workers is fair, open, and educationally sound. They fear that cheating has been a growing problem among standardized tests. An analyst from FairTest says: "It's too early to know whether the tests will contain a big enough pool of questions to prevent organized cheating."[17] Among their many other concerns regarding CBT are the following:

a. "Computers may worsen test bias between men, women, ethnic groups, and persons from different socioeconomic backgrounds."
b. "Computer anxiety is much more prevalent among females than males, with black females reporting the greatest anxiety."

c. "Computerized tests show only one item on the screen at a time, preventing test-takers from easily checking previous items and the pattern of their responses, two practices known to help test takers."

d. "Most studies show there is a higher score for paper-and-pencil exam."

Faculty members are encouraged to discuss these and other issues of concern prior to a decision to adopt CBT.

## CONCLUSION

Although the National Council of State Boards of Nursing initiated the move to a computerized licensing examination in 1994, adoption of CBT as an evaluation modality in nursing curricula is scarcely evident in the professional literature. No clear explanation for this situation exists. The benefits of CBT for students and faculty are many, and perhaps as they become more well known its use will increase.

The introduction of computerized testing into nursing curricula is highly encouraged. The technology is increasingly user friendly, and the advantages equally shared between students and faculty. Test presentation software continues to evolve with levels of sophistication and features complementing academic requirements along with the ability to emulate aspects of the NCLEX-RN. The very positive student responses that will be received are a wonderful impetus to solve the occasional challenges. Nursing school administrators and interested faculty should carefully assess current and planned resources to ensure that computerized testing is a success if introduced in their institution. In an era where computers are an ever-present and integral part of education at all levels, it is imperative that nursing faculty embrace this technology.

---

### NOTES

1. J. Graham (personal communication, April 26, 1999), Sylvan Technology Center, Augusta, GA.

2. Educational Testing Service, ETS test takers are trading pencils for computers. [On-line] Available: http://etis1.ets.org/aboutets/z2-cbt.html.

3. The Educational Society for Resource Management, Computer-Based Testing (CBT), 1998. [On-line] Available: http://www.apics.org/certification/cer4cbt.htm.

4. P.N. Halkitis and J.M. Leahy, Computerized Adaptive Testing: The Future Is Upon Us, *Nursing & Health Care* 14 (1993):378–385.

5. D. Anna, Computerized Testing in a Nursing Curriculum: A Case Study, *Nurse Educator* 23 (1998):22–26.

6. D. Anna, Computerized Testing.

7. D. Anna, Computerized Testing.

8. P.N. Halkitis and J.M. Leahy, Computerized Adaptive Testing.

9. D. Anna, Computerized Testing.

10. D. Anna, Computerized Testing.

11. D. Anna, Computerized Testing.

12. K.C. Bloom and L.B. Trice, The Efficacy of Individualized Computerized Testing in Nursing Education, *Computers in Nursing* 2 (1997):82–88.

13. J.M. Kirkpatrick, D.M. Billings, K. Hodson-Carlton, R.B. Cummings, A.C. Hanson, J. Malone, A. Miller, L. Robinson, and E.E. Zwin, Computerized Test Development Software: A Comparative Review, *Computers in Nursing* 2 (1996):113–125.

14. D. Lewis and J. Watson, Nursing Faculty Concerns Regarding the Adoption of Computer Technology, *Computers in Nursing* 2 (1997):71–76.

15. R. Hannifin and W. Sayenye, Technology in the Classroom: The Teacher's Role and Resistance to It, *Educational Technology* 33 (1993):26–30.

16. FairTest, Computerized Testing: More Questions Than Answers. [On-line] Available: http://www.fairtest.org/facts/computer.htm.

17. The GMAT Goes Digital, *USA Today*, August 3, 1998. [On-line] Available: http://www.usatoday.com/life/cyber/tech/ctb424.htm.

---

## RESOURCE

Question Designer for Windows (Version 3.20) [Computer software]. Stamford, CT: Presence Corporation; 1999.

# CHAPTER 28

# The Clinical Pathway: A Tool To Evaluate Clinical Learning

*Martha J. Bradshaw*

## DEFINITION AND PURPOSE

The clinical pathway is an abbreviated form of clinical evaluation that provides a means for the instructor to evaluate student progress using specified criteria. Clinical pathways can be used to evaluate nursing practice and clinical learning that occur in less traditional care settings. Learning activities are directed toward the same clinical outcomes as would be expected in traditionally structured patient care settings. The emphasis is on application of nursing principles in a new setting, versus gaining experience via repeated opportunities in a familiar setting. As students apply principles, they recognize the development of individual nursing judgment and decision making, and they begin to visualize themselves as professional nurses.

## THEORETICAL RATIONALE

Clinical pathways, also called critical pathways, are being used by nurses and other members of the health care team as a directed approach to goal-based outcomes; they are especially beneficial in case management.[1] Most nursing literature describes pathways for use in complex patient care situations, but pathways are also used for orientation of new nursing staff, quality improvement, and for student precepted experiences.[2-4] One of the advantages of a pathway is that it is a cost-effective means, in both time and money, by which the individual is directed to the goal(s).[5] Pathways also enable all individuals involved to know exactly what the goals are, thus clarifying expectations and making energy expenditure more efficient.[6]

## CONDITIONS

In selected situations, student clinical learning activities are one-time experiences and may deviate from the more structured patient care experiences. In addition, many clinical experiences are short term because of decrease in hospitalization and emphasis on wellness programs. Examples of these clinical experiences are community health fairs, outpatient surgery, and pediatric health screenings in day care settings. Whereas these unique clinical opportunities provide expanded observations and open up new areas of practice, one-time experiences do not always lend themselves to achievement of established clinical learning outcomes. If the learning outcomes are not readily identified, then the clinical instructor cannot easily evaluate clinical progress based on the experience. Therefore, instructors traditionally create one-time experiences as *observation-only* activities, or as task-focused activities that may not represent a professional nursing approach. In doing so, many valuable learning opportunities may be lost to the students. Instructors also lose the opportunity to determine the extent to which students are able to adapt to unique settings, apply principles, and enact new roles.

Use of a clinical pathway for student experiences enables continued learning by students and maximizes the benefits of the one-time clinical opportunities. Just as the critical pathway is an abbreviated version of a patient's plan of care, the student clinical pathway is an abbreviated version of the clinical evaluation tool.[7] Student clinical pathways are based on the same purposes as are patient- or staff-oriented pathways: they are goal directed, designed to be efficient, and effective in terms of time and energy. The components of the clinical pathway are derived directly from the clinical evaluation tool used by faculty in student evaluation.

### TYPES OF LEARNERS

Whereas the clinical pathway could be used with learners of all levels, it is most appropriate for the undergraduate student. The clinical pathway offers specific learning outcomes and can include recommended or structured activities that enable the student to meet these outcomes. Students in undergraduate clinical settings generally have more faculty supervision, which creates opportunity for direct evaluation. The clinical pathway is designed for intended learning, even though students often acquire additional personal growth during the clinical experience.

### RESOURCES

The basis for a clinical pathway is the learning outcomes for the course. Evaluation tools used by all clinical instructors are directed toward course outcomes. Instructors supervising students in selected experiences identify outcomes and expected behaviors from the evaluation tool. Based on anticipated clinical learning opportunities, the instructor develops a clinical pathway that guides the student in what will be accomplished during the experience and the activities or behaviors the instructor expects to observe in each learner.

## USING THE METHOD

Implementation of an education-focused clinical pathway enables the faculty to develop student learning experiences that are directly related to the outcomes for the total clinical course. Two examples demonstrate how pathways are derived from the clinical evaluation tool, and how components of the tool can be applied to more than one setting. Hearing and vision screening with school-age children can be conducted with nursing students at any level in the educational program. Such screenings have a place in a fundamentals course, a course on nursing care of children, or in a community nursing course. A more sophisticated version of the screening (which would include patient referral) could be developed for nurse practitioner students.

As part of a lifespan-based fundamentals clinical course, a clinical pathway was developed for use with beginning junior-level BSN students. Prior to use of a pathway, students arrived for the experience with little or no advance preparation and no clear focus of the outcomes of the experience. Therefore, students had difficulty applying the skills, working with the children, and understanding the importance of the procedure. To maximize this learning experience, a pathway was developed based on the following items from the course clinical evaluation tool:

- Demonstrates preparation for assignment.
- Performs nursing skills correctly.
- Maintains professionalism.
- Demonstrates professional inquiry activities.

As can be seen by the example in Table 28–1, other expectations are specified under the broad course outcomes. These expectations are derived from the clinical evaluation tool and applied to the situation, such as communications with children or use of critical thinking. The expectations also indicate specific behaviors related to the screening activity that must be demonstrated by the student.

Additional information is provided in the pathway for the student that leaves no room for "guess work" regarding preparation and professional behaviors. Also, the standard for acceptable behavior (Pass) is indicated as part of the directions, so that, in the event a student demonstrates unacceptable behaviors, he or she has a clear understanding of how the final evaluation was determined (see Exhibit 28–1).

An evaluation sheet provides feedback to the student regarding the experience and serves as the evaluation measure and anecdotal record for the instructor. Information regarding clinical activities and evaluation is found in the clinical section of the course syllabus. In that section is the detailed information indicating that a one-time activity, such as this screening, is a clinical day of equal importance to a day caring for a hospitalized patient. Clinical instructors use the information from the pathway when formulating a final clinical evaluation report on each student.

**Table 28–1** Course Outcomes Applied to Clinical Pathways

| *Learning Outcomes of Clinical Pathways* | *Clinical Learning Outcomes of Course* |
|---|---|
| Demonstrates professional behaviors and inquiry activities. | 1. Demonstrates professional behavior and accountability. |
| | 2. Demonstrates preparedness for assignment. |
| | 3. Provides a safe environment. |
| Demonstrates preparation and use of principles in screening techniques. | 4. Complies with the regulations of the School of Nursing and clinical agency. |
| | 5. Performs nursing skills or interventions appropriate to the patient's health. |
| Assesses behaviors of patient and family/support in ambulatory surgery and provides appropriate nursing interventions. | 6. Demonstrates safe administration of medications. |
| | 7. Establishes rapport and demonstrates good communication skills. |
| | 8. Demonstrates collaboration with other care disciplines. |
| Provides nursing interventions for a patient in the ambulatory surgery/operative unit. | 9. Demonstrates patient and family teaching. |
| | 10. Demonstrates appropriate documentation. |
| | 11. Maintains confidentiality and respect for others. |
| | 12. Completes assignments on time. |
| | 13. Seeks assistance/guidance appropriately. |
| | 14. Adapts to changing or stressful situations. |
| | 15. Uses critical-thinking skills. |
| | 16. Demonstrates professional inquiry activities. |

Exhibit 28–2 is a clinical pathway developed for use in an ambulatory surgery unit, with advanced junior-level BSN students. In addition to typical nursing activities related to an operative experience, an emphasis of this experience is: patient and caregiver interaction, alleviation of anxiety, provision of information about the procedure, and presentation of postoperative teaching prior to discharge. Although this pathway may be used for experiences with patients of all ages, it is especially beneficial for use with children and their caregivers.[8] The ambulatory surgery pathway also is constructed to indicate to the students what the expectations are for patient care. Prior to use of the pathway, students were unsure of what they were "permitted" to do, and thus missed many learning opportunities.

Items from the clinical evaluation tool include the same ones as used with the screening pathway:

- Demonstrates preparation for assignment.
- Performs nursing skills correctly.

**Exhibit 28–1** Clinical Pathway: Hearing and Vision Screening

---

The clinical pathway identifies the specific nursing activities that will enable the student to meet the objectives for this one-time clinical experience. The student will be evaluated based on completion of items on this pathway. <u>A student who fails this clinical pathway</u> (i.e., fails to pass at least **7** of the 12 items on the clinical pathway) <u>has failed the clinical day.</u>

**Objectives and Student Nursing Activities:**

*1. Demonstrates preparation and use of principles in screening techniques:*
- Attends clinical promptly, appropriately attired, and with own supplies.
- Establishes a positive working relationship with patient(s).
- Initiates and completes screening in timely manner.
- Correctly follows sequence of steps in screening assessment(s).
- Shows familiarity with equipment, screening criteria, and documentation.
- Individualizes assessments as needed based on unique attributes of each patient.

*2. Demonstrates professional behaviors and inquiry activities:*
- Uses principles of therapeutic and professional communications when interacting with patient(s).
- Shows appropriate level of independence and self-direction.
- Demonstrates critical-thinking and problem-solving skills regarding screenings or patient interactions.
- Documents or reports results of screening exam.
- Seeks guidance or advice from instructor as needed.
- Discusses screening results and/or patient responses with instructor and fellow students.

**<u>Student Preparation</u>**
- Complete check-off on hearing and vision screening equipment in the Skills Lab. If needed, practice again before clinical experience.
- You are permitted to bring your H&V booklet or some guidelines written on a card. This does not take the place of preparation and familiarity with the procedure. If you make too many references to the guidelines, your instructor will consider you unprepared. Bring these pathway sheets to give to your instructor.

---

- Maintains professionalism.
- Demonstrates professional inquiry activities.

Because the ambulatory surgery pathway is broader in scope, it uses additional evaluation tool items:

- Provides a safe environment.
- Establishes good rapport and maintains good communication.
- Recognizes skill and knowledge limitations and seeks assistance appropriately.

**Exhibit 28–2** Clinical Pathway: Ambulatory Surgery Experience

For this one-time clinical experience, the clinical pathway identifies the specific nursing care activities on which the student will be evaluated. Items on this pathway will enable the student to meet the objectives for the Ambulatory Surgery Experience for NUR (listed below). A student who fails the Ambulatory Surgery experience (i.e., receives a failing evaluation on two of the three sections of the clinical pathway) has failed a clinical day.

**Objectives and Student Nursing Activities:**

1. *Assesses behaviors of patient and family/support in ambulatory surgery and provides appropriate nursing interventions:*
   - Introduces self to patient and family/support person; establishes a working relationship.
   - Identifies behaviors related to hospitalization and surgery; discusses conclusions regarding behaviors with instructor, giving specific examples.
   - Indicates how patient behaviors influence preoperative, surgical, and postoperative periods.
   - Gives specific examples of family/support coping abilities.
   - Makes conclusions and interventions that are correctly based on patient's developmental level.

2. *Provides nursing interventions for a patient in the ambulatory surgery/operative unit:*
   - Demonstrates preparedness regarding knowledge of surgical procedure; discusses procedure and pertinent information with instructor.
   - Reviews patient's health history, lab, and other data as available on unit.
   - Teams with staff RN to provide care for patient.
   - Conducts assessments, including vital signs, in a timely manner, using correct technique.
   - Recognizes comfort and safety needs, specific for operative patients.
   - Provides interventions promptly.
   - Administers medications, based on the "5 rights" and according to School of Nursing guidelines.
   - Practices professional therapeutic communication skills in the areas of teaching, reassurance, and collaboration.

3. *Demonstrates professional behaviors and inquiry activities:*
   - Selects appropriate priorities for patient and family/support.
   - Conducts self in dignified, professional manner, including conversation and general appearance.
   - Shows organization and good use of time.
   - Demonstrates initiative to be involved in patient care and to further own learning.
   - Evaluates outcomes of patient's surgical experience; discusses patient responses and readiness for discharge/transfer with instructor.

*continues*

**Exhibit 28–2**  continued

---

**Ambulatory Surgery Experience Clinical Pathway: Evaluation**

*Note:* The student must receive a passing evaluation for at least two of the objectives in order to receive a passing grade for this clinical day.

*1. Assess behaviors of patient and family/support in ambulatory surgery and provide appropriate nursing interventions.*

PASS/FAIL                                   Comments:

_____

_____

_____

_____

*2. Provide nursing interventions for a patient in the ambulatory surgery/ operative unit.*

PASS/FAIL                                   Comments:

_____

_____

_____

_____

*3. Demonstrate professional behaviors and inquiry activities.*

PASS/FAIL                                   Comments:

_____

_____

_____

_____

Instructor _____ Date _____

---

- Demonstrates safe administration of medications.
- Uses critical thinking in decision making and applying various problem-solving methods.

The ambulatory surgery pathway is used in the same way as the hearing and vision screening pathway. Evaluation information is used by the clinical instructor as part of the final course evaluation. One benefit of using the pathway in total course evaluation is that it provides the instructor with a glimpse at behavior patterns in a student, regardless of setting.

In developing the pathway, the focus is on outcomes (student learning), not process (tasks or activities).[9] Therefore, the instructor may designate specified activities or behaviors that direct the student to the outcomes; not all behaviors must be seen in order to attain the goal. Furthermore, other activities related to the patient situation may present themselves that enable the student to meet the outcomes.

## POTENTIAL PROBLEMS

Any difficulties encountered in using the clinical pathway are related to the nature of this evaluation measure. It is intended to evaluate the student in a one-time experience, based on selected criteria.

Potential problems with this method include:

- Inability of the instructor to observe and evaluate all behaviors. The type of clinical activity and spontaneous events govern the student's participation in care and types of care provided.
- The new environment may have a negative effect on the students' behavior. Some students adapt more quickly than others to working in new settings. This is especially true of more experienced students and field-independent students who are able to sort out and select relevant information about the clinical setting. Students who are less able to adapt are therefore hampered in their performance and may appear to be weak in clinical judgment or nursing skills.
- It is easy to "rubber stamp" evaluation remarks. For the instructor who has 40 or 50 students progressing through the one-time experience, the evaluation remarks become repetitive and tiresome. Instructors must endeavor to make individual comments that are an accurate description of the student. Remarks that reflect abilities in other clinical settings will validate the student's total clinical evaluation.
- To some instructors, the clinical pathway may be seen as too "behavioral." In some cases, this is the intent of the pathway: to evaluate psychomotor skills. An immunization pathway is an example of psychomotor evaluation. The clinical pathway can be constructed in such a way to provide opportunities for the student to use critical-thinking and problem-solving abilities in ways that the instructor can readily observe and evaluate. An example is priority setting and decision making related to immediate patient care needs. This is an advantage of the pathway in that it facilitates evaluation in spontaneous situations.

## CONCLUSION

Clinical pathways are a means by which an instructor can objectively and effectively evaluate student learning and progress toward clinical outcomes. An advantage to use of pathways in one-time experiences is that the pathway serves as a criterion-based frame of reference for both the student and the instructor because the criteria are the same as for other clinical experiences in that course. The faculty member thus has an objective measure of student learning and performance, and the student always knows the measure on which he or she will be evaluated.

Clinical pathways are limited to brief experiences and are not designed to show professional growth and progress in learning over time; however, a pathway could be designed to appraise critical thinking and professional behaviors associated with spontaneous incidents, such as a problem patient. Nurse educators can use pathways as a creative means to address student responses in a variety of situations.

---

**NOTES**

1. A.P. Elizondo, Nursing Case Management in the Neonatal Intensive Care Unit, Part 2: Developing Critical Pathways, *Neonatal Network: Journal of Neonatal Nursing* 14 (1995):11–19.

2. C. Evers, S. Odom, J. Latulip-Gardner, and S. Paul, Developing a Critical Pathway for Orientation, *American Journal of Critical Care* 3 (1994):217–223.

3. C. Perez, The Next Frontier in Clinical Pathways: The Journey to Outcomes Management, *Nursing Case Management* 1 (1996):75–78.

4. A.L. Kersbergen and P.E. Hrobsky, Use of Clinical Map Guides in Precepted Clinical Experiences, *Nurse Educator* 21 (1996):19–22.

5. N.S. Kowal and M. Delaney, The Economics of a Nurse-Developed Critical Pathway, *Nursing Economics* 14 (1996):156–161.

6. Elizondo, Nursing Case Management, 13.

7. P. Wieczorek, Developing Critical Pathways for the Operating Room, *AORN Journal* 62 (1995):925–927.

8. M.A. Geeze, Pediatric Outpatient Upper Endoscopy: Perioperative Case Management, *Seminars in Perioperative Nursing* 3 (1994):27–39.

9. Perez, Next Frontier, 76.

# CHAPTER 29

# Evaluation of
# Learning Outcomes

*Katherine E. Nugent*

## INTRODUCTION

The role of faculty in a collegiate setting involves a complex set of expectations that vary depending on the institutional mission and the type of program. Regardless of the institutional mission, all educational institutions have a focus on teaching.

The teaching role of the faculty includes all aspects of facilitating student learning, including evaluation of learning; however, evaluation of learning is only one component of evaluation associated with the faculty role. Faculty members are also involved in evaluation of teaching, evaluation of their peers, and evaluation of the program. Therefore, an understanding of evaluation as it relates to the teaching-learning environment is important.

So what makes the evaluation component of education so important? There is a growing demand from consumers and stakeholders of education that colleges and universities be more accountable for the product they are graduating. Mandates from accrediting associations and education commissions state that effectiveness of educational programs be addressed, placing an emphasis on measuring student learning and documenting student learning outcomes. Historically, quality of educational programs has been measured in terms of resources, program offerings, faculty qualifications, and student services; however, these definitions of quality are being challenged, and educators are being charged with the task of documenting program effectiveness in terms of learning.

Most faculty members take little ownership of their responsibility in evaluation; however, because evaluation provides nurse educators with an avenue for demonstrating quality of teaching, as well as the effectiveness of the educational program, all faculty members must understand their role in evaluation. Through evaluation, faculty members demonstrate accountability in the education process and for the quality of education. Understanding the importance of evaluation is based on understanding the methodology and theory of evaluation as it relates to the faculty role. This chapter addresses selected concepts of teacher evaluation, evaluation of student learning, and program evaluation. In addition, some foundational concepts concerning evaluation are introduced.

## FOUNDATIONAL CONCEPTS

Before addressing specific aspects of evaluation, a brief introduction to some basic concepts of evaluation is included. These concepts are universal in nature and are applicable to any type of evaluation.

### Definition

Evaluation is traditionally defined as *the process used in determining the value or worth of something*. It involves collecting data to determine if what is observed is different than what was expected. Therefore, evaluation is conducted for the purpose of making decisions. Evaluation, as it is related to the teaching-learning environment, is defined as the process used in determining the effectiveness of teaching and/or the value of a learning opportunity in assisting students to achieve the goals of education. The inherent purpose of educational evaluation is to provide valid data on which to make educational decisions related to the program of study. Therefore, evaluation and teaching become a synergistic process in which each influences the other.

It is important to distinguish between the roles of evaluation and the goals of evaluation. The goal of evaluation is synonymous with the definition of evaluation: to determine the worth of something through the collection of data. A common mistake in evaluation is not clearly identifying or articulating the purpose of the evaluation. Defining the goal involves specifying what is to be accomplished, what decisions need to be made, and who are the intended audience or stakeholders. For example, the goal of evaluation in a school of nursing is to determine the effectiveness of the program.

The roles of evaluation depend on what that "something" is that is being evaluated and on whose standards of value the results will be analyzed. Therefore, the role of evaluation is situational and more specific. Because of this, one must be clear in the role of evaluation and the expected outcomes of conducting the evaluation. For example, one role of evaluation would be to inform students of their progress in mastering the content included in a specific course. Another role of evaluation would be to provide faculty members with feedback concerning the effectiveness of their teaching. Both roles provide data associated with the overall goal of measuring program effectiveness.

## Clarification of Terms

The terms *assessment of learning* and *measurement of learning* are sometimes used mistakenly instead of evaluation. Assessment of learning is defined as *an appraisal of changes in learner knowledge, skills, attitudes, and ways of thinking*[2] and is the first step of the evaluation process in learning. Evaluation is the compilation of information from various sources and is ongoing. These data are interpreted to determine the extent to which identified actions were successful. Assessment is different from evaluation in that evaluation is the process of making value judgments based on available information and conclusions for the purpose of improvement or revision.[3]

Similarly, measurement differs from evaluation in that no value judgments are made. Measurement is the process of assigning a quantitative or qualitative description to what is being evaluated. It helps with the value judgment by answering the question of "how much." The purpose of measurement is to provide a reference point on which to make value judgments on collected data. The concept of measurement in learning is extremely critical because we do not have a meter (machine) that attaches to the learner and tells us the level of learning that is occurring. Therefore, because this process is not observable, we must design a situation in which the desired behavior can be observed or assessed. This situation is termed *measurement*. It is a designed situation, thus the designer (evaluator) is making some assumptions and judgments. In the best constructed situation, because of the assumptions that precede the development of that situation, the measurement is only a method of estimating what the learner has learned, and unfortunately is often imprecise.[4] Therefore, we must use more than one type of measurement in conducting evaluation.

There are two major ways of interpreting test scores and other types of measurement used in evaluation: *norm-referenced* and *criterion-referenced interpretation*. A norm-referenced interpretation focuses on how learners' results compare with those of their peers. Norm-referenced data are reported in terms of percentiles, using relative standards, and allow comparisons using group or national norms. Therefore, when using norm-referenced measurement, the characteristics of the comparison group need to be clearly defined.

Criterion-referenced measurement involves interpretation based on present criteria, not in relation to another group. The focus is on the performance level of the learners and describes how well the student performs in relation to the set criteria. Criterion-referenced assessment must be based on a preestablished performance level.

### Systematic Evaluation

Because the process of decision making is inherent in evaluation, valid and reliable data must be collected. Validity and reliability can be obtained only through a systematic approach to evaluation. A systematic approach can be ensured when an evaluation design is used to guide the process. An evaluation design is defined as a plan that identifies what decisions will be made, when and from whom data will be gathered, as well as what instruments will be used to obtain the data. General considerations include what evaluation model will be used, what type of data needs to be collected, how the data will be analyzed and by whom, and how the evaluation results will be disseminated. Deliberate decisions about the evaluation design ensure that the evaluation plan is valid, reliable, timely, pervasive, and credible.

### EVALUATION MODEL

Different models of evaluation exist; however, most models are based on a decision-facilitating model that evolved from the prototype context, input, process, and product (CIPP) model by Daniel Stufflebeam.[1] This evaluation model is a comprehensive model based on the assumption that evaluation is a continuing process. The CIPP model consists of four types of evaluation that facilitate four types of decisions. The first type of evaluation is *context evaluation*. Context evaluation involves studying the environment associated with the program. It compares the actual conditions with the desired ones. Context evaluation has been described as a "situation analysis" or "the diagnostic stage of evaluation." During this stage of evaluation, planning decisions are made. Data collected during this type of evaluation include: What is the purpose of this service? What is trying to be achieved? and Is there a need for this service? The key concept associated with context evaluation is that it is a continuous process providing information throughout the evaluation design and not a one-time activity.

The second stage of the model, *input evaluation*, is designed to provide information for determining how to utilize the resources to meet the program outcomes. Input evaluation is necessary in making structural decisions in which one determines the actual and potential resources, facilities, and strategies available to the system. Structuring decisions to determine the required sources of support are made during this stage of evaluation. Data collected during this evaluation phase include: What resources are available? and How will the planned change affect the ongoing components and processes in the current structure? Input evaluation can be relatively simple or extremely complex depending on the magnitude of the program.

*Process evaluation* is the third stage of the CIPP model. This stage of evaluation addresses the implementation of the program and identifies the congruency between the planned and actual situation. Therefore, implementing decisions is associated with this stage of evaluation. Data are collected that describe the actual functioning of the system as well as identify areas of weakness. Data are collected on the following: Is the program being implemented as it was planned? and Have problems developed that were not anticipated in the original plan? Process evaluation has been described as a "piloting" project to identify the glitches in the program so that changes can be made before the final outcome.

*Product evaluation*, more currently called outcome evaluation, provides data for recycling decisions. This evaluation determines if the outcomes produced have met the objectives of the program. Evaluation data include: Has the program benefited those intended? Has the program attained its goals? and Was the outcome of the program worth the investment? A systematic evaluation design includes these four components of evaluation, each occurring at different times.

## TYPES OF EVALUATION

In addition to the four types of evaluation mentioned previously, two other terms have been used to describe the types of evaluation: *formative* and *summative*. Formative evaluation is the gathering of data to make decisions during the planning, development, and implementation of the program. Formative evaluation is frequent and periodic, and provides feedback while the program is being implemented. The purpose of formative evaluation is to assist in making changes to achieve the goals of the program or to refine or improve the outcome. Therefore, formative evaluation is considered diagnostic in nature.

The purpose of summative evaluation is to determine the effectiveness of a program after the program has been implemented. Summative evaluation measures final outcomes or results and occurs at the end of the evaluation design. Conclusions are made and information is gathered for future decisions.

## FACULTY RESPONSIBILITY IN EVALUATION

The faculty member has responsibilities in the following types of evaluation: program evaluation, teacher evaluation, and evaluation of student learning, each of which will be discussed briefly.

### Program Evaluation

A systematic evaluation design in education is usually referred to as program evaluation. Bevil defines program evaluation as the systematic and continuous process of gathering and analyzing data about all dimensions of the program and then using this information for decision making about program quality and effectiveness (p. 60).[5] The key concepts in this definition are continuous process and decision making. Program evaluation is a decision-support activity that extends beyond data collection, measurement, and dissemination of the evaluation results. It is a circular process that involves people who will assess and deliberate the findings to make program decisions, implement these decisions, and reevaluate the results.[6]

Because of the circular nature of program evaluation, it should be an integral part of any educational institution. The purposes of evaluation are to diagnose problems, assess strengths and weaknesses, and test new approaches for accomplishing and advancing the school's philosophy and outcomes. It should be practical, yielding information that is reliable and useful to the decision makers and to the stakeholders. More specifically, program evaluation helps faculty and administrators account for scarce fiscal resources, make administrative and curricular decisions, appraise faculty and staff development needs, examine both intended and actual effects of the program within the community, and provide a mechanism to ensure fulfillment of accreditation requirements.

Program evaluation includes all of the internal and external forces and constraints that impinge upon a nursing education program. It involves both a review of the past practice and a prediction of future practice. It looks at the environment, needs, resources, and deficiencies of the institution. An educational program evaluation collects data about the organization and administration, faculty, students, curriculum, and resources. Some examples of data include:

- assessment of the curriculum
- effective functioning of the organizational activities
- faculty participation in the program
- faculty qualifications
- assessment of faculty teaching, scholarship/service
- assessment of the behaviors of graduates
- comparison of graduates with past graduates and with graduates of other comparable programs
- library resources
- classroom resources

Faculty involvement in the evaluation process is an important variable in program evaluation. The first and most obvious role is in providing appropriate data as specified by the evaluation plan. The validity of the evaluation findings depends on the validity and reliability of the data collected. Other faculty responsibilities include participating in determining the type of evaluation, suggesting appropriate tools of measurement, and revising the evaluation design as the organization changes.

An important faculty role in program evaluation is participating in the analysis of data and making appropriate recommendations. It is important to objectively analyze evaluation data to prevent the formation of "false assumptions." Thus, it may be necessary in the analysis of data to clarify or validate the collected data through focus group technique. Because faculty members not only participate in the evaluation process but also respond affectively to the results, they must make recommendations based on the actual data and not on a subjective personal basis.

The most important role of faculty in program evaluation involves what is called "the feedback loop of evaluation" or the implementation of evaluation findings. Unfortunately, even though a systematic evaluation design is developed and implemented and although accurate recommendations are made, it is not uncommon for evaluation reports to be shelved. Barrett-Barrick states that promoting the use of evaluation findings among faculty is difficult because the importance of the report is often overlooked.[7] It is important to remember that the purpose of program evaluation is to improve the program outcomes. Improvement of the program can occur only if faculty members take personal accountability to implement the recommendations and continue the evaluation process to determine if recommendations did improve the program.

## EVALUATION OF LEARNING

A major component of the faculty role associated with teaching is the evaluation of student learning. In this context, the purpose of evaluation is to ascertain the learner's current level of knowledge and learning needs, to give feedback to improve learner achievement, to improve teaching effectiveness, to judge learning and teaching outcomes, and to provide data concerning program effectiveness. Much faculty time is devoted to designing measurements to collect data for measuring learning and then assigning a grade to reflect the degree of learning. Yet this process is a very small component of total program evaluation.

Evaluation of learning is defined as *the systematic process of collecting and interpreting information as a basis for decisions about learners*. It is more specific than program evaluation and obviously focuses on the learner. Evaluation of learning incorporates not only the objectives of the learning experience but also the characteristics of the learner. Evaluation of learning enables faculty members to determine the progression of students toward meeting the educational objectives. Specifically, the goal is to discover to what degree learners have attained the knowledge, attitudes, or skills emphasized in a learning experience. Because no instruments are available that can measure the student's brain to determine if learning has occurred, simulated or designed situations are developed to measure learning. Therefore, evaluation of learning is a value judgment based on the data obtained from the various designed measurements taken in the classroom and clinical settings. The evaluation methods should match the nature of the course and the outcomes. For example, if students are enrolled in a course that contains 45 clock hours of didactic and 150 clock hours of clinical, it would be important that most of the measurements used to evaluate this course would measure learning in the clinical area.

The process for evaluating learning is similar to the process for program evaluation, in that it is based on a planned design. Deliberate planning and thought are needed to decide what evaluation methods should be used in a course of study. First, faculty members need to identify what is to be evaluated. What are the outcomes of learning? Inherent in this process is the specification of the domain of learning. In nursing, learning occurs not only in the cognitive or knowledge domain, but also in the affective or value domain, and in the psychomotor or competency domain. Each domain of learning requires different evaluation measures. For example, a multiple-choice exam measures a student's cognitive understanding of a concept but does not measure the student's ability to perform a clinical skill.

In addition, in measuring the domain of a learner, the faculty must determine the complexity of the learning. Complexity of learning is determined when one considers the characteristics of the learner (i.e., level of learning, prerequisite courses, past clinical experiences). Integrated into this determination is the identification of the content or concepts associated with the learning experience. All of these factors clearly describe the behavior to be measured that indicates that learning has occurred. One should construct a matrix that identifies all of the factors to ensure that all concepts are integrated and the best measurement is chosen.

**Context-Dependent Measurement**

Nurse educators are challenged to prepare graduates to practice in a managed care health environment and to care for patients with complex health needs. This challenge involves shifting the focus of teaching from content to process. Students need more than mastery of knowledge to be successful in practice. They must be able to solve problems, make decisions, and think critically. Therefore, it becomes as important to evaluate not only a student's learning of content but also a student's ability to think critically. This requires different evaluation methods than traditionally used. Oermann and Gaberson state that in assessing students' cognitive skills, the test items and evaluation methods need to meet two criteria: (1) introduce new information not encountered by students at an earlier point in the instruction and (2) provide data on the thought process used by students to arrive at an answer.[8] This type of evaluation, called *context-dependent evaluation*, includes context-dependent test items, case method and study, discussion, debate, and other reality-based scenarios.

As stated earlier, evaluating higher-level thinking skills, although it involves more planning and time than most multiple-choice tests, is extremely important in nursing education. Ability to solve patient problems is an essential skill needed for successful nursing practice. In evaluating these skills, the faculty member introduces new material in a format similar to a patient scenario. The student is asked to analyze the data, thus providing data on the thought process used to arrive at the answer. Therefore, the material must provide sufficient data for decision making.

The intent is to evaluate the underlying thought process. Guidelines for writing context-dependent item sets include:

- Provide sufficient introductory information for the student to accurately analyze the situation.
- Have questions address the underlying thought process used to arrive at the answer, not the answer itself.
- Gear the information provided to the student's level of understanding and experience.
- Specify how the responses will be scored.[9]

For example, to test decision making, the introductory material may present a situation up to the point of the decision, then ask students to make the decision, or it may describe a situation and decision and ask whether the students agree or disagree with the decision. The question is not measuring content but the students' decision-making skills.

Grading measurements evaluating higher-order thinking is different from grading traditional tests because it requires more time and analysis. The potential for subjectivity or grading biases exists in this type of evaluation. Providing a template that has been designed based on content validity reduces some of the subjectivity.

## Classroom Assessment

Formative evaluation can provide valuable data when evaluating student learning and the teaching strategies being used. Classroom assessment is a type of formative evaluation that involves ongoing assessment of student learning and assists faculty in selecting teaching strategies.[10] This technique involves both students and instructors in the continuous monitoring of student learning. The purpose of classroom assessment parallels the purpose of formative evaluation. The purpose is to collect data during the learning experience to make adjustments so that students can benefit from the modifications before the final measurement of learning occurs. This approach is learner-centered, teacher-directed, mutually beneficial, formative, context-specific, ongoing, and firmly rooted in good practice.[11]

Classroom assessment differs from other measurements of learning in that it is usually anonymous and is never graded. It is context specific, meaning that the technique used to evaluate one class or a content-related learning experience will not necessarily work in another experience.

The use of classroom assessment provides feedback about learning not only to the faculty but to the student as well. Assessment techniques (e.g., the muddiest point, one sentence summary, chain notes, RSQC2 ) are simple to use, take little time, and yet are fun for the student. An example of a popular assessment technique is muddiest point. Close to the end of the learning session, the student is asked to write, "What was the muddiest point in this lecture?" (or whatever teaching strategy was used). The faculty then reviews the responses to determine if a concept is mentioned frequently or if a pattern emerges indicating that a concept or content was misunderstood. Based on the results, the faculty may choose to address the "muddiest point" in the next class. Answering the question also causes students to reflect on the session and identify concepts needing further study.

## Clinical Evaluation

Because nursing is a practice discipline, student learning involves more than acquiring cognitive knowledge. Learning includes the practice dimension where the student demonstrates the ability to apply theory in caring for patients. Evaluating student learning and student competency in clinical is challenging. The faculty must make professional judgments concerning the student's competencies in practice, as well as the higher-level cognitive learning associated with application. Yet, the clinical environment changes from one learning experience to another, making absolute comparisons among students even in the same clinical setting impossible. In addition, role expectations of the learners and evaluators are perceived differently. The evaluations of a student's performance frequently are influenced by one's own professional orientation and expectations. Evaluation in the clinical setting is the process of collecting data in order to make a judgment concerning the students' competencies in practice based on standards or criteria. Judgments influence the data collected; therefore, it is not an objective process. Deciding on the quality of performance and drawing inferences and conclusion from the data also involves judgment by the faculty. It is a subjective process that is influenced by the bias of the faculty and student and by the variables present in the clinical environment. These factors and others make evaluating the clinical experience a complex job.

In clinical evaluation, the faculty members observe performance and collect data associated with higher-order cognitive thinking. The judgment of a student's performance in the clinical area can either be based on norm-referenced or criterion-referenced evaluation. With norm-referenced evaluation, the student's clinical performance is compared with the performance of other students in the course, whereas criterion-referenced evaluation is the comparison of the student's performance with a set of criteria. Regardless of the type of evaluation used, providing a fair and valid evaluation is still challenging. Using multiple and varied sources of data increases the possibility that a valid evaluation occurs (i.e., observation, evaluation of written work, student comments, staff comments). Also, making observations throughout the designated experience in an effort to obtain a sampling of behaviors that will reflect quality of care provided and the extent of student learning validates the evaluation.

Because it has been established that even with the best-developed evaluation criteria clinical evaluation is subjective, the evaluation must be fair. Oermann and

Gaberson addressed the following dimensions associated with fairness in clinical evaluation:[12]

- identifying the faculty's own values, attitudes, beliefs, and biases that may influence the evaluation process
- basing clinical evaluation on predetermined objectives or competencies
- developing a supportive clinical environment
- basing judgments on the expected competency according to curriculum
- comparing the student's present behavior performance with past performance, other students' performances, or to the level of a norm reference group

The process of evaluating a student's performance in a clinical setting poses several challenges to evaluation theory. Extensive documentation exists in the literature addressing clinical evaluation and providing examples of evaluation tools. Because students are demonstrating their ability to apply nursing knowledge in caring for patients in an uncontrolled environment, it is difficult for them to hide their lack of understanding or inability to "put it all together." Although this setting is ideal for learning, the variables that exist in the setting make each learning experience different. Faculty members also struggle with the concept of when the time for learning ends and the time for evaluation begins. Again, the literature provides guidelines addressing this issue.

The solution exists within the context of clearly defining the parameters of formative and summative evaluation. Although not without its flaws, this solution worked as long as the clinical experiences existed in the hospital setting and were defined by discrete units of time; however, educating students in a managed care environment has changed the settings and the focus of the clinical experience. Faculty members no longer have the security of the familiar hospital setting and the discrete time units. Patients receive health care in a variety of settings such as day surgery, outpatient clinics, community settings, and in the home. Patients admitted to the hospital stay shorter periods, require more extensive care, and present with more complex situations. Thus, past strategies that were successful in clinical evaluation are no longer applicable.

The key to successful clinical evaluation in the present educational environment is the use of confirmative evaluation. The purpose of this type of evaluation is to collect, examine, and interpret data to determine the continuing competence of learners, thereby allowing the faculty to assess if learners remain competent.[13] Confirmative evaluation is based on the outcomes of the entire learning experience and not determined by clinical settings. Different types of evaluation tools will be needed to perform confirmative evaluation aimed at evaluating student competencies that transcend clinical settings. Therefore, it is important to select evaluation methods that provide data on the identified competencies, to use a variety of measurements, and to select measurements that are realistic for the learning experience. The following are some examples of measurements that have been used successfully in clinical evaluation.

## Clinical Concept Mapping

Clinical concept mapping was developed by an educational researcher as an instructional and assessment tool for use in science education.[14] In general, the technique is a hierarchical graphic organizer developed individually by students. It demonstrates their understanding of relationships among concepts. Key concepts are placed centrally, and subconcepts and clusters of data are placed peripherally. All concepts are linked by arrows, lines, or broken lines to demonstrate the association between and among the concepts and the data.[15]

Clinical concept mapping is applicable in evaluating students in the clinical setting because it facilitates the linking of previously learned concepts to actual patient scenarios. The diagramming of the concepts allows faculty members to evaluate the student's interpretation of collected data and how it applies to the student's patient and to management of patient care. It also provides data for faculty members to evaluate the student's ability to apply class content and concepts to implementing nursing care. Faculty members are also able to evaluate the student's ability to solve problems and to think critically. Clinical concept mapping can be applied to a variety of clinical settings[16] and to a variety of learning experiences.

## Portfolio Assessment

Portfolio analysis can serve an important component of the process of assessing student learning outcomes. When used appropriately, portfolio assessment provides valid data for clinical evaluation of students. A portfolio is a compilation of documents demonstrating learning, competencies, and achievements, usually over a period of time. Used extensively in business to demonstrate one's accomplishments, the portfolio is now used in education to track academic achievement of outcomes.[17] Although portfolios are discussed here in relation to clinical evaluation, they can also be used in different aspects of program evaluation.

Portfolios are valid measures in clinical evaluation in that students provide evidence in their portfolios to confirm their clinical competence and to document their learning. They can be used in formative and summative evaluation and are especially valid in association with confirmative evaluation. Portfolio assessments are a positive asset in clinical settings in which students are not directly supervised by faculty.

Nitko describes the use of portfolios in terms of best work and growth and learning portfolios.[18] Best work portfolios provide evidence that students have mastered outcomes and have attained the desired level of competence (summative evaluation). Growth and learning portfolios are designed to monitor students' progress (formative evaluation). Both types of portfolios reflect the philosophy of clinical evaluation.

Portfolios are constructed to match the purpose and objectives of the clinical experience. Faculty members need to clearly delineate the purpose and outcomes and to identify examples of work to be included. Likewise, the criteria by which the contents of the portfolio will be evaluated must be provided for the students. Students need to understand that portfolios are a reflection of their learning and an evaluation of their performance.

Although still in the exploratory stage, portfolios are evolving as effective measurements in outcome evaluation. If portfolios are used in clinical evaluation, then faculty members benefit from data that demonstrate the clinical progression of students through the curriculum toward the program outcomes. Portfolios can be used to evaluate faculty productivity and development. Similar to all forms of evaluation, the use of portfolios needs to be designed and implemented in a systematic manner.

## Clinical Journals

Teaching/learning in the clinical setting is broad and diverse, including much more than can be identified superficially. Journaling is a technique that has been successfully used to bring together those elusive bits of information and experience associated with the clinical experience.[19] Clinical journals provide an opportunity for students to not only document their clinical experience but also to reflect on their performance and knowledge. Journals provide an avenue for students to express their feelings of uncertainty and to engage in dialogue with the faculty concerning the experience. Journaling also can be structured to include nursing care, problem solving, and identification of learning needs. Whereas journals provide valuable evaluation data, the challenge is to obtain from the students the quality of journal entries needed.

Hodges addressed this issue in a proposed model in which four levels of journal writing were identified.[20] These levels of journal writing progressed from summarizing, describing, and reacting to clinical experience, then to analyzing and critiquing positions, issues, and views of others. Examples of journal entries that parallel this progression are moving from writing objectives or a summary to writing a critique or a focused argument. The key to this progression lies in providing a clear purpose for the journal entry. To think critically, students need to know what they are thinking about.[21] Once faculty members have identified the desired outcome of the clinical journal, they can assist the students in attaining these outcomes by providing clear guidelines.

Although keeping a journal requires a substantial commitment of time by both faculty and students, it is a valuable evaluation tool for both groups. Controversy exists concerning whether journals should be used for evaluation of students' learning or to be graded.[22] Some educators maintain that grading journals negates the students' ability to be reflective and truthful concerning clinical experiences; however, as students document their evolution of clinical experiences, their journal entries are laden with expressions of self-evaluation.[23] If journals are to be graded, then clear and concise criteria must exist that not only identify how they are graded but also what is to be included in the journal. Regardless of the decision to grade or not to grade them, clinical journals provide important evaluation data concerning the student's performance in the clinical setting and can be used effectively to monitor the student's development in terms of program outcomes.

### Clinical Pathways

Clinical pathways, also called critical pathways, are traditionally used in health care delivery to provide continuity of care in a cost-effective manner. Clinical pathways are used to evaluate quality of care by identifying critical aspects of care and benchmarks that need to occur for the patient to attain the health outcome.

The format and concept of clinical pathways can be used as a successful tool in evaluating student performance during a clinical experience.[24] The clinical pathway can be conceptualized in terms of an abbreviated clinical evaluation tool, identifying not only objectives of the clinical but also knowledge or competency needed to meet the outcomes. Therefore, the clinical pathway as an evaluation tool is criterion-referenced in that it identifies the objectives of the clinical experience and the associated behavioral performance of the student. The clinical pathway provides data concerning learning and skill acquisition in one-time clinical experiences, community experience, or other precepted experiences where faculty members may or may not be present.

In summary, evaluation of learning is an important component of the faculty teaching role. Because the purpose of evaluation is to provide valid data concerning learning in all domains, a variety of measurements are needed. The key to successful evaluation is to match the evaluation tool with the learning in order to provide reliable and valid data on which to make judgments.

In addition to making a judgment concerning a student's performance in clinical, it is important to remember that the other purpose of clinical evaluation is to provide feedback to the student regarding his or her performance and to provide the student with an opportunity to improve in the needed areas. Clinical evaluation should be a consistent and frequent means of communicating the student's progress. Using an adopted clinical evaluation tool ensures that all students are counseled using the same criteria. The evaluation process needs to be constructed so that active student participation is included. Feedback should be stated in the specific terms of the measurement tool and the outcomes of the course. Comments should be based on data and should not contain general global clichés such as "will make a good nurse." Strengths, as well as areas needing improvement, should be documented. If a student needs to improve to pass the clinical experience, then the student should be given, in writing, those areas needing improvement with specific guidelines on what behavior is required to pass. Again, all comments should be stated in terms of the criteria on the evaluation tool.

## EVALUATION OF TEACHING

Another area of evaluation in which faculty members are actively involved is in the evaluation of teaching. The purpose of this form of evaluation is to assess the quality of teaching in the classroom and in the clinical setting. Inherent in this definition is the understanding that results of the evaluation will be used to provide feedback concerning teaching for the development of faculty and refinement of teaching skills. Much has been written over the last three decades concerning evaluation of teaching. Oermann states that research in nursing education suggests five characteristics and qualities of effective teaching in nursing:[25]

- knowledge of the subject matter
- clinical competence
- teaching skill
- interpersonal relationships with students
- personal characteristics

Other skills needed include the abilities to:

- Identify students' learning needs.
- Plan instruction.
- Explain concepts and ideas clearly.
- Demonstrate procedures effectively.
- Use sound evaluation practices.[26]

These characteristics and skills should be reflected in an evaluation tool measuring teaching effectiveness.

Data collected concerning teaching effectiveness are obtained from a variety of sources. The most common source of data is derived from students. Student evaluation of teaching is achieved through a variety of methods: (1) evaluation of a teaching experience (i.e., individual lecture), (2) evaluation of a course (teaching behaviors over time), or (3) evaluation of clinical teaching. A significant amount of debate has occurred about the ability of students to provide reliable, objective evaluation data. Some educators argue that students do not know how to distinguish "good" teaching. Nothing is further from the truth. Obtaining data from students is valid because the students participate in the teaching-learning episode and can provide a perspective on the teacher's behaviors and skills. Now, having said that, it is important to briefly mention some guidelines in interpreting student evaluation.

Participating in evaluation of teaching can result in anxiety and tension for faculty. Because most faculty members strive to be "good educators," this type of evaluation is usually an emotional process. Therefore, it is important to consider some guidelines when interpreting the results of student evaluation of teaching. Consider the variables of the course (i.e., difficulty of course, number of students in the course, number of faculty) when interpreting evaluation data. Look for patterns in the evaluation responses. Match those patterns with your instinct concerning what other factors were present in the teaching-learning environment that may have influenced the data. Interpretation of the results should be focused only on clustering of responses, whether desirable or undesirable. Extreme responses should be discounted because every group of students contains a few negativists and a few who are not honest in their responses. Seek clarification of data from other faculty members, groups of students, and administrators.

It is important to be ethical in collecting data from students concerning evaluation of teaching; therefore, the following points should be considered:

- All handwritten comments should be typed by a neutral person not involved in teaching the course being evaluated and who will not recognize the student's handwriting.
- All evaluations should be anonymous.
- During the administration of an evaluation scale, the faculty member should not be present. A word of caution concerning this aspect is that some responsible person should be in the room, to prevent students from "ganging up" in their comments.
- Arrangements not involving the faculty member should be made for collecting the data and delivering them in a sealed envelope.
- Responses should never be tabulated until after final course grades are processed.

Other sources of teacher evaluation are peer evaluation and administrator evaluation. When conducting peer evaluation, it is important to remember that the definition of a peer or colleague should be determined before the evaluation. This definition is usually determined by some guidelines within the nursing education unit that may be based on academic experience, rank, and familiarity with the teaching material. It is also important to remember that peer or administrator evaluations are, at the most, an evaluation of a teaching episode. Additionally, although feedback can be given, it should be interpreted within the context of the teaching episode. A follow-up session between the evaluator and the faculty member should be planned to discuss the results of the observation. A copy of the written evaluation should be given to the faculty member for his or her portfolio.

## CONCLUSION

An important part of the faculty role is associated with evaluation because evaluations in the educational setting are undertaken to influence the actions and activities of individuals and groups, who have, or are presumed to have, an opportunity to tailor their actions on the basis of the results. An understanding of evaluation and how it impacts the teaching-learning environment is critical. Proper use of evaluation techniques requires an awareness of both their limitations and their strengths and requires matching the appropriate measurement with the purpose or role of evaluation. This chapter has addressed some aspects of the faculty role in evaluation, but this overview is not comprehensive or inclusive in nature.

Nursing is entering a new era of teaching that will alter traditional roles between faculty and students. Inherent in this new era of teaching is the mandate to evaluate teaching and learning using less traditional methods.

---

### NOTES

1. D. Stufflebeam, The Relevance of the CIPP Evaluation Model for Educational Accountability, *Journal of Research and Developmental Education* 5, no. 1 (1980):19–25.
2. M.P. Bourke and B.A. Ihrke, The Evaluation Process: An Overview, in *Teaching in Nursing,* eds. D. Billings and J. Halstead, Chapter 20 (Philadelphia: Saunders, 1998).
3. Bourke and Ihrke, The Evaluation Process.
4. N.L. Van Hoozer, B.D. Ostmoe, D. Weinholtz, M.J. Craft, C.L. Gjerde, and M.A. Albanese, *The Teaching Process: Theory and Practice in Nursing* (Norwalk, CT: Appleton-Century-Crofts, 1987).
5. C. Bevil, Program Evaluation in Nursing Education: Creating a Meaningful Plan, in *Assessing Education Outcome*, ed. M. Garbin, 363–367 (New York: National League for Nursing, 1991).
6. C. Barrett-Barrick, Promoting the Use of Program Evaluation Findings, *Nurse Educator* 18, no. 1 (1993):10–12.
7. C. Barrett-Barrick, Promoting the Use of Program Evaluation Findings.
8. K. Oermann and M. Gaberson, Evaluation of Problem-Solving, Decision-Making, and Critical Thinking: Context-Dependent Item Sets and Other Evaluation Strategies, in *Evaluation and Testing in Nursing Education,* eds. M. Oermann and K. Gaberson (New York: Springer Publishing, 1998).
9. Oermann and Gaberson, Evaluation of Problem-Solving.
10. H. Melland and C. Volden, Classroom Assessment: Linking Teaching and Learning, *Journal of Nursing Education* 37, no. 6 (1998):275–277.
11. T. Angelo and K. Cross, Classroom Assessment Techniques: A Handbook for College Teachers, 2nd ed. (San Francisco: Jossey-Bass, 1993).
12. Oermann and Gaberson, Evaluation of Problem-Solving.

13. Oermann and Gaberson, Evaluation of Problem-Solving.

14. J. Novak, Concept Mapping: A Useful Tool for Science Education, *Journal of Research in Science Teaching* 27, no. 10 (1990):937–949.

15. N. Baugh and K. Mellott, Clinical Concept Mapping as Preparation for Student Nurses' Clinical Experiences, *Journal of Nursing Education* 37, no. 6 (1998):253–256.

16. G. Bentley and K. Nugent, A Creative Student Presentation on the Nursing Management of a Complex Family, *Nurse Educator* 23, no. 3 (1998):8–9.

17. M. Ryan and K. Carlton, Portfolio Applications in a School of Nursing, *Nurse Educator* 22, no. 1 (1990):35–39.

18. A. Nitko, Educational Assessment of Students, 2nd ed. (Englewood Cliffs, NJ: Prentice Hall, 1996).

19. L. Kobert, In Our Own Voice: Journaling as a Teaching/Learning Technique for Nurses, *Journal of Nursing Education* 34, no. 3 (1995):140–142.

20. H. Hodges, Journal Writing as a Mode of Thinking for RN-BSN Students: A Leveled Approach to Learning to Listen to Self and Others, *Journal of Nursing Education* 35 (1996):137–141.

21. H. Brown and J. Sorrell, Use of Clinical Journals To Enhance Critical Thinking, *Nurse Educator* 18, no. 5 (1993):16–18.

22. V. Holmes, Grading Journals in Clinical Practice, *Journal of Nursing Education* 36, no. 10 (1997): 89–92.

23. L. Kobert, In Our Own Voice.

24. M. Bradshaw, Clinical Pathways: A Tool To Evaluate Clinical Learning, *Journal of the Society of Pediatric Nurses* 4, no. 1 (1999):37–40.

25. M. Oermann, Research on Teaching in the Clinical Setting, in *Review of Research in Nursing Education*, ed. K.R. Stevens, vol. vii, 91–126 (New York: National League for Nursing, 1996).

26. Oermann and Gaberson, Evaluation of Problem-Solving.

## SUGGESTED READING

Angelo, T., and K. Cross. 1993. *Classroom assessment techniques: A handbook for college teachers.* 2nd ed. San Francisco: Jossey-Bass.

Barrett-Barrick, C. 1993. Promoting the use of program evaluation findings. *Nurse Educator* 18, no. 1:10–12.

Baugh, N., and K. Mellott. 1998. Clinical concept mapping as preparation for student nurses' clinical experiences. *Journal of Nursing Education* 37, no. 6:253–256.

Bentley, G., and K. Nugent. 1998. A creative student presentation on the nursing management of a complex family. *Nurse Educator* 23, no. 3:8–9.

Bevil, C. 1991. Program evaluation in nursing education: Creating a meaningful plan. In *Assessing education outcome*, ed. M. Garbin, 363–367. New York: National League for Nursing.

Bradshaw, M. 1999. Clinical pathways: A tool to evaluate clinical learning. *Journal of the Society of Pediatric Nurses* 4, no. 1:37–40.

Brown, H., and J. Sorrell. 1993. Use of clinical journals to enhance critical thinking. *Nurse Educator* 18, no. 5:16–18.

Gronlund, N., and R. Linn. 1990. *Measurement and evaluation in teaching.* 6th ed. Englewood Cliffs, NJ: Macmillan.

Hodges, H. 1996. Journal writing as a mode of thinking for RN-BSN students: A leveled approach to learning to listen to self and others. *Journal of Nursing Education* 35:137–141.

Holmes, V. 1997. Grading journals in clinical practice. *Journal of Nursing Education* 36, no. 10:89–92.

Kobert, L. 1995. In our own voice: Journaling as a teaching/learning technique for nurses. *Journal of Nursing Education* 34, no. 3:140–142.

Melland, H., and C. Volden. 1998. Classroom assessment: Linking teaching and learning. *Journal of Nursing Education* 37, no. 6:275–277.

Nitko, A. 1996. *Educational assessment of students.* 2nd ed. Englewood Cliffs, NJ: Prentice Hall.

Novak, J. 1990. Concept mapping: A useful tool for science education. *Journal of Research in Science Teaching* 27, no. 10:937–949.

Oermann, M. 1996. Research on teaching in the clinical setting. In *Review of research in nursing education,* ed. K.R. Stevens, vol. vii, 91–126. New York: National League for Nursing.

Oermann, M., and K. Gaberson. 1998. Evaluation of problem-solving, decision-making, and critical thinking: Context-dependent item sets and other evaluation strategies. In *Evaluation and testing in nursing education,* eds. M. Oermann and K. Gaberson. New York: Springer Publishing.

Rossi, P., and H. Freeman. 1993. *Evaluation: A systematic approach.* Newbury Park: Sage Publications.

Ryan, M., and K. Carlton. 1990. Portfolio applications in a school of nursing. *Nurse Educator* 22, no. 1: 35–39.

Stufflebeam, D. 1980. The relevance of the CIPP evaluation model for educational accountability. *Journal of Research and Developmental Education* 5, no. 1:19–25.

# Index